THE COMPLETE
AIR FRYER COOKBOOK
FOR BEGINNERS

800 Creative and Affordable Recipes that You Can Easily Replicate. Quickly Create Your Own Tasty Dishes Every Day to the Delight of Your Whole Family

Isabelle Lauren

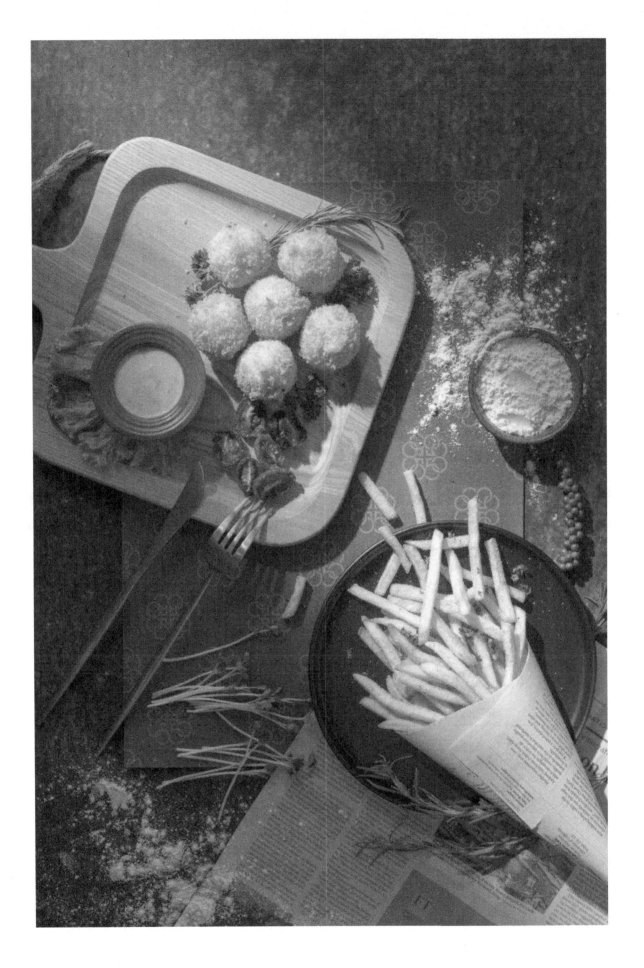

Table of Contents

HOW AN AIR FRYER WORKS? 16

Cook Tips For Beginners 16

BREAKFAST AND BRUNCH 18

1. *Asparagus Frittata* 18
2. *Air-Fried British Breakfast* 18
3. *Blueberry Cobbler* 19
4. *Grilled Ham and Cheese* 19
5. *Breakfast Potatoes* 19
6. *Scramble Casserole* 20
7. *Broccoli Stuffed Peppers* 20
8. *Cheese Soufflés* 20
9. *Chocolate-Filled Doughnuts* 21
10. *Hash Browns* 21
11. *Soufflé* 21
12. *Steak and Eggs* 22
13. *Maple-Glazed Doughnuts* 22
14. *Bagels* 22
15. *French Toast Sticks* 23
16. *Granola* 23
17. *Fried Potatoes* 23
18. *Cherry Tarts* 24
19. *Strawberry Tarts* 24
20. *Jalapeno Muffins* 25
21. *Mixed Berry Muffins* 25
22. *Mushrooms Frittata* 25
23. *Omelet* 26
24. *Puffed Egg Tarts* 26
25. *Radish Hash Browns* 26
26. *Sausage and Cream Cheese Biscuits* 27
27. *Sausage and Egg Burrito* 27
28. *Cheese and Bacon Muffins* 27
29. *Spinach Frittata* 28
30. *Vegetable Egg Cups* 28
31. *Vegetable Egg Soufflé* 28
32. *Waffles and Chicken* 28
33. *Italian Frittata* 29
34. *Zucchini Muffins* 29
35. *Zucchini Noodles* 30

BREAD, PIZZA AND PASTA 31

36. *3-Ingredients: Banana Bread* 32
37. *Apple Bread* 32
38. *Bacon and Garlic Pizzas* 32
39. *Baked Bread* 33
40. *Pizza* 33
41. *Vegan Beer Bread* 33
42. *Carrot Bread* 34
43. *Olive Bread and Rosemary* 34
44. *Carrot, Raisin & Walnut Bread* 34
45. *Cauliflower Pizza Crusts* 35
46. *Cheesy Bacon Bread* 35
47. *Cheesy Garlic Bread* 35
48. *Chicken Pizza Rolls* 36
49. *Cinnamon Sugar Toast* 36
50. *Cranberry Bread* 36
51. *Crust-less Meaty Pizza* 37
52. *Mac and Cheese* 37
53. *Fitness Bread* 37
54. *Panettone Bread Pudding* 38
55. *Chocolate Bread* 38
56. *Lemon Bread* 38
57. *Lemon-Butter Shortbread* 39
58. *Pizza Crust* 39
59. *Mushroom-Onion Eggplant Pizzas* 39
60. *Mozzarella Flatbread* 40
61. *New York Pizza* 40
62. *Nutty Bread Pudding* 40
63. *Philo Pasta Rolls* 41
64. *Pizza Bombs* 41
65. *Pumpkin Bread* 41
66. *Lunch Pizzas* 42
67. *Roasted Veggie Pasta Salad* 42
68. *Salmon with Shrimp & Pasta* 42
69. *Salted Caramel Banana Muffins (Vegan)* 43
70. *Shrimp Pasta* 43

71.	Vegan Spelled Bread	43
72.	Strawberry Bread	44
73.	Vegan Spicy Sourdough Bread	44
74.	Banana Bread (Vegan)	44
75.	Sugar-Free Pumpkin Bread	45
76.	Bread with Lentils and Millet (Vegan)	45
77.	Taco Stuffed Bread	45
78.	Corn Bread	46
79.	Walnut Bread with Cranberries	46
80.	Walnut Zucchini Bread	46
81.	Whole Wheat Toast	47
82.	Vegan Wholegrain Bread	47
83.	Yogurt Pumpkin Bread	47
84.	Chicken & Pepperoni Pizza	48
85.	Meat Lovers' Pizza	48
86.	Mozzarella, Bacon & Turkey Calzone	48
87.	Pita Bread	49
88.	Breakfast Berry Pizza	49
89.	Yogurt Banana Bread	50
90.	Flat Bread with Olive and Rosemary	50
91.	Yogurt Bread	50
92.	Caprese Sandwiches (Vegan)	51

SNACKS AND APPETIZERS 52

93.	Air Fryer Olives	52
94.	Air Fryer Nuts	52
95.	Air Fryer Buffalo Cauliflower	53
96.	Air Fryer Mini Pizza	53
97.	Air Fryer Egg Rolls	53
98.	Air Fryer Chicken Nuggets	54
99.	Chicken Tenders	54
100.	Kale & Celery Crackers	54
101.	Air Fryer Spanakopita Bites	55
102.	Air Fryer Onion Rings	55
103.	Air Fryer Delicata Squash	56
104.	Zucchini Parmesan Chips	56
105.	Air Fryer Roasted Corn	56
106.	Air-Fried Spinach Frittata	56
107.	Air Fryer Buffalo Cauliflower	57
108.	Air Fryer Sweet Potato Fries	57

109.	Air Fryer Kale Chips	57
110.	Crispy Air Fryer Brussels Sprouts	58
111.	Vegetable Spring Rolls	58
112.	Zucchini Gratin	58
113.	Asparagus Frittata	59
114.	Air Fryer Bacon-Wrapped Jalapeno Poppers	59
115.	Easy Air Fryer Zucchini Chips	59
116.	Air Fryer Avocado Fries	60
117.	Avocado Egg Rolls	60
118.	Cheesy Bell Pepper Eggs	60
119.	Air Fryer Crisp Egg Cups	61
120.	Air Fryer Lemon-Garlic Tofu	61
121.	Vegan Mashed Potato Bowl	61
122.	Vegan Breakfast Sandwich	62
123.	Crispy Fat-Free Spanish Potatoes	62
124.	Cheese and Veggie Air Fryer Egg Cups	63
125.	Low Carb Air Fryer Baked Eggs	63
126.	Easy Air Fryer Omelet	63
127.	Breakfast Bombs	64
128.	Air Fryer Breakfast Toad-in-the-Hole Tarts	64
129.	Air Fried Cheesy Chicken Omelet	64
130.	Air Fryer Spicy Chickpeas	65
131.	Apple Chips	65
132.	Air Fryer Walnuts	65
133.	Avocado Chips	65
134.	Allspice Chicken Wings	66
135.	Avocado Rolls	66
136.	Baguette Bread	66
137.	Banana Chips	67
138.	Baked Almonds	67
139.	Basil Crackers	67
140.	Banana & Raisin Bread	67
141.	Beets Chips	68
142.	Banana & Walnut Bread	68
143.	Bean Burger	68
144.	Brown Sugar Banana Bread	69
145.	Cabbage Rolls	69
146.	Butternut Squash with Thyme	69

147.	Cauliflower Crackers	70
148.	Cheesy Garlic Dip	70
149.	Cheese Brussels Sprouts	70
150.	Cheese Onion Dip	71
151.	Cheese Spinach Dip	71
152.	Chickpeas Snack	71
153.	Chocolate Banana Bread	71
154.	Cinnamon Banana Bread	72
155.	Corn Fritters	72
156.	Date & Walnut Bread	72
157.	Date Bread	73
158.	Cauliflower Hummus	73
159.	Jalapeno Poppers	74
160.	Cheesy Dip	74
161.	Sweet Potato Fries	74
162.	Zucchini Chips	74
163.	Egg Roll Wrapped with Cabbage and Prawns	75
164.	Crab Dip	75
165.	Pineapple Sticky Ribs	75
166.	Fried Ravioli	76
167.	Garlic Cauliflower Florets	76
168.	Carrot Fries	76
169.	Jalapeno Spinach Dip	76
170.	Polenta Biscuits	77
171.	Potato and Beans Dip	77
172.	Peanut Butter Banana Bread	77
173.	Mushroom Pizza	78
174.	Crispy Potatoes	78
175.	Ranch Potatoes	78
176.	Potato Chips	78
177.	Rice Balls	79
178.	Salsa Cheesy Dip	79
179.	Nuggets with Parmesan Cheese	79
180.	Sesame Garlic Chicken Wings	80
181.	Soda Bread	80
182.	Sour Cream Banana Bread	80
183.	Spicy Brussels Sprouts	81
184.	Tortilla Chips	81
185.	Spicy Cauliflower Florets	81
186.	Sunflower Seed Bread	81
187.	Potato Tots	82
188.	Cinnamon Chickpeas	82
189.	Potato Croquettes	82
190.	Veggie Sticks	83
191.	Potato Wedges	83
192.	Ricotta Dip	83
193.	Wontons	83

MAINS **85**

194.	Bacon Wrapped Shrimp	85
195.	Carrot & Potato Mix	85
196.	Air Fryer Breaded Pork Chops	86
197.	Pork Taquitos in Air Fryer	86
198.	Air Fryer Tasty Egg Rolls	86
199.	Pork Dumplings in Air Fryer	87
200.	Air Fryer Pork Chop & Broccoli	87
201.	Cheesy Pork Chops in Air Fryer	87
202.	Pork Rind Nachos	88
203.	Jamaican Jerk Pork in Air Fryer	88
204.	Pork Tenderloin with Mustard Glazed	88
205.	Balsamic Vinaigrette on Roasted Chicken	89
206.	Breaded Mushrooms	89
207.	Bang Panko Breaded Fried Shrimp	89
208.	Basil Chicken Bites	90
209.	Broccoli Stew	90
210.	Vegan Cauliflower Rice	90
211.	Chicken and Beans	90
212.	Chicken Pasta Parmesan	91
213.	Chinese Chicken Drumsticks	91
214.	Cilantro-Lime Fried Shrimp	92
215.	Cornish Game Hens	92
216.	Courgettes Casserole	92
217.	Creamy Cauliflower and Broccoli	93
218.	Curried Chicken, Chickpeas and Raita Salad	93
219.	Curried Coconut Chicken	93
220.	Eggplant Fries	94
221.	Eggplant Bake	94
222.	Fennel and Tomato Stew	94

223. Chimichanga 95
224. Garlicky Pork Stew 95
225. Gingered Chicken Drumsticks 95
226. Herbed Roasted Chicken 95
227. Honey Glazed Chicken Drumsticks 96
228. Lemon Lentils and Fried Onion 96
229. Lemony Tuna 96
230. Mexican Stuffed Potatoes 97
231. Okra Casserole 97
232. Paprika Cod 97
233. Chicken with Potatoes 98
234. Roasted Chickpeas 98
235. Rosemary Grilled Chicken 98
236. Rosemary Russet Potato Chips 99
237. Salmon Quiche 99
238. Spiced Chicken 99
239. Potato Cauliflower Patties 100
240. Spicy Chicken Legs 100
241. Tamarind Glazed Potatoes 100
242. Spinach and Olives 101
243. The Cheesy Sandwich (Vegan) 101
244. Spinach and Shrimp 101
245. Chicken Drumsticks 101
246. Tandoori Chicken Legs 102
247. Bean Dish 102
248. Thyme Eggplant and Beans 102
249. Tomato and Avocado 103
250. Paneer Pizza 103
251. Tomato and Beef Sauce 103
252. Tomatoes and Cabbage Stew 104
253. Turkey and Bok Choy 104
254. Vegan Taquito 104
255. Turkey and Broccoli Stew 105
256. Turkey and Mushroom Stew 105
257. Turkey and Quinoa Stuffed Peppers . 105
258. Chicken and Asparagus 106

POULTRY **107**

259. Air-Fried Lemon and Olive Chicken ... 107
260. Breaded Chicken Tenderloins 107
261. Parmesan Chicken Meatballs 108
262. Lemon Rosemary Chicken 108
263. Air Fryer Chicken & Broccoli 108
264. Air Fried Maple Chicken Thighs 109
265. Mushroom Oatmeal 109
266. Bell Peppers Frittata 110
267. Southwest Chicken in Air Fryer 110
268. No-Breading Chicken Breast in Air Fryer 110
269. Lemon Pepper Chicken Breast 111
270. Herb-Marinated Chicken Thighs 111
271. Air Fried Chicken Fajitas 111
272. Air Fried Blackened Chicken Breast ... 112
273. Chicken with Mixed Vegetables 112
274. Garlic Parmesan Chicken Tenders 112
275. Chicken Thighs Smothered Style 113
276. Lemon-Garlic Chicken 113
277. Buttermilk Chicken in Air-Fryer 113
278. Orange Chicken Wings 114
279. Air Fryer Brown Rice Chicken Fried .. 114
280. Chicken Cheesey Quesadilla in Air Fryer 114
281. Delicious Chicken Pie 115
282. Chicken Bites in Air Fryer 115
283. Popcorn Chicken in Air Fryer 115
284. Turkey Fajitas Platter in Air Fryer 116
285. Turkey Juicy Breast Tenderloin 116
286. Turkey Breast with Mustard Maple Glaze 116
287. Zucchini Turkey Burgers 117
288. No-breaded Turkey Breast 117
289. Almond Flour Coco-Milk Battered Chicken 117
290. Almond-Crusted Chicken 118
291. Bacon Chicken Lasagna 118
292. Baked Chicken & Potatoes 118
293. Basil Pesto Chicken 119
294. Basil-Garlic Breaded Chicken Bake 119
295. BBQ Chicken Wings 119
296. BBQ Spicy Chicken Wings 120
297. Baked Chicken 120

298. *Buffalo Chicken Wings* 120

299. *Buffalo Chicken Tenders* 120

300. *Caribbean Chicken* 121

301. *Carne Asada Tacos* 121

302. *Cheddar Turkey Bites* 121

303. *Chicken Lasagna* 122

304. *Cheesy Meatloaf* 122

305. *Chicken Breasts & Spiced Tomatoes* ..122

306. *Chicken Casserole* 123

307. *Cheesy Chicken Rice* 123

308. *Chicken Coconut Meatballs* 123

309. *Chicken Fajitas* 124

310. *Chicken Fillets, Brie & Ham* 124

311. *Chicken Kabab* 124

312. *Chicken Meatballs* 125

313. *Chicken Mushrooms Bake* 125

314. *Chicken Paillard* 125

315. *Chicken Parmesan* 126

316. *Chicken Pizza Crust* 126

317. *Chicken Pizza Crusts* 126

318. *Chicken Pram* 127

319. *Chicken Stir-Fry* 127

320. *Chicken with Oregano Chimichurri* ...127

321. *Chimichurri Turkey* 128

322. *Collard Wraps with Satay Dipping Sauce* 128

323. *Creamy Chicken Wings* 129

324. *Crisp Chicken with Mustard Vinaigrette* 129

325. *Crispy Chicken Thighs* 129

326. *Crispy Honey Garlic Chicken Wings* .130

327. *Crunchy Almond and Salad with Roasted Chicken* 130

328. *Curried Coconut Chicken* 130

329. *Fennel Chicken* 131

330. *Greek Chicken Meatballs* 131

331. *Honey Chicken Breasts* 131

332. *Chicken Drumsticks with Garlic & Thyme* 132

333. *Chicken Thighs* 132

334. *Korean Chicken Wings* 132

335. *Lemon Pepper Chicken Legs* 133

336. *Lemon Pepper Drumsticks* 133

337. *Mustard Turkey Bites* 133

338. *Nutmeg Chicken Thighs* 134

339. *Chicken Parmesan* 134

340. *Fried Chicken Roast Served with Fruit Compote* 134

341. *Roasted Chicken* 135

342. *Spiced Chicken Breasts* 135

343. *Spiced Duck Legs* 135

344. *Stir-Fried Chicken with Water Chestnuts* 136

345. *Strawberry Turkey* 136

346. *Sweet and Sour Chicken* 136

347. *Teriyaki Chicken Wings* 136

348. *Teriyaki Duck Legs* 137

349. *Turkey Turnovers* 137

350. *Crispy & Spicy Chicken Thighs* 137

351. *Zingy & Nutty Chicken Wings* 138

352. *Lemongrass Chicken* 138

353. *Salsa Chicken* 138

354. *Sweet Chicken* 139

355. *Chicken with Vegetables* 139

356. *Chicken Zucchini Casserole* 139

357. *Chinese Chicken Wings* 140

358. *Delicious Curried Chicken* 140

360. *Honey Mustard Sauce Chicken* 140

361. *Mexican Chicken Lasagna* 141

362. *Fajita Chicken* 141

363. *Garlicky Chicken Wings* 141

364. *Herb Garlic Meatballs* 142

365. *Hot Chicken Wings* 142

366. *Italian Turkey* 142

367. *Juicy Baked Chicken Wings* 142

368. *Juicy Garlic Chicken* 143

369. *Pepper Lemon Chicken Breasts* 143

370. *Pepper Lemon Baked Chicken Legs* ...143

371. *Pepper Lemon Chicken* 144

372. *Lemon Rosemary Chicken* 144

373. *Old Bay Chicken* 144

374. Olive Tomato Chicken 145

375. Parmesan Chicken & Vegetables 145

376. Parmesan Pesto Chicken 145

377. Baked Chicken Breasts 146

378. Pumpkin Chicken Lasagna 146

379. Chicken Meatballs 146

380. Simple Chicken Thighs 147

381. Simply Baked Chicken 147

382. Spicy Chicken Meatballs 147

383. Spicy Chicken Wings 147

386. Chicken Fajita Casserole 148

RED MEAT **150**

388. Lamb Kebabs 150

389. Air Fried Beef Schnitzel 150

390. Air Fryer Meatloaf 151

391. Air Fried Steak with Asparagus 151

392. Air Fryer Hamburgers 152

393. Air Fryer Steak Kabobs with Vegetables 152

394. Air Fried Empanadas 152

395. Air Fry Rib-Eye Steak 153

396. Beefsteak with Olives And Capers 153

397. Grilled Pork in Cajun Sauce 153

398. Ribs with Cajun and Coriander 153

400. Marinated Beef BBQ 154

401. Steak with Chimichurri Sauce 154

402. Egg and Bell Pepper with Beef 155

403. Spanish Rice Casserole with Beef and Cheese 155

404. Beef Roast in Worcestershire-Rosemary 155

405. Beef with Honey and Mustard 156

406. Texas Beef Brisket 156

407. Teriyaki BBQ Recipe 156

408. Beef in Almond and Eggs Crust 157

409. Beef Casserole 157

410. Beef and Pasta Casserole 157

411. Air Fry Catfish 158

412. Air Fried Fish Fillet 158

413. Salmon Cakes in Air Fryer 159

414. Coconut Shrimp 159

415. Fish Sticks in Air Fryer 160

Prep Time: 10 mins   Cook Time:15 mins   160

Serving 4 160

416. Honey-Glazed Salmon 160

417. Basil-Parmesan Crusted Salmon 160

418. Cajun Shrimp in Air Fryer 161

419. Crispy Air Fryer Fish 161

420. Air Fryer Lemon Cod 161

421. Air Fryer Salmon Fillets 161

422. Air Fryer Fish & Chips 162

423. Grilled Salmon with Lemon-Honey Marinade 162

424. Air-Fried Fish Nuggets 162

425. Garlic Rosemary Prawns 163

426. Air-Fried Crumbed Fish 163

427. Parmesan Garlic Crusted Salmon 163

428. Air Fryer Salmon with Maple Soy Glaze 164

429. Air Fried Cajun Salmon 164

430. Air Fryer Shrimp Scampi 164

431. Sesame Seeds Fish Fillet 165

432. Lemon Pepper Shrimp in Air Fryer 165

433. Lemon Garlic Shrimp in Air Fryer 165

434. Parmesan Shrimp 166

435. Juicy Air Fryer Salmon 166

436. Crispy Fish Sandwiches 166

437. Air Fried Shrimp with Chili-Greek Yogurt Sauce 167

438. Air Fryer Crab Cakes 167

439. Air Fryer Tuna Patties 167

440. Fish Finger Sandwich 168

441. Lime-Garlic Shrimp Kebabs 168

442. Air Fryer Sushi Roll 168

443. Roasted Salmon with Fennel Salad ... 169

444. Catfish with Green Beans 169

445. Honey & Sriracha Tossed Calamari ... 170

446. Scallops with Creamy Tomato Sauce. 170

447. Shrimp Spring Rolls in Air Fryer 170

448. Air Fryer Salmon 171

449. **Bacon-Wrapped Shrimp** 171

450. **Baked Salmon Rolls** 171

451. **Mahi Fillets** 172

452. **Cajun Catfish Fillets** 172

453. **Cajun Salmon** 172

454. **Cheesy Tuna Patties** 173

455. **Chili Tuna Casserole** 173

456. **Coconut Shrimp** 173

457. **Cod and Endives** 174

458. **Cod and Tomatoes** 174

459. **Crab Cakes** 174

460. **Crab Dip** 175

461. **Crispy Paprika Fillets** 175

462. **Dijon Salmon** 175

463. **Baked Tilapia** 175

464. **Garlic Lime Shrimp** 176

465. **Garlic Tilapia** 176

466. **Glazed Tuna and Fruits** 176

467. **Golden Beer-Battered Cod** 177

468. **Greek Pesto Salmon** 177

469. **Grilled Salmon** 177

470. **Fish And Chips** 178

471. **Indian Fish Fingers** 178

472. **Mustard-Crusted Sole Fillets** 178

473. **Parmesan Cod** 179

474. **Parmesan Walnut Salmon** 179

475. **Parmesan-Crusted Halibut Fillets** 179

476. **Parmesan-Crusted Salmon Patties** 180

477. **Paella** 180

478. **Salmon and Cauliflower Rice** 180

479. **Salmon with Coconut Sauce** 180

480. **Salmon and Dill Sauce** 181

481. **Salmon Dill Patties** 181

482. **Salmon Patties** 181

483. **Sesame Shrimp** 182

484. **Air Fry Salmon** 182

485. **Sole and Cauliflower Fritters** 182

486. **Spicy Shrimp** 183

487. **Spicy Tilapia** 183

488. **Sticky Hoisin Tuna** 183

489. **Sweet and Savory Breaded Shrimp** ...184

490. **Shrimp Fajitas** 184

491. **Tilapia and Salsa** 184

492. **Tilapia with Vegetables** 185

493. **Trout with Mint** 185

494. **Tuna Veggie** 185

495. **Bacon Shrimps** 186

496. **Cajuned Salmon** 186

497. **Coconut Chili Shrimp** 186

498. **Creamed Cod** 187

499. **Garlic Lemon Shrimp** 187

501. **Fennel Cod** 188

502. **Air Fryer Salmon (2nd Version)** 188

503. **Air Fryer Salmon Patties** 188

504. **Bang Panko Breaded Fried Shrimp** ...189

505. **Flying Fish** 189

506. **Grilled Salmon** 189

507. **Soy Salmon Fillets** 190

508. **Lemony Tuna** 190

509. **Shrimp Po Boy** 190

510. **Old Bay Crab Cakes** 191

511. **Pistachio-Crusted Lemon-Garlic Salmon** 191

512. **Salmon Noodles** 191

513. **Salmon Quiche** 192

514. **Scallops and Vegetables** 192

515. **Tuna Stuffed Potatoes** 192

VEGETABLES **194**

516. **Air Fried Asparagus** 194

517. **Air Fried Brussels Sprouts** 194

518. **Air Fried Carrots, Squash & Zucchini** 195

519. **Cauliflower in an Almond Crust with Avocado Ranch Dip** 195

520. **Air Fried Kale Chips** 195

521. **Cauliflower Rice** 196

522. **Steamed Broccoli** 196

523. **Pasta with Artichoke Pesto and Chickpeas (Vegan)** 196

524. **Almond Asparagus** 197

525. **Onion Rings with Almond Four Battered** 197

526.	Coconut Artichokes	197
527.	Baby Potatoes	198
528.	Baked Eggplant with Marinara and Cheese	198
529.	Polenta Roll with Cheese Sauce	198
530.	Baked Vegan Eggplant	199
531.	Baked Potato with Cream Cheese (Vegan)	199
532.	Baked Egg Tomato	199
533.	Baked Macaroni with Cheese	200
534.	Baked Zucchini with Cheese	200
535.	Baked Sweet Potatoes	200
536.	Baked Salad (Vegan)	200
537.	Balsamic Mushrooms	201
538.	Asparagus and Prosciutto	201
539.	Balsamic Cabbage	201
540.	Basil Tomatoes	202
541.	Beet Salad	202
542.	Beet Salad and Parsley	202
543.	Beets and Arugula Salad	203
544.	Tortilla with Bell Pepper-Corn Wrapped	203
545.	Bell Peppers and Kale Leaves	203
546.	Jalapeño Poppers	204
547.	Tomato Chili and Black Beans	204
548.	Brown Rice, Spinach and Frittata	204
549.	Broccoli Salad	205
550.	Brussels Sprouts with Pine Nuts	205
551.	Brussels Sprouts And Tomatoes	205
552.	Burritos	206
553.	Cajun Asparagus	206
554.	Buttery Potatoes	206
555.	Cajun Mushrooms and Beans	207
556.	Carrot Mix	207
557.	Cheddar Muffins	207
558.	Cauliflower, Chickpea, and Avocado Mash	208
559.	Cheese and Bean Enchiladas	208
560.	Cauliflower Chickpea Tacos	208
561.	Cheesy Broccoli Casserole	209
562.	Cherry Tomatoes Skewers	209
563.	Cheesy Macaroni Balls	210
564.	Cherry Tomato Salad	210
565.	Cheesy Asparagus and Potatoes	210
566.	Cheesy Spinach	211
567.	Chinese Beans	211
568.	Chili Potatoes	211
569.	Coconut Mix	211
570.	Indian Cilantro Potatoes with Pepper	212
571.	Collard Green Mix	212
572.	Corn and Cabbage Salad	212
573.	Broccoli with Cream Cheese	213
574.	Creamy Spinach Quiche	213
588.	Polenta Roll with Cheese	217
589.	Potato with Cheese	217
590.	Banana with Tofu 'n Spices	218
591.	Vegetables with Tandoori Spice	218
592.	Honey Seasoned Vegetables	218
593.	Carrots and Zucchinis with Mayo Butter	219
594.	Easy Brussels Sprouts	219
595.	Yellow Squash 'n Zucchini	219
596.	Veggie Burger with Spices	220
597.	Buffalo Sauce Cauliflower	220
599.	Potatoes with Tofu	220
600.	Gold Ravioli	221
601.	Mediterranean Vegetables	221
602.	Veg Rolls	221
603.	Rice and Eggplant	222
605.	Mushrooms with Mascarpone	222
606.	Chickpea, Fig, and Arugula Salad	223
607.	Sriracha Cauliflower	223
608.	Roasted Apple Potatoes	223
610.	Garlicky Cauliflower	224
611.	Green Beans	224
612.	Potato Casserole	224
613.	Baked Zucchini Egg	225
614.	Roasted Broccoli	225
615.	Vegetable Tots	225
616.	Delicious Potato Fries	226

11

617. *Parmesan Potatoes* 226
618. *Masala Gallettes* 226
619. *Potato Samosa* 227
620. *Veggie Kebab* 227
621. *Sago Galette* 227
622. *Stuffed Peppers Baskets* 228
623. *Macaroni Samosa* 228
624. *Greek Potato* 228
625. *Mushroom Cakes* 229
626. *Green Salad* 229
627. *Tomatoes Salad* 229
628. *French Mushroom* 230
629. *Zucchini and Pumpkin Salad* 230
630. *Squash Stew* 230
631. *Stew of Okra and Eggplant* 231
632. *White Beans Stew* 231
633. *Spinach and Lentils* 231
634. *Winter Green Beans* 231
635. *Green Beans Casserole* 232
636. *Chinese Cauliflower Rice* 232
637. *Artichokes Dish* 232
638. *Yellow Lentil* 233
639. *Vegetables Lasagna* 233
640. *Onion Pie* 233
641. *Vegetables Pizza* 234
642. *Vegetable Stew* 234
643. *Spinach Dish* 235
644. *Vegetable Burger* 235
645. *Potatoes with Zucchini* 235
646. *Ratatouille* 236
647. *Potato and Broccoli with Tofu Scramble* 236
648. *Summer Rolls* 236
649. *Veg Rolls* 237
650. *Potatoes with Tofu* 237
651. *Rice and Eggplant* 238
652. *Mushroom and Pepper Pizza Squares* 238
653. *Green Beans with Shallot* 238
654. *Herbed Chips* 239

655. *Lemony Pear Chips* 239
656. *Fishless Tacos With Chipotle Cream* .239
657. *Thai-Style Crab Cakes* 240
658. *Vegan Spring Rolls* 240
659. *Popcorn (Vegan)* 241
660. *Stuffed Eggplant* 241
661. *Potato Air Fried Hash Browns* 242
662. *Kale Salad Sushi Rolls* 242
663. *Jackfruit Taquitos* 243
664. *Ginger Tofu Sushi Bowl* 243
665. *Spicy Cauliflower* 243
666. *Italian Eggplant Parmesan* 244
667. *Stuffed Potatoes* 244
668. *Turmeric Cauliflower Steaks* 245
669. *Garlic Beans* 245
670. *Oregano Eggplants* 245
671. *Garlic Parsnips* 245
672. *Pomegranate and Florets* 246
673. *Lime Broccoli* 246
674. *Green Cayenne Cabbage* 246
675. *Tomato and Balsamic Greens* 246
676. *Lime Endives* 247
677. *Artichokes with Oregano* 247
678. *Green Veggies* 247
679. *Flavored Green Beans* 248
680. *Herbed Eggplant and Zucchini* 248
681. *Okra and Corn Salad* 248
682. *Chard Salad* 248
683. *Garlic Tomatoes* 249
684. *Eggplant and Garlic Sauce* 249
685. *Stuffed Peppers* 249
686. *Green Beans and Tomatoes* 249
687. *Pumpkin Oatmeal* 250
688. *Yellow Squash, Zucchini and Carrots* 250
689. *Hasselback Potatoes* 250
690. *Sriracha Honey Brussels Sprouts* 250
691. *Roasted Carrots* 251
692. *Parmesan Broccoli Florets* 251
693. *Baked Potatoes* 251

694. Parmesan Green Beans 252

695. Roasted Asparagus 252

696. Healthy Veggies 252

697. Parmesan Breaded with Zucchini Chips 252

698. Spicy Potato Fries 253

699. Vegetarian Frittata 253

700. Paprika Onion 254

701. Parsnip & Potato Bake with Parmesan 254

702. Spicy Cheese Lings 254

703. Green Paneer Ginger Cheese Balls 255

705. Coconut & Spinach Chickpeas 255

706. Cauliflower, Olives, and Chickpeas ...255

707. Fruit and Vegetable Skewers 256

708. Roasted Potatoes with Rosemary 256

709. Spicy Broccoli with Garlic 256

710. Roasted Carrots with Garlic 257

711. Roasted Balsamic Vegetables 257

712. Pesto Tomatoes 257

713. Stuffed Tomatoes 257

714. Parmesan Asparagus 258

715. Spicy Butternut Squash 258

716. Sweet & Spicy Parsnips 258

SOUPS 259

717. Chicken Soup 259

718. Leek, Rice, and Potato Soup 259

719. Mushroom and Kale Soup 260

720. Italian Chicken Soup 260

721. Chicken and Broccoli Soup 260

722. Vegetable and Beef Soup 260

723. Beef Soup 261

724. Bean Soup 261

DESSERTS 262

725. Banana Split 262

726. Sugar-Free Chocolate Soufflé 263

727. Sugar-Free Air Fried Carrot Cake 263

728. Sugar-Free Low Carb Cheesecake Muffins 263

729. Sugar-Free Chocolate Donut Holes ...264

730. Low Carb Peanut Butter Cookies 264

731. Air Fryer Blueberry Muffins Recipe ..264

732. Air Fryer Lemon Slice & Bake Cookies 265

733. Brownies 265

734. Air Fryer Cookies 266

735. Air Fryer Apple Fritter 266

736. Berry Cheesecake 266

737. Grain-Free Cakes 267

738. Tahini Oatmeal Chocolate Chunk Cookies 267

739. Eggless & Vegan Cake 268

740. Banana Muffins in Air Fryer 268

741. Apple Cider Vinegar Donuts 268

742. Banana Slices 269

743. Pineapple Bites 269

744. Cheesecake Bites 270

745. Chocolate Bites 270

746. Blueberry Tacos 270

747. Shortbread Sticks 271

748. Apple Pastries 271

749. Cinnamon Toast 271

750. Chocolate Mug Cake 271

751. Strawberry Cake 272

752. Fried Peaches 272

753. Apple Dumplings 272

754. Apple Pie 273

755. Air Fryer Chocolate Cake 273

757. Banana-Choco Brownies 274

758. Chocolate Donuts 274

759. Air Fryer Donuts 274

760. Chocolate Soufflé 274

761. Fried Bananas with Chocolate Sauce 275

762. Chocolate Banana Muffins 275

763. Air Fryer Apple Pies 275

764. Air Fryer Churros 276

765. Spicy Cardamom Crumb Cake 276

766. Peach Cobbler 277

767. Apple Cider Donuts 277

768. Apple Pudding 277

769. Cinnamon Rolls 278

770. Lava Cake 278

771. Cheesecake Egg Rolls 278

772. Brazilian Pineapple 279

773. Chocolate Chunk Walnut Blondies 279

774. Mexican Brownies 279

775. Chocolate Chip Cookie Blondies 280

776. Blueberry Bars 280

777. Potato Cream Cheese Bars 280

778. Raspberry Crumble Cake 281

779. Carrot Cake 281

780. Pineapple Orange Cake 281

781. Chocolate Strawberry Cobbler 282

782. Leches Cake 282

783. Caramel Apple Crisp 282

784. Gingerbread with Lemon Cream 283

785. Tiramisu Cheesecake 283

786. Pumpkin Cheesecake 283

787. Cinnamon Bread Pudding 284

788. Chocolate Croissant Pudding 284

FRUITS 285

789. Cocoa and Coconut Bars (Vegan) 285

790. Vanilla Cake 285

791. Vegan Apple Cupcakes 286

792. Vegan Orange Bread and Almonds ... 286

793. Vegan Tangerine Cake 286

794. Maple Tomato Bread (Vegan) 287

795. Vegan Lemon Squares 287

796. Dates and Cashew Sticks (Vegan) 287

797. Vegan Grape Pudding 288

798. Pumpkin and Coconut Seeds Bars (Vegan) 288

799. Vegan Cinnamon Bananas 288

800. Coffee Pudding 289

801. Vegan Blueberry Cake 289

802. Peach Cinnamon Cobbler 289

Conversion Tables 290

INDEX 324

HOW AN AIR FRYER WORKS?

An air fryer is comparable to an oven in the way it roasts and bakes. However, the distinction is that the heating elements are only located on the top and supported by a strong, large fan, which results in very crispy food in a short amount of time. The air fryer uses the rotation of heated air to easily and evenly cook food instead of using a pan of hot oil. The meal is placed in a metal basket (mesh) or rack to encourage the hot air to flow evenly around the food, producing the same light browning and crispness as frying in oil. Air fryers are easy to use, cook food faster than frying, and clean up quickly. You can prepare a selection of healthy foods like fruit, beef, seafood, poultry, and more, as well as make beneficial variations of your favorite fried foods like chips, onion rings, or fries.

It's also super quick to clean, and most systems include dishwasher-safe components.

Cook Tips For Beginners

- Shake the basket: Be sure to move the food around as it cooks in the device's tray. Shake it every 5-10 mins for the best performance.

- Don't overcrowd the basket: Give plenty of space for foods so that air circulates efficiently. This will ensure that you get crispy results.

Gently brush the food with cook spray.

- Keep food dry: To avoid splattering and excessive smoke, make sure food is dry before frying (even if you've marinated it). Likewise, be sure to regularly remove grease from the bottom of the machine while preparing high-fat items such as chicken wings.

- Cut food into equal-sized pieces for even cook.

- Other functions of air frying: The air fryer is not just for frying; it is also perfect for other healthier cook methods, such as grilling, baking and roasting. It's also valuable for reheating foods.

Since most beef meats are moist, they don't need additional oil:

- Season them with salt and your favorite herbs and spices.

- Be sure to stick to dry seasonings; less moisture contributes to crispier results.

- Wait until the last few mins of cook, whether you choose to baste the beef with any sauce or barbecue sauce.

- Lean cuts of meat, or items that contain little or no fat, need to brown, and the crispiness needs a splash of oil. Before frying, clean pork chops, boneless chicken breasts and drizzle with a touch of oil. Because of the higher smoke point, vegetable or canola oil is generally preferred, which ensures survival in the extreme heat of the air fryer.

- Before air frying, vegetables often need to be sprayed with oil. Sprinkle them with salt. Use less than you usually would. Crispy air-fried pieces have great flavor.

BREAKFAST AND BRUNCH

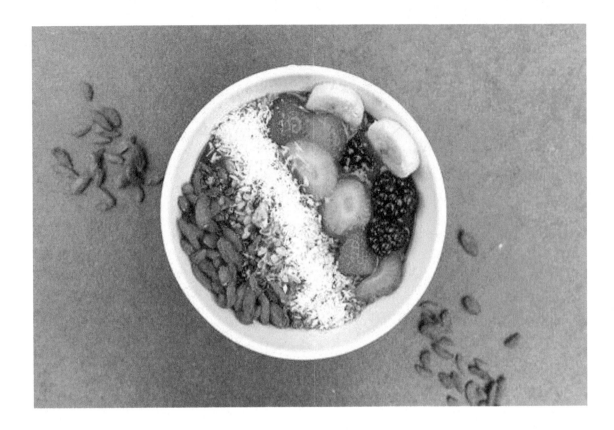

1. Asparagus Frittata

Prep Time: 10 mins
Servings: 4

Cook Time: 10 mins

Ingredients:
- *Six eggs*
- *Three mushrooms, sliced*
- *2 tsp butter, melted*
- *Ten asparagus, chopped*
- *1/4 cup half and half*
- *One cup mozzarella cheese, shredded*
- *1 tsp pepper*
- *1 tsp salt*

Directions: Stir mushrooms and asparagus with melted butter and add into the air fryer basket. Cook mushrooms and asparagus at 350 degrees F for five mins. Shake basket twice.
Meanwhile, in a bowl, whisk together eggs, half and half, salt and pepper. Transfer cook mushrooms and asparagus into the air fryer baking dish. Pour egg mixture over mushrooms and asparagus.
Place dish in the air fryer and bake at 350 degrees F for five.

Nutrition: Cal 211 Fat 13 g Carbs 4 g Protein 16 g

2. Air-Fried British Breakfast
Prep Time: 5 mins
Servings: 4

Cook Time: 20 mins

Ingredients:
- *Eight sausages*
- *Eight bacon slices*
- *Four eggs*
- *1 (16-ounce) can of baked beans*
- *Eight slices of toast*

Directions: Add sausages and bacon slices to an air fryer and cook them for ten mins at a 320 degrees F.

Using a ramekin, add the baked beans, then place another ramekin and add the eggs and whisk.
Increase the temperature to 290 degrees F.
Place it inside your oven and cook it for an additional ten mins.

Nutrition: Cal 850 Fat 40 g Carbs 20 g Protein 48 g

3. Blueberry Cobbler

Prep Time: 5 mins
Servings: 4

Cook Time: 15 mins

Ingredients:
- ⅓ cup whole-wheat pastry flour
- ¾ teaspoon baking powder
- Dash sea salt
- ½ cup fresh blueberries

- ¼ cup Granola, or plain store-bought granola
- ½ cup 2% milk

- 2 tablespoons pure maple syrup

- ½ teaspoon vanilla extract
- Cook oil spray

Directions: In a medium bowl, whisk the baking powder, flour, and salt. Add milk, maple syrup, and vanilla and gently whisk, just until thoroughly combined.
Preheat the oven by selecting BAKE, setting the temperature to 350 degrees F, and setting the time to three mins Select START.
Spray a 6-by-2-inch round baking pan with cook oil and pour the batter into the pan. Top with blueberries and granola.
Once the oven is preheated, place the pan into the basket.
Select BAKE, set the temperature to 350 degrees F, and set the time to fifteen mins Select START to begin.
When the cook is complete, the cobbler should be nicely browned and a knife inserted into the middle should come out clean. Enjoy topped with a little vanilla yogurt.

Nutrition: Cal 112 Fat 1 g Carbs 23 g Protein 3 g

4. Grilled Ham and Cheese

Prep Time: 5 mins
Servings: 2

Cook Time: 10 mins

Ingredients:
- 1 teaspoon butter
- Four slices bread

- Four slices smoked country ham
- Four slices Cheddar cheese

- Four thick slices tomato

Directions: Spread ½ teaspoon of butter onto one side of 2 slices of bread. Each sandwich will have one slice of bread with butter and one slice without.
Assemble each sandwich by layering two slices of Cheddar, two slices of ham, and two slices of tomato on the unbuttered pieces of bread. Top with the other bread slices, buttered side up.
Place the sandwiches in the oven buttered-side down. Cook for four mins
Open the air fryer. Flip the grilled cheese sandwiches. Bake for an additional four mins
Cool before serving. Cut each sandwich in half.

Nutrition: Cal 525 Fat 25 g Carbs 34 g Protein 41 g

5. Breakfast Potatoes

Prep Time: 10 mins
Serving: 6

Cook Time: 20 mins

Ingredients:
- 1½ teaspoons olive oil, divided
- Four large potatoes, skins on, cut into cubes

- 2 teaspoons seasoned salt, divided
- 1 teaspoon minced garlic, divided

- ½ onion, diced
- Two large green peppers, cut into 1-inch chunks

Directions: Lightly mist the fryer basket with olive oil.
In a bowl, mix the potatoes with ½ teaspoon of oil. Sprinkle with 1 teaspoon of seasoned salt and ½ teaspoon of minced garlic. Mix to coat.

Place the seasoned potatoes in the air fryer basket in a single layer. Cook for five mins. Shake the basket and cook for another five mins.
Meanwhile, in a bowl, stir the green peppers and onion with the remaining ½ teaspoon of oil.
Sprinkle the peppers and onions with the remaining 1 teaspoon of salt and ½ teaspoon of minced garlic. Stir to coat.
Add peppers and onions to the air fryer basket with the potatoes. Cook for five mins. Shake the basket and cook for an additional five mins.

Nutrition: Cal 199 Fat 1 g Carbs 43 g Protein 5 g

6. Scramble Casserole

Prep Time: 20 mins   **Cook Time:** 10 mins
Servings: 4

Ingredients:
- Six slices bacon
- Six eggs
- Cook oil
- ½ cup chopped red bell pepper
- ½ cup chopped green bell pepper
- ½ cup chopped onion
- ¾ cup shredded Cheddar cheese
- Salt and pepper

Directions: In a pan, over medium heat, cook the bacon, five to seven mins, flipping to evenly crisp. Dry out on paper towels, crumble, and set aside. In a bowl, whisk the eggs. Add salt and pepper.
Spray a barrel pan with cook oil. Add the beaten eggs, crumbled bacon, red bell pepper, green bell pepper, and onion to the pan.
Place in the oven. Cook for six mins. Open the air fryer and sprinkle the cheese over the casserole. Cook for an additional two mins.

Nutrition: Cal 348 Fat 26 g Carbs 4 g Protein 25 g

7. Broccoli Stuffed Peppers

Prep Time: 10 mins   **Cook Time:** 40 mins
Servings: 2

Ingredients:
- four eggs
- 1/2 cup cheddar cheese, grated
- 1/2 tsp garlic powder
- 1 tsp dried thyme
- 2 bell peppers cut in half
- 1/4 cup feta cheese, crumbled
- 1/2 cup broccoli, cooked
- 1/4 tsp pepper
- 1/2 tsp salt

Directions: Preheat the air fryer to 325 degrees F.
Stuff feta and broccoli into the bell peppers halved.
Beat egg in a bowl with seasoning and pour egg mixture into the pepper halved over feta and broccoli.
Place bell pepper halved into the basket and cook for 35-40 mins. Top with grated cheddar and cook until cheese melted.

Nutrition: Cal 340 Fat 22 g Carbs 12 g Protein 22 g

8. Cheese Soufflés

Prep Time: 10 mins   **Cook Time:** 6 mins
Servings: 8

Ingredients:
- Six large eggs, separated
- 3/4 cup heavy cream
- 1/4 tsp cayenne pepper
- 1/2 tsp xanthan gum
- 1/4 tsp cream of tartar
- 2 tbsp chives, chopped
- Two cups cheddar cheese, shredded
- 1 tsp salt
- 1/2 tsp pepper

Directions: Preheat the air fryer to 325 degrees F.
Spray eight ramekins with cook spray. Set aside.
In a medium bowl, whisk together cayenne pepper, pepper, almond flour, salt, and xanthan gum.
Slowly add heavy cream and stir to combine.
Whisk in egg yolks, chives, and cheese until well combined.
In a bowl, add egg whites and cream of tartar and beat until stiff peaks form.
Fold egg white mixture into the almond flour until combined.
Pour mixture into the prepared ramekins. Divide ramekins in batches.

Place the first batch of ramekins into the air fryer basket.
Cook soufflé for twenty mins.

Nutrition: Cal 210 Fat 16 g Carbs 1 g Protein 12 g

9. Chocolate-Filled Doughnuts

Prep Time: 10 mins
Servings: 12

Cook Time: 30 mins

Ingredients:
- 1 (8-count) can refrigerated biscuits
- Cook oil spray
- Forty-eight semisweet chocolate chips
- 3 tablespoons melted unsalted butter
- ¼ cup confectioners' sugar

Directions: Separate the biscuits and cut each into thirds, for twenty-four pieces.
Flatten each biscuit piece slightly and put two chocolate chips in the center. Wrap the dough around the chocolate and seal the edges.
Insert the crisper plate into the basket. Preheat the oven selecting air fry, setting the temperature to 330 degrees F, and setting the time to three mins. Select start to begin.
Once the oven is preheated, spray the crisper plate with cook oil. Brush doughnut holes with a bit of the butter and place it into the basket. Select air fry, set the temperature to 330 degrees F, and set the time between eight and twelve mins Select start.
When the cook is complete, place the doughnut holes on a plate and dust with the confectioners' sugar.

Nutrition: Cal 393 Fat 17 g Carbs 55 g Protein 5 g

10. Hash Browns

Prep Time: 15 mins
Servings: 4

Cook Time: 20 mins

Ingredients:
- Four russet potatoes
- 1 teaspoon paprika
- Salt
- Pepper
- Cook oil

Directions: Peel the potatoes. Using a cheese grater shred the potatoes.

Put the shredded potatoes in a bowl of cold water. Let sit for five mins. Toss to help dissolve the starch.
Dry out the potatoes and with paper towels. Make sure the potatoes are completely dry.
Season the potatoes with the paprika, salt and pepper.
Spray the potatoes with cook oil and transfer them to the air fryer. Cook for twenty mins and shake the basket every five mins (for four times).

Nutrition: Cal 150 Carbs 34 g Protein 4 g

11. Soufflé

Prep Time: 5 mins
Servings: 4

Cook Time: 15 mins

Ingredients:
- Six eggs
- 1/3 of cup of milk
- ½ cup of shredded mozzarella cheese
- 1 tablespoon of freshly chopped parsley
- ½ cup of chopped ham
- ½ teaspoon of garlic powder
- 1 teaspoon of salt
- 1 teaspoon of pepper

Directions: Grease four ramekins with a nonstick cook spray. Preheat the air fryer to 350 degrees F.
Using a bowl, add and mix all the ingredients properly.
Pour the egg mixture into the greased ramekins and place it inside your air fryer.
Cook it inside your oven for eight mins. Then carefully remove the soufflé from your air fryer and allow it to cool off.

Nutrition: Cal 195 Fat 15 g Carbs 6 g Protein 9 g

12. Steak and Eggs

Prep Time: 10 mins

Cook Time: 30 mins

Servings: 4

Ingredients:
- Cook oil spray
- 4 (4-ounce) New York strip steaks
- 1 teaspoon granulated garlic, divided
- Four eggs
- 1 teaspoon salt, divided
- 1 teaspoon freshly ground black pepper, divided
- ½ teaspoon paprika

Directions: Insert the crisper plate into the basket. Preheat the Air Fryer and select air fry, setting the temperature to 360 degrees F, and setting the time to three mins Select start to begin.
Spray the crisper plate with cook oil. Place two steaks into the basket; do not oil or season them at this time.
Select air fry, set the temperature to 360 degrees F, and set the time to nine mins Select start.
After five mins, open the unit and flip the steaks. Sprinkle each with ¼ teaspoon of salt, ¼ teaspoon of granulated garlic, and ¼ teaspoon of pepper. Resume cook until the steaks register at least 145 degrees F on a food thermometer.
When the cook is complete, transfer the steaks to a plate and tent with foil to keep warm. Repeat steps 2, 3, and 4 with the remaining steaks.
Spray four ramekins with oil. Crack one egg into each ramekin. Sprinkle the eggs with the paprika and remaining ½ teaspoon each of salt and pepper. Work in batches, place two ramekins into the basket.
Select BAKE, set the temperature to 330 degrees F, and set the time to five mins Select start to begin. When the cook is complete and the eggs are cooked to 160 degrees F, remove the ramekins and repeat step 7 with the remaining two ramekins.
Serve the eggs with the steaks.

Nutrition: Cal 304 Fat 19 g Carbs 2 g Protein 31 g

13. Maple-Glazed Doughnuts

Prep Time: 10 mins

Cook Time: 14 mins **Servings:** 8

Ingredients:
- 1 (8-count) can jumbo flaky refrigerator biscuits
- Cook oil spray
- ½ cup light brown sugar
- ¼ cup butter
- 3 tablespoons milk
- 2 teaspoons pure maple syrup

Directions: Insert the crisper plate into the basket. Preheat the oven by selecting air fry, setting the temperature to 350 degrees F, and setting the time to three mins.
Cut out the center of the buscuits with a small, round cookie cutter.
Once the unit is preheated, spray the crisper plate with cook oil. Work it in batches, place four doughnuts into the basket.
Select air fry, set the temperature to 350 degrees F, and set the time to five mins Select start.
When the cook is complete, place the donuts on a plate. Repeat steps 3 and 4 with the remaining donuts.
In a saucepan heat, combine the butter, brown sugar, and milk. Heat until butter is melted and sugar is dissolved, about four mins. Remove the pan and whisk in the confectioners' sugar and maple syrup until smooth.
Dip the slightly cooled doughnuts into the maple glaze. Place them on a wire rack. Let rest just until the glaze sets.

Nutrition: Cal 219 Fat 10 g Carbs 30 g Protein 2 g

14. Bagels

Prep Time: 10 mins

Cook Time: 10 mins **Servings:** 2

Ingredients:
- One egg
- ½ cup self-rising flour, plus more for dusting
- ½ cup plain Greek yogurt
- 1 tablespoon water
- 4 teaspoons everything bagel spice mix
- Cook oil spray
- 1 tablespoon butter, melted

Directions: In a bowl, using a wooden spoon, mix together the flour and yogurt until a tacky dough forms. Transfer the dough to a lightly floured work surface and roll the dough into a ball.
Cut into two pieces and roll each piece into a log. Form each log into a bagel shape, pinching the ends together.
In a bowl, whisk the water and egg. Brush the egg wash on the bagels.

Sprinkle 2 teaspoons of the spice mix on each bagel and press it into the dough.

Insert the crisper plate into the basket and then the basket into the unit. Preheat by selecting bake, setting the temperature to 330 degrees F, and setting the time to three mins Select start.

Spray the crisper plate with cook spray. Drizzle with the bagels with the butter and place them into the basket.

Select BAKE, set the temperature to 330 degrees F, and set the time to ten mins Select START.

When the cook is complete, the bagels should be lightly golden on the outside.

Nutrition: Cal 271 Fat 13 g Carbs 28 g

15. French Toast Sticks

Servings: 12
Prep Time: 5 mins

Cook Time: 15 mins

Ingredients:

- *Four slices Texas toast*
- *1 tablespoon butter*
- *1 teaspoon stevia*
- *1 teaspoon ground cinnamon*
- *One egg*
- *¼ cup milk*
- *1 teaspoon vanilla extract*
- *Cook oil*

Directions: Cut each slice of bread into 3 pieces.

Place the butter in a microwave-safe bowl. Heat for fifteen seconds, or until the butter has melted.

Remove the bowl from the microwave. Add the egg, milk, stevia, cinnamon, and vanilla extract. Whisk until fully combined.

Sprinkle the air fryer basket with cook oil.

Dredge each of the bread sticks in the egg mixture.

Place the toast sticks in the oven. It is okay to stack them. Spray the French toast sticks with cook oil. Cook for eight mins. Open the air fryer and flip each of the toast sticks. Cook for an additional four mins.

Cool before serving.

Nutrition: Cal 52 Fat 2 g Carbs 7 g

16. Granola

Servings: 2
Prep Time: 5 mins

Cook Time: 40 mins

Ingredients:

- *One cup rolled oats*
- *3 tablespoons pure maple syrup*
- *1 tablespoon sugar*
- *1 tablespoon neutral-flavored oil*
- *¼ teaspoon salt*
- *¼ teaspoon ground cinnamon*
- *¼ teaspoon vanilla extract*

Directions: Insert the crisper plate into the basket. Then, the basket into the unit. Preheat the unit by selecting BAKE, setting the temperature to 250 degrees F, and setting the time to 3 mins. Select START.

In a bowl, mix together the oats, oil, salt, cinnamon, maple syrup, sugar, and vanilla until thoroughly combined. Transfer the granola to a 6-by-2-inch round the pan.

Once the unit is preheated, place the pan into.

Select BAKE, set the temperature to 250 degrees F and set the time to forty mins. Select START. After ten mins, mix the granola.

Resume cook, stirring the granola every ten mins, for a total of forty mins.

Place the granola on a plate to cool, when the cook is complete. It will become crisp as it cools. Store the completely cooled granola in an airtight container in a cool, dry place for 1 to 2 weeks.

Nutrition: Cal 165 Fat 5 g Carbs 27 g

17. Fried Potatoes

Servings: 4
Prep Time: 5 mins

Cook Time: 25 mins

Ingredients:

- *Three large russet potatoes*
- *1 tablespoon canola oil*
- *1 tablespoon extra-virgin olive oil*
- *1 teaspoon paprika*
- *One cup chopped onion*
- *One cup chopped red bell pepper*
- *One cup chopped green bell pepper*
- *Salt*
- *Pepper*

Directions: Cut the potatoes into ½-inch cubes. Place the potatoes in a bowl of cold water and allow them to soak for at least thirty mins, preferably an hour.

Dry out the potatoes and wipe thoroughly with paper towels. Return them to the empty bowl.

Add the canola and paprika, olive oils, and salt and pepper to flavor. Stir to fully coat the potatoes.

Transfer the potatoes to the air fryer. Cook for twenty mins, shaking the basket every five mins (a total of four times).

Put the onion and peppers to the basket. Fry for an additional three to four mins.

Nutrition: Cal 279 Fat 8 g Carbs 50 g

18. Cherry Tarts

Servings: 6
Prep Time: 15 mins

Cook Time: 20 mins

Ingredients:

For the tarts:
- *Two refrigerated piecrusts*
- *⅓ Cup cherry preserves*
- *1 teaspoon cornstarch*
- *Cook oil*

For the frosting:
- *½ cup vanilla yogurt*
- *1-ounce cream cheese*
- *1 teaspoon stevia*
- *Rainbow sprinkles*

Directions: Place the piecrusts on a flat surface. Make use of a knife or pizza cutter, cut each piecrust into three rectangles, for six in total. (I discard the unused dough left from slicing the edges.)

In a bowl, combine the preserves and cornstarch. Stir well.

Scoop 1 tablespoon of the preserve mixture onto the top half of each piece of piecrust.

Fold the bottom of each piece up to close the tart. Press along the edges of each tart to seal using the back of a fork.

Sprinkle the breakfast tarts with cook oil and place them in the oven. I do not recommend piling the breakfast tarts. They will stick together if piled. You may need to prepare them in two batches. Cook for ten mins

Allow the breakfast tarts to cool fully before removing from the air fryer.

If needed, repeat steps 5 and 6 for the remaining breakfast tarts.

To make the frosting: In a bowl, mix the cream cheese, yogurt, and stevia. Mix well.

Spread the breakfast tarts with frosting and top with sprinkles.

Nutrition: Cal 119 Fat 4 g Carbs 19 g

19. Strawberry Tarts

Servings: 6
Prep Time: 15 mins

Cook Time: 20 mins

Ingredients:
- *Two refrigerated piecrusts*
- *½ cup strawberry preserves*
- *1 teaspoon cornstarch*
- *Cook oil spray*
- *½ cup low-fat vanilla yogurt*
- *1-ounce cream cheese, at room temperature*
- *3 tablespoons confectioners' sugar*
- *Rainbow sprinkles, for decorating*

Directions: Place the piecrusts on a flat surface. Cut each piecrust into three rectangles using a knife or pizza cutter, for six in total. Discard any unused dough from the piecrust edges.

In a bowl, mix the preserves and cornstarch.

Scoop 1 tablespoon of the strawberry mixture onto the top half of each piece of piecrust.

Fold the bottom of each piece up to enclose the filling. Press along the edges of each tart to seal using the back of a fork.

Insert the crisper plate into the basket and then into the unit. Preheat by selecting bake, setting the temperature to 375 degrees F, and setting the time to three mins Select start to start.

Spray the crisper plate with cook oil. Work in batches, spray the breakfast tarts with cook oil and place them into the basket in a single layer. Do not stack the tarts.

Select bake, set the temperature to 375 degrees F, and set the time to ten mins Select start. When the cook is complete, the tarts should be light golden. Repeat steps 5, 6, 7, and 8 for the remaining breakfast tarts.

In a bowl, mix yogurt, cream cheese, and confectioners' sugar. Spread the breakfast tarts with the frosting and top with sprinkles.

Nutrition: Cal 408 Fat 20.5 g Carbs 56 g

20. Jalapeno Muffins

Servings: 8
Prep Time: 10 mins **Cook Time:** 15 mins

Ingredients:
- Five eggs
- 1/3 cup coconut oil, melted
- 2 tsp baking powder
- 3 tbsp erythritol
- 1/4 cup unsweetened coconut milk
- 2/3 cup coconut flour
- 3 tbsp jalapenos, sliced
- 3/4 tsp sea salt

Directions: Preheat the air fryer to 325 degrees F.
In a large bowl, stir coconut flour, erythritol, baking powder, and sea salt.
Mix eggs, jalapenos, coconut milk, and coconut oil until well combined.
Pour batter into the silicone muffin molds and place into the air fryer basket.
Cook muffins for fifteen mins.

Nutrition: Cal 125 Fat 12 g Carbs 7 g

21. Mixed Berry Muffins

Servings: 8
Prep Time: 15 mins **Cook Time:** 15 mins

Ingredients:
- 1⅓ cups and 1 tablespoon all-purpose flour, divided
- ¼ cup granulated sugar
- 2 tablespoons light brown sugar
- 2 teaspoons baking powder
- Two eggs
- ⅔ Cup whole milk
- ⅓ Cup safflower oil
- One cup mixed fresh berries

Directions: In a bowl, mix together 1⅓ cups of flour, brown sugar, the granulated sugar, and baking powder until mixed well.
In a small bowl, whisk eggs, milk, and oil until combined. Mix the egg mixture into the dry ingredients just until combined.
In another bowl, toss the mixed berries with the left over 1 tablespoon of flour until coated. Stir the berries into the batter.
Two times the 16 foil muffin cups to make 8 cups.
Insert the crisper plate into the basket and then the basket into the unit. Preheat the unit (select BAKE), setting the temperature to 315 degrees F, and setting the time to 3 mins Select START to start.
Once the unit is preheated, place 4 cups into the basket and fill each three-quarter full with the batter.
Select BAKE, set the temperature to 315°F, and set the time for 17 mins Select START/STOP to begin.
After about twelve mins, check the muffins.
When the cook is done, transfer the muffins to a wire rack to cool. Repeat steps 6, 7, and 8 with the remaining muffin cups and batter. Let the muffins cool for ten mins before serving.

Nutrition: Cal 230 Fat 11g Carbs 30g

22. Mushrooms Frittata

Servings: 1
Prep Time: 10 mins **Cook Time:** 13 mins

Ingredients:
- One cup egg whites
- One cup spinach, chopped
- Two mushrooms, sliced
- 2 tbsp parmesan cheese, grated
- Salt

Directions: Sprinkle pan with cook spray and heat over medium heat. Add mushrooms and sauté for 2-3 mins Add spinach and cook for 1-2 mins. Transfer mushroom spinach mixture into the air fryer.
Beat egg whites in a mixing bowl until frothy and season it with a pinch of salt.
Pour egg white mixture into the spinach mixture and sprinkle with parmesan. Place pan in the basket and cook at 350 degrees F for eight mins.

Nutrition: Cal 176 Fat 3 g Carbs 4 g

23. Omelet

Servings: 2
Prep Time: 10 mins

Cook Time: 6 mins

Ingredients:
- *Three eggs, lightly beaten*
- *2 tbsp cheddar cheese, shredded*
- *2 tbsp heavy cream*
- *2 mushrooms, sliced*
- *1/4 small onion, chopped*
- *1/4 bell pepper, diced*
- *Pepper*
- *Salt*

Directions: In a medium bowl, whisk eggs with cream, vegetables, pepper, and salt.
Preheat the air fryer to 400 degrees F.
Pour egg mixture into the air fryer pan. Place pan in the basket and cook for five mins
Add shredded cheese on top of the frittata and cook for one minute more.

Nutrition: Cal 160 Fat 10 g Carbs 4 g

24. Puffed Egg Tarts

Servings: 4
Prep Time: 10 mins

Cook Time: 20 mins

Ingredients:
- *⅓ Sheet frozen puff pastry, thawed*
- *Cook oil spray*
- *½ cup shredded Cheddar cheese*
- *Two eggs*
- *¼ teaspoon salt, divided*
- *1 teaspoon minced fresh parsley*

Directions: Insert the crisper plate into the basket and the basket into the unit. Preheat the unit (selecting bake), setting the temperature to 390 degrees F, and setting the time to three mins Select start to begin.
Lay the puff pastry sheet on a piece of parchment paper and cut it in half.
Once the unit is preheated, spray the crisper plate with cook oil. Transfer the two squares of pastry to the basket, keeping them on the parchment paper.
Select bake, set the temperature to 390 degrees F, and set the time to twenty mins Select start.
After ten mins, use a metal spoon to press down the center of each pastry square to make a well. Divide the cheese equally between the baked pastries. Crack an egg on top of the cheese, and sprinkle each with the salt. Resume cook for seven to ten mins
When the cook is complete, the eggs will be cooked through. Sprinkle each with parsley.

Nutrition: Cal 322 Fat 24 g Carbs 12 g

25. Radish Hash Browns

Servings: 4
Prep Time: 10 mins

Cook Time: 13 mins

Ingredients:
- *1 lb. radishes, washed and cut off roots*
- *1 tbsp olive oil*
- *1/2 tsp paprika*
- *1/2 tsp onion powder*
- *1/2 tsp garlic powder*
- *One medium onion*
- *1/4 tsp pepper*
- *3/4 tsp sea salt*

Directions: Slice onion and radishes. Add in a mixing bowl and toss with olive oil.
Transfer onion and radish slices in air fryer basket and cook at 360 degrees F for eight mins. Shake basket.
Return onion and radish slices in a mixing bowl and stir with seasonings.
Cook onion and radish slices in air fryer basket for five mins at 400 degrees F. Shake the basket halfway through.

26. Sausage and Cream Cheese Biscuits

Serving: 5
Prep Time: 5 mins   **Cook Time:** 15 mins

Ingredients:

- 12 ounces chicken breakfast sausage
- 1 (6-ounce) can biscuits
- ⅛ cup cream cheese

Directions: Form the sausage into five small patties. Place the sausage patties in the air fryer and cook for five mins.
Open the oven. Flip the patties. Cook for an additional five mins.
Remove the sausages from the air fryer.
Separate the biscuit dough into five biscuits. Place the biscuits in the oven. Cook for three mins.
Flip the biscuits. Cook for an additional two mins.
Split each biscuit in half. Spread 1 teaspoon of cream cheese onto the bottom of each biscuit. Top with a sausage patty and the other half of the biscuit.

Nutrition: Cal 240 Fat 13 g Carbs 20 g

27. Sausage and Egg Burrito

Servings: 6
Prep Time: 5 mins   **Cook Time:** 30 mins

Ingredients:

- Six eggs
- Salt
- Pepper
- Cook oil
- ½ cup chopped red bell pepper
- ½ cup chopped green bell pepper
- 8 ounces ground chicken sausage
- ½ cup salsa
- Six medium (8-inch) flour tortillas
- ½ cup shredded Cheddar cheese

Directions: In a bowl, whisk the eggs, add salt and pepper.
Place a skillet on medium-high heat. Spray with cook oil. Add the eggs. Scramble for two to three mins, until the eggs are fluffy. Remove the eggs and set aside.
Add the chopped bell peppers. Cook for two to three mins, once the peppers are soft.
Add the ground sausage to the skillet. Break the sausage into smaller pieces using a spoon. Cook for three to four mins, until the sausage is brown.
Add the salsa and scrambled eggs and stir to combine. Remove the skillet from heat.
Spoon the mixture onto the tortillas.
To form the burritos, fold the sides of tortillas toward the center and roll up from the bottom. You can secure each burrito with a toothpick.
Spray the burritos with cook oil and place in the air fryer. Cook the burritos for eight mins.
Open the oven and flip the burritos. Heat it for an additional 2 mins.
Sprinkle the Cheddar over the burritos.

Nutrition: Cal 236 Fat 13 g Carbs 16 g

28. Cheese and Bacon Muffins

Servings: 4
Prep Time: 5 mins   **Cook Time:** 17 mins

Ingredients:

- 1 ½ cup of all-purpose flour
- 2 teaspoons of baking powder
- ½ cup of milk
- Two eggs
- 1 tablespoon of freshly chopped parsley
- Four cooked and chopped bacon slices
- 1 thinly chopped onion
- ½ cup of shredded cheddar cheese
- ½ teaspoon of onion powder
- 1 teaspoon of salt
- 1 teaspoon of black pepper

Directions: Turn on your air fryer to 360 degrees F.
Using a large bowl, add and mix all the ingredients until it mixes properly.
Then grease the muffin cups with a nonstick cook spray or line it with a parchment paper. Pour the batter proportionally into each muffin cup.
Place it inside your air fryer and cook it for fifteen mins.
Thereafter, carefully remove it from your oven and allow it to chill.

Nutrition: Cal 180 Fat 18 g Carbs 16 g

29. Spinach Frittata

Prep Time: 5 mins
Servings: 1

Cook Time: 8 mins

Ingredients:
- Three eggs
- One cup spinach, chopped
- One small onion, minced
- 2 tbsp mozzarella cheese, grated
- Salt and Pepper

Directions: Preheat the air fryer to 350 degrees F. Spray air fryer pan with cook spray.
In a bowl, whisk eggs with remaining ingredients until well combined.
Pour egg mixture into the prepared pan and place pan in the air fryer basket.
Cook frittata for eight mins or until set.

Nutrition: Cal 384 Fat 23.3 g Carbs 10.7 g

30. Vegetable Egg Cups

Prep Time: 10 mins
Servings: 4

Cook Time: 20 mins

Ingredients:
- Four eggs
- 1 tbsp cilantro, chopped
- 4 tbsp half and half
- One cup cheddar cheese, shredded
- One cup vegetables, diced
- Salt and Pepper

Directions: Sprinkle four ramekins with cook spray and set aside.
In a mixing bowl, whisk eggs with cilantro, half and half, vegetables, 1/2 cup cheese, salt and pepper.
Pour egg mixture into the four ramekins.
Place ramekins in the basket of the air fryer and cook at 300 degrees F for twelve mins.
Top with remaining 1/2 cup cheese and cook for two mins more at 400 degrees F.

Nutrition: Cal 194 Fat 11.5 g Carbs 6 g

31. Vegetable Egg Soufflé

Prep Time: 10 mins
Servings: 4

Cook Time: 20 mins

Ingredients:
- Four eggs
- 1 tsp onion powder
- 1 tsp garlic powder
- 1 tsp red pepper, crushed
- 1/2 cup broccoli florets, chopped
- 1/2 cup mushrooms, chopped

Directions: Sprinkle four ramekins with cook spray and set aside.
In a bowl, whisk eggs with garlic powder, onion powder, and red pepper.
Add mushrooms and broccoli and mix well.
Pour egg mixture into the prepared ramekins and place ramekins into the air fryer basket.
Cook at 350 degrees F for fifteen mins. Make sure soufflé is cooked if soufflé is not cooked then cook for five mins more.

Nutrition: Cal 91 Fat 5.1 g Carbs 4.7 g

32. Waffles and Chicken

Servings: 4
Prep Time: 15 mins

Cook Time: 30 mins

Ingredients:
- Eight whole chicken wings
- 1 teaspoon garlic powder
- Chicken seasoning, for preparing the chicken
- Freshly ground black pepper
- ½ cup all-purpose flour

- *Cook oil spray*
- *Eight frozen waffles*
- *Pure maple syrup, for serving*

Directions: In a medium bowl, combine the garlic powder and chicken, and season with chicken seasoning and pepper. Stir to coat.

Transfer the chicken to a re-sealable plastic bag. Add the flour. Seal the bag and shake it to coat the chicken thoroughly.

Insert the crisper plate into the basket and the basket into the unit. Preheat the unit (selecting AIR FRY), setting the temperature to 400 degrees F, and setting the time to 3 mins. Select START to begin.

When the oven is preheated, spray the crisper plate with cook oil. Transfer chicken from bag to basket. Spray the chicken with cook oil.

Select air fry, set the temperature to 400 degrees F, and set the time to twenty mins. Select start.

After five mins, remove the basket and shake the wings. Reinsert the basket to resume cook. Remove and shake the basket every five mins until the chicken is fully cooked.

When the cook is complete, remove the cooked chicken from the basket; cover to keep warm.

Rinse the basket and crisper plate with hot water. Insert them back into the unit.

Select air fry, set the temperature to 360 degrees F, and set the time to three mins. Select start.

Once the unit is preheated, spray the crisper plate with cook spray. Work in batches, place the frozen waffles into the basket. Do not stack them. Spray the waffles with cook oil.

Select air fry, set the temperature to 360 degrees F, and set the time to six mins. Select start.

Repeat steps 10 and 11 with remaining waffles when the cook is complete.

Serve waffles with chicken and a touch of maple syrup.

Nutrition: Cal 461 Fat 22 g Carbs 45 g

33. Italian Frittata

Servings: 6
Prep Time: 5 mins

Cook Time: 10 mins

Ingredients:
- *Six eggs*
- *1/3 cup of milk*
- *4-ounces of chopped Italian sausage*
- *Three cups of stemmed and roughly chopped kale*
- *One red deseeded and chopped bell pepper*
- *½ cup of a grated feta cheese*
- *One chopped zucchini*
- *1 tablespoon of freshly chopped basil*
- *1 teaspoon of garlic powder*
- *1 teaspoon of onion powder*
- *1 teaspoon of salt*
- *1 teaspoon of black pepper*

Directions: Turn on your air fryer to 360 degrees F.

Grease the air fryer pan with a nonstick cook spray.

Add the Italian sausage to the pan and cook it inside your air fryer for five mins.

While doing that, add and toss in the remaining ingredients until it mixes properly.

Add the egg mixture and allow it to cook inside your air fryer for five mins.

Thereafter carefully remove the pan and allow it to cool off until it gets chill enough to serve.

Nutrition: Cal 225 Fat 14 g Carbs 4.5 g

34. Zucchini Muffins

Servings: 8
Prep Time: 10 mins

Cook Time: 20 mins

Ingredients:
- *Six eggs*
- *Four drops stevia*
- *One cup zucchini, grated*
- *1/4 cup Swerve*
- *1/3 cup coconut oil, melted*
- *3/4 cup coconut flour*
- *1/4 tsp ground nutmeg*
- *1 tsp ground cinnamon*
- *1/2 tsp baking soda*

Directions: Preheat the air fryer to 325 degrees F.

Add all ingredients except zucchini in a bowl and mix well. Add zucchini and stir well.

Pour batter into the silicone muffin molds and place into the basket of air fryer.

Cook muffins for twenty mins.

Nutrition: Cal 136 Fat 12 g Carbs 1 g

35. Zucchini Noodles

Servings: 3
Prep Time: 10 mins

Cook Time: 44 mins

Ingredients:

- One egg
- 1/2 cup parmesan cheese, grated
- 1/2 cup feta cheese, crumbled
- 1 tbsp thyme
- One garlic clove, chopped
- One onion, chopped
- Two medium zucchinis, trimmed and spiralized
- 2 tbsp olive oil
- One cup mozzarella cheese, grated
- 1/2 tsp pepper
- 1/2 tsp salt

Directions: Preheat the air fryer to 350 degrees F.

Add spiralized zucchini and salt in a colander and set aside for ten mins. Wash zucchini noodles and pat dry with a paper towel. Heat the oil in a pan over medium heat. Add garlic and onion and sauté for 3-4 mins. Add zucchini noodles and cook for 4-5 mins until softened. Add zucchini mixture into the air fryer baking pan. Add thyme, egg, cheeses. Stir well and season. Place pan in the air fryer and bake for 30-35 mins.

Nutrition: Cal 435 Fat 29 g Carbs 10.4 g

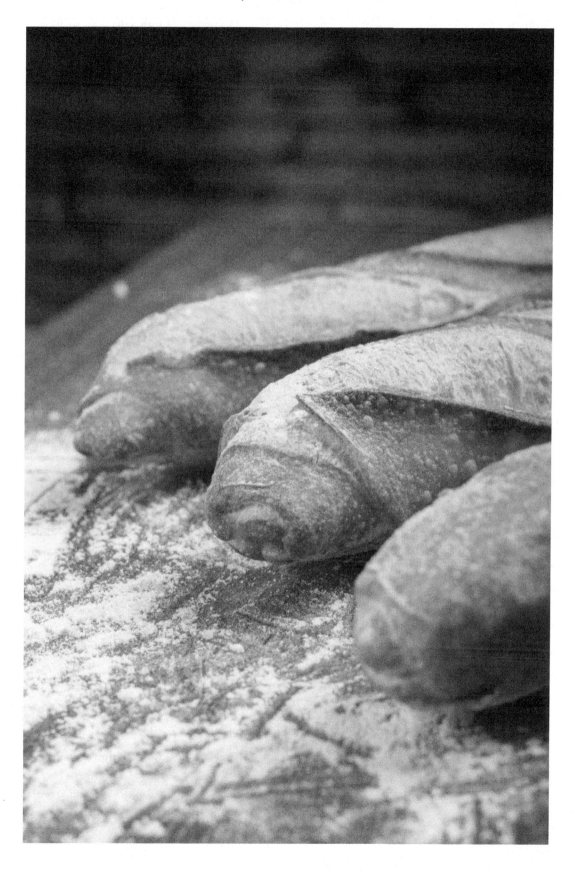

36. 3-Ingredients: Banana Bread

Prep Time: 10 mins
Servings: 6

Cook Time: 20 mins

Ingredients:
- 2 (6.4-oz.) banana muffin mix
- 1 cup water
- 1 ripe banana, peeled and mashed

Directions: In a bowl, add all the Ingredients.
Place the mixture into a loaf pan.
Press "Power Button" of Air Fryer and turn the dial to select the Bake mode.
Press the Time button and turn the dial to set the cook time to twenty mins.
Push the Temp button and rotate the dial to set the temperature at 360°F. Press Start button.
Open the lid when the unit beeps to show that it is preheated.
Arrange the pan in the Air Fry Basket and insert in the oven.
Place the pan onto a wire rack to cool for ten mins.
Carefully, invert the bread onto wire rack to cool completely before slicing.
Cut the bread into desired-sized slices.

Nutrition: Cal 144 Fat 3.8 g Carbs 25.5 g

37. Apple Bread

Prep Time: 15 mins
Servings: 6

Cook Time: 45 mins

Ingredients:
- One cup all-purpose flour
- 1/3 cup brown sugar
- 1 teaspoon ground nutmeg
- 1 teaspoon ground cinnamon
- ½ teaspoon baking soda
- Salt
- One egg
- 5 tablespoons plus 1 teaspoon vegetable oil
- ¾ teaspoon vanilla extract
- Two cups apples, peeled, cored and chopped

Directions: In a bowl, mix together the flour, spices, baking soda, sugar, and salt.
In another bowl, add the oil and egg, and whisk until smooth. Add the vanilla extract and whisk well.
Slowly, add the flour mixture, whisking continuously until well combined.
Fold in the chopped apples.
Lightly, grease a cake pan. Place mixture evenly into.
With a piece of foil, cover the pan and poke some holes using a fork.
Press "Power Button" of Air Fryer and turn the dial to select the "Air Fry" mode.
Set the cook time to forty-five mins. Push Temp button and rotate the dial to set the temperature at 330° F.
Press "Start button.
When the unit beeps, open the lid. Arrange the pan in "Air Fry Basket" and insert in the oven. After forty mins of cook, remove the foil piece from pan. Place the pan onto a wire rack for about 10-15 mins.
Carefully, invert the bread onto wire rack to cool completely before slicing.
Cut the bread into desired-sized slices and serve.

Nutrition: Cal 260 Fat 12.5 g Carbs 34.7 g

38. Bacon and Garlic Pizzas

Servings: 4

Prep Time: 10 mins

Cook Time: 10 mins

Ingredients:
- Four dinner rolls, frozen
- One cup tomato sauce
- Four garlic cloves minced
- 1/2 teaspoon oregano dried
- 1/2 teaspoon garlic powder
- Eight bacon slices, cooked and chopped
- 1 and ¼ cups cheddar cheese, grated
- Cook spray

Directions: Place dinner rolls on a working surface and press them to obtain four ovals.
Spray each oval with cook spray, transfer them to your oven and cook them at 370° F for two mins.

Spread tomato sauce on each oval, divide garlic, sprinkle oregano and garlic powder and top with bacon and cheese. Return pizzas to your heated air fryer and cook them at 370° F for eight mins more.

Nutrition: Cal 217 Fat 5 g Carbs 12 g

39. Baked Bread

Prep Time: 1hr 15 m
Servings: 1

Cook Time: 50 mins

Ingredients:
- Three Eggs
- 250 g low fat quark
- 30 g Green grain meal, wheat meal or oat meal
- 11/2 teaspoon ammonium bicarbonate
- 11/2 teaspoon salt
- Bread spice mix
- 1 teaspoon honey
- 100 g Spelled flour, possibly more
- 70 g Psyllium or flax seeds
- 30 g Poppy
- 1 teaspoon Vinegar
- 50g Sunflower seeds

Directions: Mix all the ingredients in sequence using an electric beater with a dough hook. If the mixture is flaky, take it out and knead again. Form an even loaf and bake in the air fryer at 165 degrees C for fifty mins.

Nutrition: Cal: 299 Fat: 11 g Carbs: 20 g

40. Pizza

Prep Time: 5 mins
Serving: 1

Cook Time: 8 mins

Ingredients:
- Two large eggs
- ¼ cup unsweetened, unflavored almond milk
- ¼ teaspoon acceptable sea salt
- ¼ cup shredded Parmesan cheese
- Six pepperoni slices
- 1/8 teaspoon ground black pepper
- ¼ cup diced onions
- ¼ teaspoon dried oregano leaves
- ¼ cup pizza sauce, warmed, for serving

Directions: Preheat the air fryer to 350 degrees F. Grease a six by 3-inch cake pan.
In a bowl, use a fork to whisk together the almond milk, eggs, salt, and pepper. Add the onions and stir to mix. Pour the mixture into the greased pan—top with the cheese, oregano and pepperoni slices. Cook for eight mins, until the eggs are cooked to your liking.
Loosen the eggs from the pan's sides with a spatula and place them on a serving plate. Drizzle the pizza sauce on top.

Nutrition: Cal 357; Fat 25 g; Carbs 9 g

41. Vegan Beer Bread

Prep time: 10 mins
Servings: 4

Cook time: 45 mins

Ingredients:
- 225 g wheat flour
- 150 ml dark beer or malt beer
- 75 g sourdough
- 10 g yeast
- tbsp. salt
- For the rye sourdough:
- 75 g rye flour
- 75 ml water

Directions: Mix rye flour and lukewarm water into a dough and cover and leave to rest in a warm place for twelve hours.
As soon as the sourdough is left to rest, dissolve the yeast and salt in 3 tbsp. Of dark beer until bubbles form. Then add the sourdough, wheat flour and the remaining dark beer and knead for eight mins.
Cover again the dough and then let it rest in a warm place for 1-2 hours. Then either put the dough in the hot air fryer's baking pan without further processing or shape it like a loaf and place it on the grid insert. Cook bread for 5 mins at 390° F, then reduce the baking temperature to 390° F and bake for another twenty-five mins.
Now and then, brush the bread with a little water to have excellent, shiny crust forms.

Nutrition: Cal: 326 kcal Fat: 1.31 g Carbs: 67.31 g

42. Carrot Bread

Prep Time: 15 mins
Servings: 6

Cook Time: 30 mins

Ingredients:
- One cup all-purpose flour
- 1 teaspoon baking soda
- ½ teaspoon ground cinnamon
- ¼ teaspoon ground cloves
- ¼ teaspoon ground nutmeg
- ½ teaspoon salt
- 2 eggs
- ¾ cup vegetable oil
- 1/3 cup white sugar
- 1/3 cup light brown sugar
- ½ teaspoon vanilla extract
- 1½ cups carrots, peeled and grated

Directions: In a bowl, mix together the baking soda, flour, spices and salt.
In another bowl, add the eggs, sugars, oil, and vanilla extract and beat until well combined. Add the flour mixture and mix. Fold in the carrots.
Place the mixture into a greased baking pan.
Press "Power Button" of Air Fryer. Turn the dial to select the "Air Fry". Press the Time button and turn the dial to set the cook time to thirty mins. Push the Temp button and rotate the dial to set the temperature at 320° F. Press Start.
When the unit beeps (to show that it is preheated), open the lid.
Arrange the pan in "Air Fry Basket" and insert in the oven. Place the pan onto a wire rack to cool for about ten mins.
Carefully, invert the bread onto wire rack to cool completely before slicing.
Cut the bread into desired-sized slices and serve.

Nutrition: Cal 426 Fat 29.2 g Carbs 38 g

43. Olive Bread and Rosemary

Prep time: 60 mins
Servings: 4

Cook time: 40 mins

Ingredients:
- lb. Wheat flour
- 1 cup of water
- Garlic powder
- Rosemary
- 4 tsp. fresh yeast
- Pitted black olives
- Parsley to taste
- Olive oil
- Salt

Directions: Mix the flour with the 4 tsp. of fresh yeast, a tsp. of garlic powder, ½ of parsley, and two rosemary. Mix well. Stir the yeast and spices with the flour that will give flavor to the black olive bread.
Next, add 3 tbsps. of olive oil. Mix well, ensuring that there are a few lumps as possible. Add 1 cup of water.
With a shovel, toss all ingredients and distribute the wet ingredients among the dry ones.
Mix well until the dough acquires a manageable texture. Flour the table and smear your hands with more flour.
Remove the dough from the bowl and knead with force for eight mins.
Now, shape and mold the dough into a ball and place it on a baking sheet and its greaseproof paper.
Stretch with a roller's help gives it an elongated shape, with rounded edges and a thickness of more or less 1 cm. Note that it will double in size, approximately. Let it rise for 1 hour. on the tray with the baking paper and covered with a cloth.
After the hour, paint the surface with generous olive oil so that the base is well greased.
On top, decorate with the sliced black olives, rosemary, salt and more garlic powder.
Now, put it in the air fryer at 360 degrees F for about forty mins.
When it begins to toast, after about thirty mins, if the bread is drying, you can repaint the top of the black olive bread with more oil.

Nutrition: Cal: 138 Carbs: 22 g Fat: 3.7 g

44. Carrot, Raisin & Walnut Bread

Prep Time: 15 mins
Servings: 8

Cook Time: 35 mins

Ingredients:
- 2 cups all-purpose flour
- 1½ teaspoons ground cinnamon
- 2 teaspoons baking soda
- ½ teaspoon salt
- Three eggs
- ½ cup sunflower oil
- ½ cup applesauce
- ¼ cup honey
- ¼ cup plain yogurt
- 2 teaspoons vanilla essence
- 2½ cups carrots, peeled and shredded
- ½ cup raisins
- ½ cup walnuts

Directions: Line the bottom of a greased baking pan with parchment paper.
In a medium bowl, sift together the baking soda, flour, cinnamon and salt.
In another bowl, add the eggs, oil, applesauce, honey and yogurt and with a hand-held mixer, mix on medium speed until well combined. Add the eggs, one at a time and beat well. Add the vanilla and mix well. Add the flour mixture and mix until just combined. Fold in the carrots, raisins and walnuts.
Place the mixture into a greased baking pan.
With a piece of foil, cover the pan.
Press "Power Button" of the oven, turn the dial to select the "Air Fry". Press Time button and rotate the dial to set the cook time to thirty mins. Press the Temp button and turn the dial to set the temperature at 347° F. Press Start button.
When the unit beeps to show that it is preheated, open the lid.
Place the pan in "Air Fry Basket" and insert in the oven. After twenty-five mins of cook, remove the foil.
Place the pan to cool for about ten mins.
Carefully, invert the bread onto wire rack to cool completely before slicing.
Cut the bread into desired-sized slices.

Nutrition: Cal 441 Fat 20.3 g Carbs 57.6 g

45. Cauliflower Pizza Crusts

Prep time: 10 mins
Servings: 2

Cook time: 30 mins

Ingredients:
- One cup cauliflower rice
- 1/2 tbsp. Tapioca starch
- 1/2 cup vegan grated mozzarella
- 1/8 tsp. salt
- One clove garlic, peeled and minced
- tsp. Italian seasoning

Directions: Preheat and set the air fryer's temperature to 400 degrees F for three mins.
In a medium bowl, combine all ingredients.
Divide mixture in half and spread into two pizza pans lightly greased with preferred cook oil.
Place one pan in an air fryer basket and cook for twelve mins. Once done, remove the pan from the basket and repeat with the second pan.
Top crusts with your favorite toppings and cook an additional three mins.

Nutrition: Cal: 86 kcal Fat: 0.16 g Carbs: 11.33 g

46. Cheesy Bacon Bread

Prep time: 10 mins
Servings: 4

Cook time: 15 mins

Ingredients:
- ¼ cup pickled jalapenos, chopped
- Four slices sugar-free bacon, cooked and chopped
- Two eggs
- ¼ cup parmesan cheese, grated
- Two cups mozzarella cheese, shredded

Directions: Add all of the ingredients in a bowl and mix together.
Cut out a piece of parchment paper that will fit the base of your fryer's basket. Place it inside the oven.
Roll the mixture into a circle. You may have to form two circles to cook in separate batches, depending on the size of your fryer.
Place the circle on top of the parchment paper inside your fryer. Cook at 320 degrees F for ten mins.
Turn the bread over and cook for another five mins.

Nutrition: Cal: 374 Carbs: 57 g Fat: 4 g

47. Cheesy Garlic Bread

Prep time: 10 mins
Servings: 4

Cook time: 15 mins

Ingredients:
- 1/2 tsp. garlic powder
- One egg
- ¼ cup parmesan cheese, grated
- 1 cup mozzarella cheese, shredded

Directions: Stir all the ingredients together in a large bowl. Cut a piece of parchment to fit the bottom of your fryer's basket. Pour the mixture onto the paper to form a circle. Transfer this to the oven.

Cook for ten mins at 350 degrees F.

Slice up the bread.

Nutrition: Cal: 374 Carbs: 57 g Fat: 4 g

48. Chicken Pizza Rolls

Prep time: 10 mins   **Cook time: 30 mins**

Servings: 4

Ingredients:

- Two chicken breasts, skinless, boneless and sliced
- 2 teaspoons olive oil
- One yellow onion, sliced
- 1 tablespoon Worcestershire sauce
- 14 ounces pizza dough
- 11/2 cups parmesan cheese, grated
- 1/2 cup tomato sauce
- Salt and black pepper

Directions: Preheat your air fryer at 400° F, and add the onion and half of oil.

Fry for eight mins, shaking the fryer halfway.

Add the chicken, salt, pepper and Worcestershire sauce; stir and fry for eight mins more, stirring once, and then transfer to a bowl.

Roll the pizza dough on a working surface and shape into a rectangle.

Spread the cheese all over, then the chicken and onion mix, then the tomato sauce.

Roll the dough, place it in the air fryer's basket, and brush the roll with the rest of the oil.

Bake at 370° F for 14 mins, flipping the roll halfway.

Slice your roll.

Nutrition: Cal 270, Fat 8 g, Carbs 16 g

49. Cinnamon Sugar Toast

Prep time: 10 mins   **Cook time: 8 mins**

Servings: 2

Ingredients:

- 1/4 cup granulated sugar
- 11/2 tsp. ground cinnamon
- 2 tbsp. vegan butter, room temperature
- Four slices gluten-free sandwich bread

Directions: In a prepared bowl, combine cinnamon and sugar.

Preheat the air fryer and set the temperature at 375 degrees F for three mins.

Spread butter over bread slices. Evenly sprinkle buttered slices with cinnamon-sugar mix.

Place 2 bread slices in an ungreased air fryer basket and cook for four mins. Transfer to a plate. Repeat with remaining pieces.

Nutrition: Cal: 193 Fat: 7.54 g Carbs: 26.89 g

50. Cranberry Bread

Prep Time: 15 mins   **Cook Time: 30 mins**

Servings: 10

Ingredients:

- Four eggs
- Three cups flour
- 2/3 cups sugar
- 2/3 cup vegetable oil
- ½ cup milk
- 1 teaspoon vanilla extract
- 2 teaspoons baking powder
- 2 cups fresh cranberries

Directions: In a bowl, add all the Ingredients except for cranberries and stir until well combined.

Gently, fold in the cranberries.

Place the mixture into a lightly greased baking pan evenly. Select the "Air Fry" mode.

Press the Time button and set the cook time to thirty mins.

Then push the Temp button and rotate the dial to set the temperature at 320° F.

Press Start button.

When the unit beeps, open the lid.

Arrange the pan in the basket of the Air Fryer and insert in the oven.

Place the pan onto a wire rack for about 10-15 mins.

Carefully, invert the bread onto wire rack to cool completely before slicing.

Cut the bread into desired-sized slices.

Nutrition: Cal 436 Total Fat 16.9 g Carbs 65.4 g

51. Crust-less Meaty Pizza

Prep time: 10 mins

Cook time: 15 mins

Servings: 4

Ingredients:
- 1/2 cup mozzarella cheese, shredded
- Two slices sugar-free bacon, cooked and crumbled
- ¼ cup ground sausage, cooked
- Seven slices pepperoni
- 1 tbsp. parmesan cheese, grated

Directions: Spread the mozzarella across the bottom of a six-inch cake pan. Throw on the sausage, bacon, and pepperoni, then add a sprinkle of the parmesan cheese on top. Place the pan inside your oven.

Cook at 400 degrees F for five mins. The cheese is ready once brown in color and bubbly.

Nutrition: Cal: 374 Carbs: 57 g Fat: 4 g.

52. Mac and Cheese

Prep Time: 10 mins

Cook Time: 30 mins

Serve: 6

Ingredients:
- 2 1/2 cups pasta, uncooked
- 1/2 cup cream
- 2 tbsp. flour
- 1 cup vegetable broth
- 1/2 cup parmesan cheese, grated
- 1/2 cup Velveeta cheese, cut into small cubes
- Two cups Colby cheese, shredded
- 2 tbsp. butter
- 1 tsp. salt

Directions: Cook pasta according to the packet Directions. Drain well.

Melt butter in a pan over medium heat. Slowly whisk in flour.

Whisk constantly and slowly add the broth. Slowly pour the cream and whisk constantly.

Slowly add Velveeta cheese, parmesan cheese, and Colby cheese and whisk until smooth.

Add cooked pasta to the sauce and mix well to coat.

Transfer pasta into the greased casserole dish.

Set to bake at 350 degrees F for thirty-five mins. After five mins, place the casserole dish in the preheated oven.

Nutrition: Cal 410 Fat 21.8 g Carbs 34 g

53. Fitness Bread

Prep time: 10 mins

Cook time: 80 mins

Servings: 1 bread

Ingredients:
- 150 g whole wheat flour
- 150 g whole meal rye flour
- tbsp. agave syrup, alternatively also maple syrup
- 25 g yeast
- tsp. salt
- tbsp. flaxseed oil
- 40 g chopped walnuts
- 35 g chopped pumpkin seeds
- 50 g dried fruit of your choice cut into pieces (dates, raisins, etc.)
- Water

Directions: Sieve wheat and rye flour and add salt. Dissolve the yeast in lukewarm water and mix in agave syrup. Add the flour and oil and knead everything into a soft dough. Then cover a clean kitchen towel with the dough and let it rest in a warm position for 30 mins.

In the meantime, stir the chopped nuts and kernels with the dried fruit cut into pieces and, after the resting time, knead well into the dough.

Place the dough in the baking pan of the air fryer and cover it for another fifteen mins. Then program the oven to 390 degrees F and bake the loaf for five mins. Reduce the temperature to 350 degrees F and bake for another fifty-five mins. Brush the bread with a little water now and then to create a shiny crust.

Nutrition: Cal: 927 Fat: 31.24 g Carbs: 147.53 g

54. Panettone Bread Pudding

Prep Time: 5 mins
Servings: 4

Cook Time: 15 mins

Ingredients:
- Four slices of panettone bread, crusts trimmed, bread cut into 1-inch cubes
- 4 tablespoons dried cranberries
- 2 tablespoons amaretto liqueur
- 1 cup coconut milk
- 1/2 cup whipping cream
- Two eggs
- 1/2 teaspoon ground cloves
- 1/2 teaspoon ground cinnamon
- 1 tablespoon agave syrup
- 1/2 vanilla extract

Directions: Place the panettone bread cubes in a lightly greased baking pan. Scatter the dried cranberry over the top. In a mixing bowl, thoroughly combine the remaining ingredients.
Pour the custard over the bread cubes. Let it stand for thirty mins, occasionally pressing with a wide spatula to submerge. Cook in the preheated Air Fryer at 370° F for seven mins; check to ensure even cook and bake an additional five to six mins.

Nutrition: 279 Cal, 8.7 g Fat, 37.9 g Carbs

55. Chocolate Bread

Prep time: 60 mins
Servings: 4

Cook time: 40 mins

Ingredients:
- lbs. Of flour
- tsp. fresh yeast
- ¾ cup vegetable milk
- bar of dark chocolate
- Orange peel
- Lemon peel
- tbsp. of vegetable margarine
- Cinnamon powder
- A vanilla flavored soy yogurt
- Agave syrup

Directions: Put the flour in a bowl.
Put the crumbled yeast with your hands. Beat with a fork until undo. Afterwards, cut a piece of orange peel and another lemon and let it marinate in the milk.
Add a minimum of ½ tsp. of cinnamon.
On the other hand, heat until the 3 tbsp. Of margarine is melted. When it is melted, add it to the flour and mix well. Add the yogurt, 2 tbsp. Of syrup and the flavored vegetable milk, it has previously removed the lemon and orange peels and beaten with a fork to distribute the yeast well through the milk.
Knead well until the ingredients are properly mixed.
Take the chocolate bar and chop it with a knife into small cubes. Add everything to the dough and knead for three mins, with energy.
Sprinkle a little amount of flour on the table, put the dough on top, and knead for five more mins.
Now, make a 'churro' and cut it into parts. Take each of the cuts, knead it and roll it.
Place the buns on the baking tray with the baking paper on. Let it rise for 60 mins. Afterwards, paint them with a little agave syrup, and with a spoon, spread it well over the entire surface of the bread.
Put in the air fryer at 360 degrees F for 35-45 mins. But check them after thirty-five mins, try to be aware.

Nutrition: Cal: 146 Carbs: 2 g Fat: 5 g

56. Lemon Bread

Prep Time: 15 mins
Servings: 10

Cook Time: 30 mins

Ingredients:
- 3 cups all-purpose flour
- 3 tablespoons poppy seeds
- Three eggs
- 2 cups sugar
- 1½ cups milk
- 1½ teaspoon baking powder
- 1 teaspoon salt
- one cup vegetable oil
- 2 teaspoons fresh lemon juice
- 1 teaspoon pure vanilla extract
- 2 tablespoons lemon zest, grated

Directions: In a bowl, stir together the poppy seeds, flour, baking powder and salt.

In another bowl, add the eggs, oil, lemon juice, sugar, milk, and vanilla extract and beat until well combined.

Add the flour mixture and toss until just combined. Fold in the lemon zest.

Place the mixture into a greased baking pan evenly. Select the "Air Fry" mode. Press the Time button and set the cook time to thirty mins. Set the temperature at 310° F. Press Start button.

When the unit beeps, open the lid.

Arrange the pan in the Air Fryer Basket and insert in the oven.

Place the pan on the top a wire rack for about 10-15 mins.

Carefully, invert the bread onto wire rack to cool completely before slicing.

Cut the bread into desired-sized slices.

Nutrition: Cal 533, Fat 25.4 g, Carbs 71.8 g

57. Lemon-Butter Shortbread

Prep Time: 10 mins
Servings: 4

Cook Time: 40 mins

Ingredients:
- *1 tablespoon grated lemon zest*
- *1 cup granulated sugar*
- *1 pound (454 g) unsalted butter, at room temperature*
- *¼ teaspoon fine salt*
- *Four cups all-purpose flour*
- *1/3 cup cornstarch*
- *Cook spray*

Directions: Add the lemon zest and sugar to a stand mixer fitted with the paddle attachment and beat on medium speed for 2 mins. Let stand for about 5 mins. Fold in the butter and salt and blend until fluffy.

Stir together the flour and cornstarch in a bowl. Add to the butter mixture and mix to combine.

Spritz the sheet pan with cook spray and spread a piece of parchment paper onto the pan. Scrape the dough into the pan until even and smooth.

Select Bake, Convection, set temperature to 325 degrees F, and set time to 36 mins. Select Start to begin preheating.

Once the unit has preheated, place the pan on the bake position.

After 20 mins, check the shortbread, rotating the pan if it is not browning evenly. Continue cook for another 16 mins until lightly browned.

When done, remove the pan from the oven. Slice and allow to cool for 5 mins before serving.

Nutrition: Cal: 230 Fat: 12.8 g Carbs: 1.2 g

58. Pizza Crust

Prep time: 10 mins
Servings: 4

Cook time: 15 mins

Ingredients:
- *tbsp. full-fat cream cheese*
- *1/2 cup whole-milk mozzarella cheese, shredded*
- *tbsp. blanched finely ground almond flour*
- *One egg white*

Directions: In a microwave-safe bowl, combine the mozzarella, cream cheese, and almond flour and heat in the microwave for half a minute. Mix well to create a smooth consistency. Add in the egg white and stir to form a soft ball of dough. With slightly wet hands, press the dough into a pizza crust about six inches in diameter.

Place a sheet of parchment paper in the bottom of the Air Fryer and lay the crust on top. Cook for ten mins at 350 degrees F, turning the crust over halfway through the cooking time.

Nutrition: Cal: 374 Carbs: 57 g Fat: 4 g

59. Mushroom-Onion Eggplant Pizzas

Prep time: 5 mins
Servings: 4

Cook time: 16 mins

Ingredients:
- *2 tsp. + 2 tbsp. olive oil, divided*
- *1/4 cup small-diced peeled yellow onion*

- 1/2 cup small-diced white mushrooms
- 1/2 cup marinara sauce
- One small eggplant, sliced into 8 (1/2") circles
- cup vegan shredded mozzarella
- 1/4 cup chopped fresh basil
- tsp. salt

Directions: In a prepared medium skillet over medium heat, heat 2 tsp. olive oil 30 seconds. Add onion and mushrooms. Cook for 5 mins until onions are translucent. Add marinara sauce and stir. Remove skillet from heat.
Preheat the air fryer at 375°F for 3 mins.
Rub remaining olive oil over both sides of eggplant circles. Lay circles on a large plate and season top evenly with salt—top with marinara sauce mixture, followed by shredded mozzarella.
Place half of the eggplant pizzas in an ungreased air fryer basket. Cook 5 mins.
Transfer cooked pizzas to a large plate. Repeat with remaining pizzas. Garnish with chopped basil and serve warm.

Nutrition: Cal: 111 Fat: 3.15 g Carbs: 11.74 g

60. Mozzarella Flatbread

Prep Time: 5 mins
Servings: 10

Cook Time: 5 mins

Ingredients:
- One tube prepared pizza dough
- 1/2 cup butter
- 1 teaspoon garlic
- Pinch of dried parsley
- Two cups mozzarella cheese, shredded

Directions: Open and unroll the pizza dough. From the long side, reroll the dough. Cut 1-inch rolls from dough and then flatten each roll.
In a bowl, add garlic, butter, and parsley and mix well. Brush the top of dough with butter mixture.
Select the "Air Fry" mode. Press the Time button and set the cook time to five mins. Set the temperature at 350° F.
Press Start button. When the unit beeps, open the lid.
Arrange the rolls in greased "Air Fry Basket" and insert in the oven. Place the rolls onto a wire rack for about five mins before serving.

Nutrition: Cal 126 Fat 12.1 g Carbs 2.8 g

61. New York Pizza

Prep Time: 5 mins
Servings: 4

Cook Time: 15 mins

Ingredients:
- One pizza dough
- One cup tomato sauce
- 14 ounces mozzarella cheese, freshly grated
- 2 ounces parmesan, freshly grated

Directions: Stretch your dough on a pizza peel lightly dusted with flour. Spread with a layer of tomato sauce.
Top with mozzarella and parmesan cheese. Place on the baking tray.
Bake in the preheated Air Fryer at 395° F for five mins. Rotate the baking tray and bake for a further five mins.

Nutrition: 308 Cal, 4.1 g Fat, 25.7 g Carbs

62. Nutty Bread Pudding

Prep Time: 15 mins
Servings: 3

Cook Time: 30 Mins

Ingredients:
- Eight slices of bread
- 1/2 cup buttermilk
- ¼ cup honey
- ¼ cup of sugar
- 4 tablespoon raisins
- One cup milk
- Two eggs
- 1/2 teaspoon vanilla extract
- 2 tablespoon butter, softened
- 2 tablespoon chopped hazelnuts
- Cinnamon for garnish

Directions: Preheat the Air fryer to 310 degrees F.

Beat the eggs along with the honey, milk, buttermilk, vanilla, sugar, and butter.

Mix in raisins and hazelnuts.

Cut the bread into cubes and place them in a bowl.

Pour the milk mixture over the bread. Let soak for ten mins. Cook the pudding for thirty mins and garnish with cinnamon.

Nutrition: Cal 432, Fat 21 g, Carbs 54 g

63. Philo Pasta Rolls

Prep Time: 4 mins

Cook Time: 5 mins

Servings: 20

Ingredients:

- *1/2 -pound flour for 4 sheets of philo paste*
- *Two small cans of tuna*
- *One onion*
- *One green pepper*
- *Fried tomato sauce*
- *1/2 oz. of white cabbage*
- *Olive oil*
- *Salt*
- *Ground pepper*

Directions: Put in a frying pan a bottom of olive oil. Add the pepper onion, and white cabbage, all very chopped. Start to make the sofrito and wait to have the tender vegetables; add the drained and crumbled tuna.

Link and add the tomato sauce, just enough to leave a thick and not very liquid dough.

Rectify with salt and let it cool down. Spread the sheets of philo paste and distribute the filling between them. Tie the rolls so that they are well sealed. Place on the appetizer tray of your oven.

Paint with a little olive oil and a brush.

We select twenty mins at 350 degrees F.

Nutrition: Cal: 197, Carbs: 53 g, Fat: 1 g

64. Pizza Bombs

Prep time: 5 mins

Cook time: 12 mins

Servings: 9 pizza bites

Ingredients:

- *1/3 cup gluten-free all-purpose flour*
- *1/4 tsp. salt*
- *1/4 tsp. baking powder*
- *1/2 cup small-diced pepperoni*
- *2 ounces Tofutti, room temperature*
- *1/4 cup shredded mozzarella cheese*
- *1/2 tsp. Italian seasoning*
- *2 tbsp. Almond Milk*
- *1 tsp. olive oil*
- *1/2 cup marinara sauce, warmed*

Directions: Preheat the air fryer at 325 degrees F for five mins.

In a bowl, combine salt, flour, and baking powder.

In a prepared bowl, combine the remaining ingredients, except marinara sauce, stir until smooth. Add dry ingredients to bowl and mix well.

Form mixture into nine (1") balls and place on an ungreased pizza pan. It's okay if pizza balls are touching. Put the pan in then basket of the air fryer and cook twelve mins.

Transfer balls to a plate. Serve warm with marinara sauce for dipping.

Nutrition: Cal: 112 Fat: 3.94 g Carbs: 14.85 g

65. Pumpkin Bread

Prep Time: 15 mins

Cook Time: 40 mins

Servings: 10

Ingredients:

- *1 1/3 cups all-purpose flour*
- *One cup sugar*
- *Two eggs*
- *¾ teaspoon baking soda*
- *1 teaspoon pumpkin pie spice*
- *1/3 teaspoon ground cinnamon*
- *½ cup pumpkin puree*
- *1/3 cup vegetable oil*
- *¼ cup water*
- *¼ teaspoon salt*

Directions: In a bowl, mix together the flour, spices sugar, baking soda, and salt

In another bowl, add the eggs, oil pumpkin, and water and beat until well combined.

In a large mixing bowl, add the flour mixture and stir until just combined.

Place the mixture into a lightly greased loaf pan. With a piece of foil, cover the pan.

Select Bake mode of the Air Fryer. Press the Time button and set the cook time to forty mins. Now push the Temp button and set the temperature at 325° F. Press Start button.

Arrange the pan in the "Air Fry Basket" and insert in the oven.

After twenty-five mins of cook, remove the foil.

Place the pan onto a wire rack to cool for about ten mins.

Carefully, invert the bread onto wire rack to cool completely before slicing.

Cut the bread into desired-sized slices.

Nutrition: Cal 217, Fat 8.4 g, Carbs 34 g

66. Lunch Pizzas

Prep time: 10 mins

Cook time: 7 mins

Servings: 4

Ingredients:
- Four pitas
- tablespoon olive oil
- ¾ cup pizza sauce
- 4 ounces jarred mushrooms, sliced
- 1/2 teaspoon basil, dried
- Two green onions, chopped
- Two cup mozzarella, grated
- One cup grape tomatoes, sliced

Directions: Spread pizza sauce on each pita bread, sprinkle basil and green onions, and divide mushrooms and top with cheese.

Arrange pizzas in your air fryer and cook them at 400° F for seven mins.

Top each pizza with tomato slices.

Nutrition: Cal 200 Fat 4 g Carbs 7 g

67. Roasted Veggie Pasta Salad

Prep time: 10 mins

Cook time: 15 mins

Servings: 6

Ingredients:
- One Yellow squash
- 4 oz Brown mushrooms
- One Zucchini
- each Red - Green - Orange bell peppers
- one Red onion
- 1 pinch each Fresh ground pepper and salt
- 1 tsp. Italian seasoning
- One cup Grape tomatoes
- Five cups Pitted Kalamata olives
- 1 lb. Cooked Rigatoni or Penne Rigate
- 25 cups Olive oil
- tbsp. Fresh chopped basil
- tbsp. Balsamic vinegar

Directions: Preheat the Air Fryer to 380 degrees F.

Cut the peppers into large chunks and slice the red onion. Slice the tomatoes and olives into halves. Cut the squash and zucchini into half-moons.

Put the mushrooms, red onion, squash, peppers, and zucchini in a large container. Drizzle with some of the oil, tossing well using the salt, pepper, and Italian seasoning.

Prepare in the Air Fryer until the veggies are softened - not mushy (12 to 15 min.). Stir the fixings in the basket about halfway through the cook cycle for even frying.

Toss the cooked pasta, olives, roasted veggies, and tomatoes into a large container. Pour in the vinegar, and toss.

Keep it refrigerated until ready to serve—adding the fresh basil as serving time.

Nutrition: Cal: 374 Carbs: 57 g Fat: 4 g

68. Salmon with Shrimp & Pasta

Prep Time: 20 mins

Cook Time: 18 mins

Servings: 4

Ingredients:
- 14 ounces pasta
- 4 tablespoons pesto, divided
- 4 (4-ounces) salmon steaks
- 2 tablespoons olive oil
- 1/2 pound cherry tomatoes, chopped

- *Eight large prawns, peeled and deveined*
- *2 tablespoons fresh lemon juice*
- *2 tablespoons fresh thyme, chopped*

Directions: In a pan of salted boiling water, add the pasta and cook for about 8-10 mins.
Meanwhile, in the bottom of a baking dish, spread 1 tablespoon of pesto.
Place salmon steaks and tomatoes over pesto in a single layer and drizzle evenly with the olive oil. Add the prawns on top in a single layer. Drizzle with lemon juice and sprinkle with thyme.
Set the temperature of the oven to 390° F. Arrange the baking dish in air fryer and air fry for about eight mins.
Once done, remove the salmon mixture from the oven.
Drain the pasta and transfer into a bowl. Add the remaining pesto and stir to coat well. Add the pasta with salmon mixture.

Nutrition: Cal: 592 Carbs: 58.7 g Fat: 23.2 g

69. Salted Caramel Banana Muffins (Vegan)

Servings: 8
Prep time: 10 mins

Cook time: 14 mins

Ingredients:
- *A cup gluten-free all-purpose flour*
- *1/2 tsp. baking soda*
- *1/3 cup granulated sugar*
- *1/4 tsp. salt*
- *1/3 cup mashed banana, about one large ripe banana*
- *1/2 tsp. vanilla extract*
- *Silken tofu*
- *tbsp. vegetable oil*
- *1/4 cup salted caramel chips*

Directions: Preheat the air fryer set the temperature at 375 degrees F for three mins.
In a bowl, combine sugar, flour, baking soda, and salt. In a separate medium bowl, combine mashed banana, tofu, vanilla, and oil.
Pour all wet ingredients into dry ingredients and combine. Fold in salted caramel chips. Do not overmix. Spoon mixture into 8 silicone cupcake liners lightly greased with preferred cook oil.
Place 4 muffins in an air fryer basket. Cook for seven mins, then transfer to a cooling rack. Repeat with remaining muffins.

Nutrition: Cal: 103 Fat: 1.93 g Carbs: 19.71 g

70. Shrimp Pasta

Servings: 4
Prep time: 10 mins

Cook time: 15 mins

Ingredients:
- *5 ounces spaghetti, cooked*
- *8 ounces shrimp, peeled and deveined*
- *1 tablespoon butter, melted*
- *2 tablespoons olive oil*
- *Salt and black pepper to taste*
- *Five garlic cloves, minced*
- *1 teaspoon chili powder*

Directions: Put 1 tablespoon of the olive oil, along with the butter, in your oven.
Preheat the air fryer at 350° F, add the shrimp, and cook for ten mins.
Add all other ingredients, including the remaining 1 tablespoon of oil, stir, and cook for five mins more.

Nutrition: Cal 270, Fat 7 g, Carbs 15 g

71. Vegan Spelled Bread

Prep time: 10 mins
Servings: 1

Cook time: 45 mins

Ingredients:
- *500 g spelled flour*
- *tbsp. salt*
- *One yeast cube*
- *250 ml of lukewarm water*
- *One pinch of sugar*
- *1 tsp. anise*

Directions: Put flour, anise and salt in a bowl and mix. Make a well in the middle and crumble the yeast into it. Pour a pinch of sugar over it. Cover the yeast and sugar with lukewarm water and let rest for ten mins so that the yeast dissolves.

Stir all ingredients in the bowl and knead into a dough. Cover with a clean kitchen towel and let rise in a warm place for about sixty mins.

Line the breadbasket of the oven with baking paper or grease and dust with flour. Put the dough in the breadbasket of the Air fryer and bake for 30-35 mins at 360 degrees F.

Nutrition: Cal: 182 Fat: 5.23 g Carbs: 38.6 g

72. Strawberry Bread

Prep Time: 15 mins   **Cook Time: 30 mins**
Servings: 8

Ingredients:
- 2½ cups all-purpose flour
- 1 cup sugar
- 2 teaspoons baking powder
- 1 teaspoon salt
- 1 large egg
- 1 cup whole milk
- 2 tablespoons vegetable oil
- 1 teaspoon vanilla extract
- 1½ cups fresh strawberries, hulled and sliced

Directions: In a bowl, mix together the flour, baking powder, sugar, and salt.

In another bowl, add the milk, egg, oil and vanilla and beat until well combined. Add the flour mixture and stir well.

Fold in the strawberry slices. Place the mixture into a lightly greased baking pan evenly.

Select the "Air Fry" mode. Set the cook time to thirty mins. Now push the Temp button and set the temperature at 310° F. Press Start button to start.

Arrange the pan in "Air Fry Basket" and insert in the oven. Place the pan onto a wire rack for about 10-15 mins.

Carefully, invert the bread onto wire rack to cool completely before slicing.

Cut the bread into desired-sized slices.

Nutrition: Cal 320 Fat 7.2 g Carbs 59.3 g

73. Vegan Spicy Sourdough Bread

Prep time: 10 mins   **Cook time: 40 mins**
Servings: 1

Ingredients:
- 500 g flour
- 75 g ready-made sourdough
- ½ yeast cube
- tbsp. salt
- 375 ml of water
- ½ tsp. rosemary
- ½ tsp. marjoram
- ½ tsp. tarragon

Directions: Mix the flour with salt, marjoram rosemary, and tarragon. Crumble the yeast and dissolve in lukewarm water. Mix with the flour and herbs. Add the sourdough and knead everything into a dough. Cover with a clean kitchen towel and let rise for about an hour.

Grease the bread pan and then sprinkle with flour, or line with baking paper. Pour in the dough and let it rest for another thirty mins. Now sprinkle the dough with a little flour and bake in the air fryer for thirty-five mins at 390 degrees F.

Nutrition: Cal: 188 kcal Fat: 6.34 g Carbs: 31.03 g

74. Banana Bread (Vegan)

Prep time: 15 mins   **Cook time: 65 mins**
Servings: 12

Ingredients:
- Three very ripe bananas
- 2 cups of whole wheat flour
- ¾ cup brown sugar
- tsp. ground cinnamon
- tsp. baking soda
- ¼ tsp. of salt
- One flax egg
- ½ cup unsweetened non-dairy milk
- 1/3 cup coconut oil, melted
- tsp. vanilla extract

Directions: Preheat the air fryer to 350 degrees F.

Using a fork, you can mash the bananas.

In a bowl, mix flour, cinnamon, sugar, baking soda and salt until they are well integrated.

Add the bananas, milk, oil flax egg, and vanilla extract. Stir until well-integrated.

Grease a pan with parchment paper and bake for about 60-70 mins.

Take out the banana bread and leave it in the mould for at least fifteen mins, then you can move it to a wire rack. Ideally, let it cool completely before slicing it, but you can also have it hot if you want.

Nutrition: Cal: 209.3 Carbs: 43.4 g Fat: 3.1 g

75. Sugar-Free Pumpkin Bread

Prep Time: 15 mins   **Cook Time: 25 mins**
Servings: 4

Ingredients:
- ¼ cup coconut flour
- 2 tablespoons stevia blend
- teaspoon baking powder
- ¾ teaspoon pumpkin pie spice
- ¼ teaspoon ground cinnamon
- 1/8 teaspoon salt
- ¼ cup canned pumpkin
- 2 large eggs
- 2 tablespoons unsweetened almond milk
- 1 teaspoon vanilla extract

Directions: In a bowl, add the flour, baking powder, stevia blend, spices and salt and mix well.

In another bowl, add the pumpkin, almond milk, eggs, and vanilla extract and beat until well combined.

Add the flour mixture and stir until just combined.

Line a baking pan with greased parchment paper. Place the mixture into the prepared pan. Select the "Air Fry" mode.

Set the cook time to twenty-five mins. Set the temperature at 350° F and press the Start button.

Carefully, invert the bread onto wire rack to cool completely before slicing.

Cut the bread into desired-sized slices.

Nutrition: Cal 52 Fat 2.8 g Carbs 3 g

76. Bread with Lentils and Millet (Vegan)

Prep time: 25 mins   **Cook time: 45 mins**
Servings: 2-4

Ingredients:
- 1 lb. coral lentils
- ½ lb. of millet
- 1 tbsp. of vinegar or lemon
- 1 tsp. salt
- Water
- Spices

Directions: Place the lentils and millet in a bowl. Cover them with water and then let stand for 12 hours. After that time, rinse the grains, discarding the soaking water.

Crush the lentils and millet with a mini primer or food processor to form a sticky dough. Add the vinegar or the lemon, the salt and the chosen spices and mix.

Let the dough rest in a bowl and then covered with plastic wrap or with a kitchen cloth at room temperature for two days. After that time, the dough begins to rise, and you will feel an acidic smell due to the grains' fermentation. Place the dough in a previously oiled bread pan or upholstered with vegetable paper.

Take in a preheated air fryer at 360 degrees F for about 30-40 mins.

Nutrition: Cal: 80 Carbs: 14 g Fat: 2 g

77. Taco Stuffed Bread

Prep Time: 5 mins   **Cook Time:** 15 mins
Servings: 4

Ingredients:
- 1 loaf French bread
- 1/2 pound ground beef
- 1 onion, chopped
- 1 teaspoon garlic, minced
- 1 package taco seasoning
- 1 1/2 cups Queso Panela, sliced

- *Salt and ground black pepper*
- *3 tablespoons tomato paste*
- *2 tablespoons fresh cilantro leaves, chopped*

Directions: Cut the top off of the loaf of bread; remove some of the bread from the middle creating a well and reserve.
In a skillet, cook the ground beef with the onion and garlic until the onion is translucent.
Add the taco seasoning, salt, pepper, cheese, and tomato paste. Place the taco mixture into your bread.
Bake in the preheated Air Fryer at 380° F for five mins. Garnish with fresh cilantro leaves.

Nutrition: 472 Cal, 21.9 g Fat, 37.6 g Carbs

78. Corn Bread

Prep time: 10 mins
Servings: 9

Cook time: 25 mins

Ingredients:
- *1 cup white flour*
- *1 cup polenta*
- *½ cup brown sugar*
- *¼ tsp of salt*
- *½ tsp baking soda*
- *1 tbsp. baking powder*
- *¼ cup of melted butter*
- *1 flax eggs*
- *buttermilk*
- *1/3 cup unsweetened non-dairy milk*

Directions: Preheat the air fryer to 400 degrees F.
In a bowl, add the white flour, salt, bicarbonate, cornmeal, sugar, yeast, and mix until they are integrated.
Put the rest of the ingredients to the bowl. Stir again until all the ingredients have been integrated.
Pour the dough into a pre-greased baking pan and bake for about twenty-five mins. Brown on the outside, and when you put a knife, it comes out clean.
Take the cornbread out of the oven and let it cool for a few mins before slicing.

Nutrition: Cal: 68.7 Carbs: 13.1 g Fat: 0.7 g

79. Walnut Bread with Cranberries

Prep time: 10 mins
Servings: 1

Cook time: 40 mins

Ingredients:
- *500 g of wheat flour*
- *One yeast cube*
- *250 ml of lukewarm water*
- *tbsp. salt*
- *100 g walnuts*
- *100 g cranberries, dried*

Directions: In a prepared bowl, mix the flour and salt and create a well in the middle. Pour the yeast into the well and pour lukewarm water over it. Let rest for ten mins.
Then add walnuts and cranberries and knead everything into a dough. Grease the bread pan and dust with flour. Alternatively line with baking paper.
Now cover the bread pan with a clean kitchen towel and let rise in a warm place for 60 mins.
Then bake for 30-35 mins at 390 degrees F.

Nutrition: Cal: 632 Fat: 17.55 g Carbs: 102.2 g

80. Walnut Zucchini Bread

Prep Time: 15 mins
Servings: 8

Cook Time: 20 mins

Ingredients:
- *1½ cups all-purpose flour*
- *½ teaspoon baking soda*
- *½ teaspoon baking powder*
- *½ tablespoon ground cinnamon*
- *½ teaspoon salt*
- *2¼ cups white sugar*
- *½ cup vegetable oil*
- *1½ eggs*
- *1½ teaspoons vanilla extract*
- *cup zucchini, grated*
- *½ cup walnuts, chopped*

Directions: In a bowl and stir together the flour, baking soda, baking powder, cinnamon, and salt.

In another bowl, add the sugar, eggs, oil, and vanilla extract and whisk until combined. Add the flour mixture and stir. Gently, fold in the zucchini and walnuts. Place the mixture into a lightly greased loaf pan.

Select the "Air Fry" mode. Set the cook time to twenty mins. Set the temperature at 320° F and press Start button. Arrange the pan in "Air Fry Basket" and insert in the oven. Place the pan onto a wire rack to cool for about ten mins. Carefully, invert the bread onto wire rack to cool completely before slicing.

Cut the bread into desired-sized slices.

Nutrition: Cal 483 Fat 19.3 g Carbs 76 g

81. Whole Wheat Toast

Prep time: 5 mins   **Cook time: 10 mins**
Servings: 3

Ingredients:
- 1 Loaf of sliced whole wheat bread
- Two Ripe bananas
- One Can of coconut milk
- 2 Tsp. of vanilla
- 1 Tsp. of cinnamon
- ¼ Tsp. of salt
- ½ Cup of dry roasted pecans
- Cook spray

Directions: Start by cutting the whole-wheat bread into equal-sized slices.

In a blender, stir the coconut milk, the cinnamon, the pecan, the vanilla, and salt. Pour your obtained mixture into a deep bowl; then add bread and let soak for about two mins.

Grease a baking tray and preheat your air fryer to about 350 degrees F. Lay the soaked bread into the greased tray and put it in the air fryer basket. Close the lid and then set the timer to about eight mins and the temperature to 360 degrees F.

When the timer beeps, remove the bread toasts from the air fryer; then set it aside to cool for about five mins.

Nutrition: Cal 110 Fat 0.9 g Carbs 21.1 g

82. Vegan Wholegrain Bread

Prep time: 10 mins   **Cook time: 1 hour**
Servings: 1

Ingredients:
- 500 g whole wheat flour
- 150 g ready-made sourdough
- 100 g grain mixture
- 300 ml of lukewarm water
- One packet of dry yeast
- 2 tbsp. salt

Directions: Put the flour, sourdough, water, salt, dry yeast and 2/3 of the grain mixture in a prepared bowl and knead into a dough. Cover the dough in the bowl with a clean kitchen towel and leave in a warm place for 60 mins.

Line the air fryer with parchment paper and place the loaf on top. Brush the loaf surface with water and carefully press the rest of the grain mixture into the loaf.

Bake bread for ten mins at 390 degrees F, and then reduce the temperature to 300 degrees F and cook for another forty mins. Let the bread cool down well before eating.

Nutrition: Cal: 542 Fat: 5.02 g Carbs: 114.68 g

83. Yogurt Pumpkin Bread

Prep Time: 10 mins   **Cook Time: 15 mins**
Servings: 4

Ingredients:
- Two large eggs
- 8 tablespoons pumpkin puree
- 6 tablespoons banana flour
- 4 tablespoons honey
- 4 tablespoons plain Greek yogurt
- 2 tablespoons vanilla essence
- Pinch of ground nutmeg
- 6 tablespoons oats

Directions: In a bowl, add in all the ingredients except oats and with a hand mixer, mix until smooth.

Add the oats and with a fork, stir well.

Grease and flour a loaf pan.

Place the mixture into the prepared loaf pan.

Select the "Air Fry" mode. Set the cook time to fifty mins. Set the temperature at 360° F and press the Start button.
Arrange the pan in "Air Fry Basket" and insert in the oven.
Carefully, invert the bread onto wire rack to cool completely before slicing.
Cut the bread into desired-sized slices.

Nutrition: Cal 232 Fat 8.33 g Carbs 29.3 g

84. Chicken & Pepperoni Pizza

Prep Time: 20 mins
Servings: 2

Cook Time: 30 mins

Ingredients:
- 2 cups cooked chicken, cubed
- 20 slices pepperoni
- cup sugar-free pizza sauce
- cup mozzarella cheese, shredded
- ¼ cup parmesan cheese, grated

Directions: Place the chicken into the base of a four-cup baking dish and add the pepperoni and pizza sauce on top. Stir well to coat the meat with the sauce thoroughly.
Add the parmesan and mozzarella on top of the chicken, then place the baking dish into your fryer.
Cook for fifty mins at 375 degrees F.
When everything is bubbling and melted, remove from the oven.

85. Meat Lovers' Pizza

Prep Time: 10 mins
Serving: 2

Cook Time: 12 mins

Ingredients:
- 1 pre-prepared 7-inch pizza crust, defrosted if necessary.
- 1/3 cup of marinara sauce.
- 20ounces of grilled steak, sliced into bite-sized pieces
- 20ounces of salami, cut fine
- 20ounces of pepperoni, cut fine
- ¼ cup of American cheese
- ¼ cup of shredded mozzarella cheese

Directions: Preheat the Air Fryer Oven to 350° F. Lay the pizza dough flat on a sheet of parchment paper or tin foil, cut large enough to hold the entire pie crust but small enough that it will leave the edges of the air fryer basket uncovered to allow for air circulation.
Using a fork, stab the pizza dough several times across the surface – piercing the pie crust will allow air to circulate throughout the crust and ensure even cook. With a deep soup spoon, scoop the marinara sauce onto the pizza dough, and spread evenly in expanding circles over the pie-crust surface.
Be sure to leave at least 1/2 inch of bare dough around the edges to ensure that extra-crispy crunchy first bite of the crust!
Distribute the steak pieces and the slices of salami and pepperoni evenly over the sauce-covered dough, then sprinkle the cheese in an even layer on top.
Set the air fryer timer to twelve mins, and place the pizza with foil or paper on the fryer's basket surface. Again, be sure to leave the edges of the basket uncovered to allow for proper air circulation, and don't let your bare fingers touch the hot surface. After twelve mins, when the Air Fryer Oven shuts off, the cheese should be perfectly melted and lightly crisped, and the pie crust should be golden brown. If necessary, using a spatula – or two, remove the pizza from the air fryer basket and set on a serving plate. Wait a few mins until the pie is cool enough to handle, then cut into slices.

86. Mozzarella, Bacon & Turkey Calzone

Prep Time: 20 mins
Servings: 4

Cook Time: 10 mins

Ingredients:
- Pizza dough
- 4 oz cheddar cheese, grated
- 1 oz mozzarella cheese
- 1 oz bacon, diced
- 2 cups cooked and shredded turkey
- One egg, beaten
- 1 teaspoon thyme
- 4 tablespoon tomato paste
- 1 teaspoon basil
- 1 teaspoon oregano
- Salt and pepper

Directions: Preheat the Air fryer oven to 350° F.

Divide the pizza dough into 4 equal pieces so you have the dough for 4 small pizza crusts. Combine the tomato paste, oregano, basil, and thyme, in a bowl.

Brush the mixture onto the crusts just make sure not to go all the way and avoid brushing near the edges on one half of each crust, place 1/2 turkey, and season the meat with salt and pepper.

Top the meat with some bacon. Combine the cheddar and mozzarella and divide it between the pizzas, making sure that you layer only one half of the dough.

Brush the edges of the crust with the beaten egg. Fold the crust and seal with a fork. Cook for ten mins.

Nutrition: Cal 435.4 Fat 15.6 g Carbs 53.6 g

87. Pita Bread

Prep time: 10 mins
Servings: 4

Cook time: 15 mins

Ingredients:
- 1 tbsp. Pizza sauce
- 1 Pita bread
- 25 cup Mozzarella cheese
- Olive oil
- 1 Stainless-steel short-legged trivet
- 7 slices Pepperoni
- 5 tsp. Fresh minced garlic
- 25 cup Sausage
- 1 tbsp. Thinly sliced onions

Directions: Heat the Air Fryer in advance to 350 degrees F.

Spoon the sauce onto the bread.

Mince the garlic and thinly slice the onions. Toss on the toppings using a drizzle of oil.

Arrange it in the Air Fryer and place the trivet.

Set the timer for 6 mins. Serve when it's nicely browned.

Nutrition: Cal: 374, Carbs: 57 g, Fat: 4 g

88. Breakfast Berry Pizza

Prep time: 7 mins
Servings: 6

Cook time: 15 mins

Ingredients:
- 1 sheet of frozen puff pastry
- 1 Container of Strawberry Cream
- 6 Oz of fresh raspberries
- 6 Oz of fresh blueberries
- 6 Oz of fresh blackberries
- 8 Oz of fresh strawberries
- ½ Tsp. of vanilla bean paste
- ¼ Tsp. of almond extract
- 2 Tsp. of maple syrup

Directions: Preheat your air fryer to about 390 degrees F.

Thaw 1 of your pastry sheets according to the directions on the pack.

Cut your pastry into its half and make fine cuts, with a knife, right on the top of each of the pastry sheet or poke it with a toothpick.

Repeat the same process with the remaining quantity of the pastry.

Put the pastry sheet in a greased baking tray and put it in the air fryer basket; then close the lid.

Set the timer set to fifteen mins and the temperature to 390 degrees F.

Remove the pastries from the air fryer and set them aside to cool for ten mins; meanwhile, prepare the topping by mixing the Strawberry Cream into a bowl.

Add the raspberries and mash the strawberries; then mix it with the raspberries, the vanilla paste, the almond extract and the maple syrup.

Mix the mixture very well and when your crust becomes cool, pour the mixture over it with a spatula.

Top with the berries and the fresh strawberries.

Nutrition: Cal 247.8 Fat 6.1 g Carbs 21 g

89. Yogurt Banana Bread

Prep Time: 15 mins   **Cook Time: 28 mins**
Servings: 5
Ingredients:

- 1 medium very ripe banana, peeled and mashed
- 1 large egg
- 1 tablespoon canola oil
- 1 tablespoon plain Greek yogurt
- ¼ teaspoon pure vanilla extract
- ½ cup all-purpose flour
- ¼ cup granulated white sugar
- ¼ teaspoon ground cinnamon
- ¼ teaspoon baking soda
- 1/8 teaspoon sea salt

Directions: In a bowl, add the mashed banana, oil, yogurt egg, and vanilla and beat until well combined.
Add the flour, sugar, cinnamon baking soda, and salt and mix until just combined.
Place the mixture into a lightly greased mini loaf pan.
Select the Bake mode. Set the cook time to twenty-eight mins. Set the temperature at 350° F and press the Start button. When the unit beeps, open the lid.
Arrange the pan in "Air Fry Basket" and insert in the oven. Place the pan onto a wire rack to cool for about ten mins.
Invert the bread onto wire rack to cool completely before slicing.
Cut the bread into desired-sized slices.

Nutrition: Cal 145 Fat 4 g Carbs 25 g

90. Flat Bread with Olive and Rosemary

Prep time: 15 mins   **Cook time: 20 mins**
Servings: 5

Ingredients:

- One and ½ tsp. of active dry yeast
- One and ½ tsp. of unrefined cane sugar
- ½ Tsp. of kosher salt
- One and ½ cups of all-purpose flour
- One and ½ cups of whole spelt flour
- Tbsp. of finely cut fresh rosemary leaves
- Tbsp. of extra-virgin olive oil
- Tbsp. of thyme
- ½ Cup of pitted and cut olive

Directions: In a deep mixing bowl, mix a little bit of olive oil with a little bit of yeast, salt, sugar and pour in about 1 cup of water (Make sure the water is warm).
Set aside the mixture and let rest for about 11 mins.
Add in the flours and the chopped rosemary; then blend the ingredients on a deficient speed.
Use the dough hook to knead your dough, and once you obtain a smooth one; divide it into about two balls.
Put the dough balls over a floured baking paper and let rest for about 3 hours.
Put the pizza over a greased baking tray and use your hands and fingers to spread it into a circle.
Cover your bread with a kitchen towel and set it aside to rest for about 12 mins.
Brush the bread with olive oil and put it in the basket of the air fryer; close the lid and set the timer to about 10 mins. and the temperature to about 365° F.
When the timer beeps, remove the bread from the air fryer and sprinkle a little bit of pepper, olive oil and salt.

Nutrition: Cal 156.4 Fat 10.1 g Carbs 4.6 g

91. Yogurt Bread

Prep Time: 20 mins   **Cook Time: 40 mins**
Servings: 10

Ingredients:

- 1½ cups warm water, divided
- 1½ teaspoons active dry yeast
- teaspoon sugar
- cups all-purpose flour
- cup plain Greek yogurt
- teaspoons kosher salt

Directions: Add ½ cup of the warm water, yeast and sugar in the bowl of a stand mixer, fitted with the dough hook attachment and mix well.
Set aside for about five mins.
Add the flour, yogurt, and salt and mix on medium-low speed until the dough comes together.
Then, mix on medium speed for five mins.
Place the dough into a bowl.

With a plastic wrap, cover the bowl and place in a warm place for about 2-3 hours or until doubled in size.
Transfer the dough onto a lightly floured surface and shape into a smooth ball.
Place the dough onto a greased parchment paper-lined rack.
With a kitchen towel, cover the dough and let rest for fifteen mins.
With a very sharp knife, cut a 4x½-inch deep cut down the center of the dough.
Select the "Bake" mode.
Set the cook time to forty mins.
Set the temperature at 325° F.
Carefully, arrange the dough onto the "Wire Rack" and insert in the oven.
Carefully, invert the bread onto wire rack to cool completely before slicing.
Cut the bread into desired-sized slices and serve.

Nutrition: Cal 157 Fat 0.7 g Carbs 31 g

92. Caprese Sandwiches (Vegan)

Prep time: 10 mins
Servings: 2

Cook time: 10 mins

Ingredients:
- 2 tbsp. balsamic vinegar
- 4 slices gluten-free sandwich bread
- 2 ounces vegan mozzarella shreds
- Two medium Roma tomatoes, sliced
- Eight fresh basil leaves
- 2 tbsp. olive oil

Directions: Preheat the air fryer and set the temperature at 350 degrees F for three mins.
Prepare sandwiches by drizzling balsamic vinegar on bottom bread slices: layer mozzarella, tomatoes, and basil leaves on top. Add top bread slices.
Brush outside the top and bottom of each sandwich lightly with oil. Place one sandwich in an ungreased air fryer basket and cook for three mins. Flip and cook an additional two mins—transfer the sandwich to a large serving plate and repeat with the second sandwich.

Nutrition: Cal: 440 Fat: 22.6 g Carbs: 41.19 g

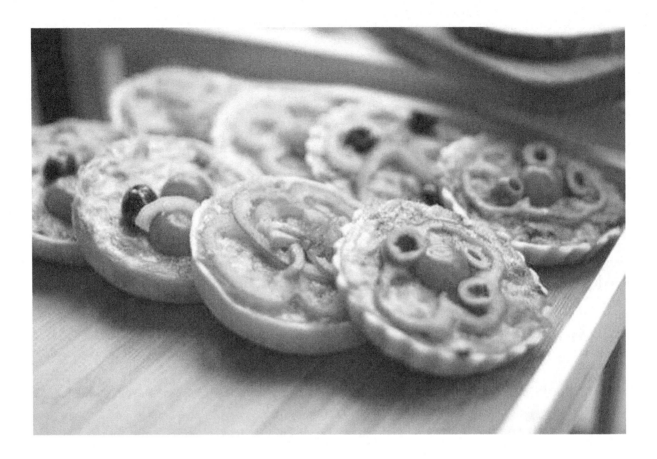

93. Air Fryer Olives

Prep Time: 10 Mins
Servings: 4

Cook Time: 5 mins

Ingredients:
- 2 cups olives
- 2 teaspoon garlic, minced
- 2 tablespoon olive oil
- 1/2 teaspoon dried oregano
- Salt and Pepper

Directions: Add olives and remaining ingredients into the bowl and stir well. Add olives to the air fryer basket then place an air fryer basket in baking pan. Place a baking pan on the oven rack. Set to air fry at 300 F for 5 mins.

Nutrition: Cal 140 Fat 14.2 g Carbs 4.8 g

94. Air Fryer Nuts

Prep Time: 10 Mins
Servings: 2

Cook Time: 4 mins

Ingredients:
- 2 cup mixed nuts
- tablespoon olive oil
- 1/4 teaspoon cayenne
- teaspoon ground cumin
- teaspoon pepper
- teaspoon salt

Directions: In a bowl, add all ingredients and stir well.
Add the nuts mixture to the air fryer basket
Place a baking pan on the oven rack. Set to air fry at 350 degrees F for four mins.

Nutrition: Cal 953 Fat 88.2 g Carbs 33.3 g

95. Air Fryer Buffalo Cauliflower

Prep Time: 5 mins   Cook Time:15 mins
Servings: 4

Ingredients:

- *Homemade buffalo sauce: 1/2 cup*
- *One head of cauliflower, cut bite-size pieces*
- *Butter melted: 1 tablespoon*
- *Olive oil*
- *Kosher salt & pepper, to taste*

Directions: Spray cook oil on the air fryer basket.
In a bowl, add buffalo sauce, melted butter, pepper, and salt. Mix well.
Put the cauliflower bits in the air fryer and spray the olive oil over it. Let it cook at 400 F for 7 mins.
Remove the cauliflower from the air fryer and add it to the sauce. Coat the cauliflower well.
Put the sauce coated cauliflower back into the air fryer.
Cook at 400 F, for 7-8 mins or until crispy.
Take out from the air fryer and serve with dipping sauce.

Nutrition: per serving: Cal 101kcal | Carbs 4g | Protein 3g | Fat: 7g

96. Air Fryer Mini Pizza

Prep Time: 2 mins   Cook Time:5 mins
Servings: 1

Ingredients:
- *Sliced olives: 1/4 cup*
- *One pita bread*
- *One tomato*
- *Shredded cheese: 1/2 cup*

Directions: Let the air fryer preheat to 350 F.
Lay pita flat on a plate. Add cheese, slices of tomatoes, and olives.
Cook for five mins at 350 F.
Take the pizza out of the air fryer.
Slice it and enjoy.

Nutrition: Cal: 344 Carbs: 37 g Protein: 18 g Fat: 13 g

97. Air Fryer Egg Rolls

Prep Time: 10 mins   Cook Time:20 mins
Servings: 3

Ingredients:
- *Coleslaw mix: half bag*
- *Half onion*
- *Salt: 1/2 teaspoon*
- *Half cups of mushrooms*
- *Lean ground pork: 2 cups*
- *One stalk of celery*
- *Wrappers (egg roll)*

Directions: Put a skillet over medium flame, add onion and lean ground pork and cook for 5-7 mins.
Add salt, mushrooms, coleslaw mixture, and celery to skillet and cook for almost five mins.
Lay egg roll wrapper flat and add filling, roll it up, seal with water.

Spray with oil the rolls. Put in the air fryer for 6-8 mins at 400F, flipping once halfway through.

Nutrition: Cal 245 Fat: 10 g Carbs: 9 g Protein: 11 g

98. Air Fryer Chicken Nuggets

Prep Time: 15 mins   **Cook Time:15 mins**
Servings: 4

Ingredients:
- Olive oil spray
- Skinless boneless: 2 chicken breasts, cut into bite pieces
- Half tsp. of kosher salt& freshly ground black pepper to taste
- Grated parmesan cheese: 2 tablespoons
- Italian seasoned breadcrumbs: 6 tablespoons (whole wheat)
- Whole wheat breadcrumbs: 2 tablespoons
- olive oil: 2 teaspoons

Directions: Let the air fryer preheat for 8 mins, to 400 F.
In a big mixing bowl, add panko, parmesan cheese, and breadcrumbs and mix well.
Sprinkle kosher salt and pepper on chicken and olive oil, mix well.
Take a few pieces of chicken, dunk them into breadcrumbs mixture.
Put these pieces in an air fryer and spray with olive oil.
Cook for 8 mins, turning halfway through.
Enjoy with kale chips.

Nutrition: Cal: 188, Carbs: 8 g, Protein: 25 g, Fat: 4.5 g

99. Chicken Tenders

Prep Time: 10 mins   **Cook Time:20 mins**
Servings: 3

Ingredients:
- Chicken tenderloins: 4 cups
- Eggs: one
- Superfine Almond Flour: ½ cup
- Powdered Parmesan cheese: ½ cup
- Kosher Sea salt: ½ teaspoon
- (1-teaspoon) freshly ground black pepper
- (1/2 teaspoon) Cajun seasoning

Directions: On a small plate, pour the beaten egg.
Mix all ingredients in a ziploc bag. Almond flour freshly ground black pepper & kosher salt and other seasonings.
Spray the air fryer with oil spray.
To avoid clumpy fingers with breading and egg. Use different hands for egg and breading. Dip each tender in egg and then in bread until they are all breaded.
Using a fork to place one tender at a time. Bring it in the ziploc bag and shake the bag forcefully. make sure all the tenders are covered in almond mixture.
Using the fork to take out the tender and place it in your air fryer basket.
Spray oil on the tenders.
Cook for 12 mins at 350F, or before 160F registers within. Raise temperature to 400F to shade the surface for 3 mins.
Serve with sauce.

Nutrition: Cal 280 Proteins 20 g Carbs 6 g Fat 10 g

100. Kale & Celery Crackers

Prep time: 10 min   **Cook time: 20 mins**
Servings: 6

Ingredients:
- One cups flax seed, ground

- 1 cups flax seed, soaked overnight and drained
- 2 bunches kale, chopped
- 1 bunch basil, chopped
- ½ bunch celery, chopped
- 2 garlic cloves, minced
- 1/3 cup olive oil

Directions: Mix the ground flaxseed with the celery, kale, basil, and garlic in your food processor and mix well.

Add the oil and soaked flaxseed, then mix again, scatter in the pan of your air fryer, break into medium crackers and cook for 20 mins at 380 degrees F.

Serve as an appetizer and break into cups.

Nutrition: Cal 143 Fat 1 g Carbs 8 g Protein 4 g

101. Air Fryer Spanakopita Bites

Prep Time: 10 mins
Servings: 4

Cook Time:15 mins

Ingredients:
- 4 sheets phyllo dough
- Baby spinach leaves: 2 cups
- Grated Parmesan cheese: 2 tablespoons
- Low-fat cottage cheese: 1/4 cup
- Dried oregano: 1 teaspoon
- Feta cheese: 6 tbsp. crumbled
- Water: 2 tablespoons
- One egg white only
- Lemon zest: 1 teaspoon
- Cayenne pepper: 1/8 teaspoon
- Olive oil: 1 tablespoon
- Kosher salt and freshly ground black pepper: 1/4 teaspoon, each

Directions: In a pot over high heat, add water and spinach, cook until wilted.

Drain it and cool for ten mins. Squeeze out excess moisture.

In a bowl, mix cottage cheese, Parmesan cheese, oregano, salt, cayenne pepper, egg white, freshly ground black pepper, feta cheese, spinach, and zest. Mix it well or in the food processor.

Lay one phyllo sheet on a flat surface. Spray with oil. Add the second sheet of phyllo on top—spray oil. Add a total of 4 oiled sheets.

Form 16 strips from these four oiled sheets. Add one tbsp of filling in one strip. Roll it around the filling.

Spray the air fryer basket with oil. Put eight bites in the basket, spray with oil. Cook for 12 mins at 375°F until crispy and golden brown. Flip halfway through.

Nutrition: Cal 82 Fat 4 g Protein 4 g Carbohydrate 7 g

102. Air Fryer Onion Rings

Prep Time: 105 mins
Servings: 4

Cook Time:10 mins

Ingredients:
- 1 egg whisked
- One large onion
- Whole-wheat breadcrumbs: 1 and 1/2 cup
- Smoked paprika: 1 teaspoon
- Flour: 1 cup
- Garlic powder: 1 teaspoon
- Buttermilk: 1 cup
- Kosher salt and pepper to taste

Directions: Cut the stems of the onion. Then cut into half-inch-thick rounds.

In a bowl, add flour, pepper, garlic powder, smoked paprika, and salt. Then add egg and buttermilk. Mix to combine.

In another bowl, add the breadcrumbs.

Coat the onions in buttermilk mix, then in breadcrumbs mix.

Freeze these breaded onions for 15 mins. Spray the fryer basket with oil spray.

Put onions in the air fryer basket in one single layer. Spray the onion with cook oil.

Cook at 370 degrees for 10-12 mins. Flip only, if necessary.

Serve with sauce.

Nutrition: Cal 205 Fat 5.5 g Carbs 7.5 g Protein 18 g

103. Air Fryer Delicata Squash

Prep Time: 5 mins
Servings: 2

Cook Time:10 mins

Ingredients:
- Olive oil: 1/2 Tablespoon
- One delicata squash
- Salt: 1/2 teaspoon
- Rosemary: 1/2 teaspoon

Directions: Chop the squash in slices of 1/4 thickness. Discard the seeds.
In a bowl, add olive oil, salt, rosemary with squash slices. Mix well.
Cook the squash for ten mins at 400 F. flip the squash halfway through.
Make sure it is cooked completely.

Nutrition: Cal: 69 Fat: 4 g Carbs: 9 g Protein 1 g

104. Zucchini Parmesan Chips

Prep Time: 10 mins
Servings: 6

Cook Time:20 mins

Ingredients:
- Seasoned, whole wheat Breadcrumbs: ½ cup
- Thinly slices of two zucchinis
- Parmesan Cheese: ½ cup (grated)
- 1 Egg whisked
- Kosher salt and pepper, to taste

Directions: Pat dry the zucchini slices so that no moisture remains.
In a bowl, whisk the egg with a few tsp. of water and salt, pepper. In another bowl, mix the grated cheese, smoked paprika (optional), and breadcrumbs.
Coat zucchini slices in egg mix then in breadcrumbs. Put all in a rack and spray with olive oil.
In a single layer, add in the air fryer, and cook for 8 mins at 350 F. add kosher salt and pepper on top if needed, enjoy as a mid-day snack.

Nutrition: Cal 101 Fat: 8 g Carbs: 6 g Protein: 10 g

105. Air Fryer Roasted Corn

Prep Time: 10 mins
Servings: 4

Cook Time:10 mins

Ingredients:
- 4 corn ears
- Olive oil: 2 to 3 teaspoons
- Kosher salt and pepper to taste

Directions: Clean the corn, wash, and pat dry. Fit in the basket of air fryer, cut if need to.
Top with olive oil, kosher salt, and pepper. Cook for ten mins at 400 F.
Enjoy crispy roasted corn.

Nutrition: Cal 28 Fat 2 g Carbs 0 g Protein 7 g

106. Air-Fried Spinach Frittata

Prep Time: 5 mins
Servings: 4

Cook Time:10 mins

Ingredients:
- 1/3 cup of packed spinach
- One small chopped red onion
- Shredded mozzarella cheese

- *Three eggs*
- *Salt, pepper*

Directions: Let the air fryer preheat to 370°F.
In a skillet over a medium flame, add oil, onion, cook until translucent, add spinach and sauté until half cooked.
Beat eggs and season with kosher salt and pepper—mix spinach mixture in it.
Cook in the air fryer for 8 mins or until cooked. Slice and Serve hot.

Nutrition: Cal 124 Fat: 10.9 g Carbs: 14.1 g Protein: 16.9 g

107. Air Fryer Buffalo Cauliflower

Prep Time: 5 mins
Servings: 4

Cook Time: 10 mins

Ingredients:
- *One egg*
- *Half head of cauliflower*
- *Whole wheat breadcrumbs: one cup*
- *Salt: 1/2 teaspoon*
- *Garlic powder: 1/2 teaspoon*
- *One cup of low-fat ranch dressing*
- *Freshly ground black pepper*
- *Hot sauce: 1/2 cup*

Directions: Cut cauliflower into floret. In a bowl, mix the egg with garlic powder, salt, and pepper.
Coat floret in eggs, then in breadcrumbs. Add them to the air fryer and cook for 8-10 mins at 400 °F.
Mix hot sauce with ranch and serve with fried cauliflower.

Nutrition: Cal: 94, Carbs: 14 g, Protein: 4 g, Fat: 2 g

108. Air Fryer Sweet Potato Fries

Prep Time: 5 mins
Servings: 2

Cook Time: 8 mins

Ingredients:
- *One sweet potato*
- *Pinch of kosher salt and freshly ground black pepper*
- *1 tsp olive oil*

Directions: Cut the peeled sweet potato in French fries. Coat with salt, pepper, and oil.
Cook in the air fryer for 8 mins, at 400 degrees. Cook potatoes in batches, in single layers. Shake once or twice.
Serve with your favorite sauce.

Nutrition: Cal: 60, Carbs: 13 g, Protein: 1 g, Fat 6 g

109. Air Fryer Kale Chips

Prep Time: 3 mins
Servings: 2

Cook Time: 5 mins

Ingredients:
- *One bunch of kale*
- *Half tsp. of garlic powder*
- *One tsp. of olive oil*
- *Half tsp. of salt*

Directions: Let the air fryer preheat to 370 degrees.
Cut the kale into small pieces without the stem.
In a bowl, add all ingredients with kale pieces.
Add kale to the air fryer.
Cook for three mins. Toss it and cook for two mins more.

Nutrition: Cal: 37, Carbs: 6 g, Protein: 3 g, Fat: 1 g

110. Crispy Air Fryer Brussels Sprouts

Prep Time: 5 mins
Servings: 4

Cook Time: 10 mins

Ingredients:

- Almonds sliced: 1/4 cup
- Brussel sprouts: 2 cups
- Kosher salt
- Parmesan cheese: 1/4 cup grated
- Olive oil: 2 Tablespoons
- Everything bagel seasoning: 2 Tablespoons

Directions: In a saucepan, add Brussel sprouts with two cups of water and let it cook over medium flame for almost ten mins. Drain the sprouts and cut in half.
In a mixing bowl, add sliced brussel sprout with crushed almonds, oil, salt, parmesan cheese, and everything bagel seasoning. Completely coat the sprouts.
Cook in the air fryer for 12-15 mins at 375 F or until light brown.

Nutrition: Cal: 155, Carbs: 3 g Protein: 6 g Fat: 3 g

111. Vegetable Spring Rolls

Prep Time: 10 mins
Servings: 4

Cook Time: 15 mins

Ingredients:

- Toasted sesame seeds
- Large carrots – grated
- Spring roll wrappers
- One egg white
- Gluten-free soy sauce, a dash
- Half cabbage: sliced
- Olive oil: 2 tbsp.

Directions: In a pan over high flame heat, 2 tbsp. of oil and sauté the chopped vegetables. Then add soy sauce. Do not overcook the vegetables.
Turn off the heat and add toasted sesame seeds.
Lay spring roll wrappers flat on a surface and add egg white with a brush on the sides.
Add some vegetable mix in the wrapper and fold.
Spray the spring rolls with oil spray and air dry for 8 mins at 200 C.
Serve with dipping sauce.

Nutrition: 129 Cal Fat 16.3 g Carbs 8.2 g Protein 12.1 g

112. Zucchini Gratin

Prep Time: 10 mins
Servings: 4

Cook Time: 15 mins

Ingredients:

- Olive oil: 1 tablespoon
- Chopped fresh parsley: 1 tablespoon
- Whole wheat bread crumbs: 2 tablespoons
- Medium zucchini
- Freshly ground black pepper & kosher salt to taste
- Grated Parmesan cheese: 4 tablespoons

Directions: Let the air fryer preheat to 370°F.
Cut zucchini in half, and a further cut in eight pieces.
Place pieces in the air fryer, but do not start frying.
In a bowl, add cheese, freshly ground black pepper, parsley, bread crumbs, and oil. Mix well.
Add the mixture on top of the zucchini. Then cook the pieces for 15 mins.
Until light golden brown, serve hot and enjoy.

Nutrition: 81.7 Cal Protein 3.6 g Carbs 6.1 g Fat 5.2 g

113. Asparagus Frittata

Prep Time: 10 mins
Servings: 2

Cook Time: 5 mins

Ingredients:

- 4 eggs, whisked
- 3 Tablespoons parmesan, grated
- 2 Tablespoons milk
- Salt and black pepper to the taste
- Ten asparagus tips, steamed
- Cooking spray

Directions: Mix the eggs with the parmesan, butter, salt, pepper, and whisk well in a pot.
Heat your air fryer to 400 degrees F and spray with grease.
Add asparagus, mix the eggs, toss a little, and cook for 5 mins.
Separate frittata into plates and serve breakfast.

Nutrition: Cal 312 Fat 5g Carbs 14 g Protein 2 g

114. Air Fryer Bacon-Wrapped Jalapeno Poppers

Prep Time: 10 mins
Servings: 10

Cook Time: 8 mins

Ingredients:

- Cream cheese: 1/3 cup
- Ten jalapenos
- Thin bacon: 5 strips

Directions: Wash and pat dry the jalapenos. Cut them in half and take out the seeds.
Add the cream cheese in the middle, but do not put too much.
Let the air fryer preheat to 370 F. cut the bacon strips in half.
Wrap the cream cheese filled jalapenos with slices of bacon.
Secure with a toothpick.
Place the wrapped jalapenos in an air fryer, cook at 370 F and cook for 6-8 mins or until the bacon is crispy.

Nutrition: Cal: 76 Carbs: 1 g Protein: 2 g Fat: 7 g

115. Easy Air Fryer Zucchini Chips

Prep Time: 10 mins
Servings: 2

Cook Time: 12 mins

Ingredients:

- Parmesan Cheese: 3 Tbsp.
- Garlic Powder: 1/4 tsp
- Zucchini: 1 Cup (thin slices)
- Corn Starch: 1/4 Cup
- Onion Powder: 1/4 tsp
- Salt: 1/4 tsp
- Whole wheat Bread Crumbs: 1/2 Cup

Directions: Let the Air Fryer preheat to 390 F. cut the zucchini into thin slices, like chips.
In a food processor bowl, mix garlic powder, kosher salt, whole wheat bread crumbs, parmesan cheese, and onion powder.
Blend into finer pieces.
In three separate bowls, add corn starch in one, egg mix in another bowl, and whole wheat breadcrumb mixture in the other bowl.
Coat zucchini chips into corn starch mix, in egg mix, then coat in whole wheat bread crumbs.
Spray the air fryer basket with olive oil. Add breaded zucchini chips in a single layer in the air fryer and spray with olive oil.
Air fry for six mins at preheated temperature. Cook for another four mins after turning or until zucchini chips are golden brown.
Serve with any dipping sauce.

Nutrition: 219 Cal Fat 26.9 g Carbs 11.2 g Protein 14.1 g

116. Air Fryer Avocado Fries

Prep Time: 10 mins
Servings: 2

Cook Time: 10 mins

Ingredients:

- One avocado
- One egg
- Whole wheat bread crumbs: 1/2 cup
- Salt: 1/2 teaspoon

Directions: Avocado should be firm and firm. Cut into wedges.
In a bowl, beat egg with salt. In another bowl, add the crumbs.
Coat wedges in egg, then in crumbs.
Air fry them at 400 °F for 8-10 mins. Toss halfway through.

Nutrition: Cal: 251 Carbs: 19 g Protein: 6 g Fat: 17 g

117. Avocado Egg Rolls

Prep Time: 15 mins
Servings: 10

Cook Time: 15 mins

Ingredients:

- Ten egg roll wrappers
- Diced sundried tomatoes: ¼ cup oil drained
- Avocados, cut in cube
- Red onion: 2/3 cup chopped
- 1/3 cup chopped cilantro
- Kosher salt and freshly ground black pepper
- Two small limes: juice

Directions: In a bowl, add sundried tomatoes, avocado, cilantro, lime juice, pepper, onion, and kosher salt mix well gently.
Lay egg roll wrapper flat on a surface, add ¼ cup of filling in the wrapper's bottom.
Seal with water and make it into a roll.
Spray the rolls with olive oil.
Cook at 400 F in the air fryer for six mins. Turn halfway through.
Serve with dipping sauce.

Nutrition: 160 Cal Fat 19 g Carbs 5.6 g Protein 19.2 g

118. Cheesy Bell Pepper Eggs

Prep time: 10 mins
Servings: 4

Cook Time: 15 mins

Ingredients:

- 4 medium green bell peppers
- 3 ounces cooked ham, chopped
- 1/4 medium onion, peeled and chopped
- 8 large eggs
- 1 cup mild Cheddar cheese

Directions: Cut each bell pepper from its tops. Pick the seeds with a small knife and the white membranes. Place onion and ham into each pepper.
Break two eggs into each chili pepper. Cover with 1/4 cup of peppered cheese. Put the basket into the air fryer.
Set the temperature to 390 ° F and change the timer for 15 mins.
Peppers will be tender when fully fried, and the eggs will be solid. Serve hot.

Nutrition: Cal: 314 Protein: 24.9 g Carbs: 4.6 g Fat: 18.6 g

119. Air Fryer Crisp Egg Cups

Prep Time: 10 mins
Servings: 4

Cook Time: 10 mins

Ingredients:

- Toasted bread: 4 slices (whole-wheat)
- Cook spray, nonstick
- Large eggs: 4
- Margarine: 1 and a half tbsp. (trans-fat free)
- Ham: 1 slice
- Salt: 1/8 tsp
- Black pepper: 1/8 tsp

Directions: Let the air fryer Preheat to 375 F, with the air fryer basket.
Take four ramekins, spray with cook spray.
Trim off the crusts from bread, add margarine to one side.
Put the bread down, into a ramekin, margarine-side in.
Press it in the cup. Cut the ham in strips, half-inch thick, and add on top of the bread.
Add one egg to the ramekins. Add salt and pepper.
Put the custard cups in the air fryer. Air fry at 375 F for 10–13 mins.
Remove the ramekin from the air fryer and serve.

Nutrition: Cal 150 Fat 8 g Carbs 6 g Protein 12 g

120. Air Fryer Lemon-Garlic Tofu

Prep Time: 20 mins
Servings: 2

Cook Time: 10 mins

Ingredients:

- Cooked quinoa 2 cups
- Lemons: two zest and juice
- Sea salt & white pepper: to taste
- Tofu: one block - pressed and sliced into half pieces
- Garlic – minced: 2 cloves

Directions: Add the tofu into a deep dish.
In another small bowl, add the garlic, lemon juice, lemon zest, salt, pepper.
Pour this marinade over tofu in the dish. Let it marinate for at least 15 mins.
Add the tofu to the air fryer basket.
Keep the leftover marinade safe. Let it air fry at 370F for 15 mins. Shake the basket after 8 mins of cook.
In a big deep bowl, add the cooked Quinoa with the Lemon-Garlic Tofu.

Nutrition: Cal 187 Fat 9 g Protein 20 g Carbs 8 g

121. Vegan Mashed Potato Bowl

Prep Time: 10 mins
Servings: 4

Cook Time: 20 mins

Ingredients:

- Mashed potatoes
- Olive oil
- Red potatoes: large, three pieces cooked with the skin on, cut into one-inch pieces
- 1/4 tsp of salt
- Sea salt and black pepper - to taste
- Half cup of unsweetened soy milk or vegan milk

For the Tofu:

- One teaspoon of garlic powder
- One block of extra firm tofu: pressed, cut into one-inch pieces
- Light soy sauce: 2 tablespoons

Directions: To make the Mashed Potatoes: Add the cooked potatoes to a large bowl, mash with masher with butter. Mash until pretty lumpy. Then add the soy milk and keep crushing until you mash till desired consistency.
Cover the bowl with plastic wrap, so it will keep warm and let it rest.

Meanwhile, add the tofu in one even layer in the air fryer, add the garlic powder and soy sauce, and make sure to cover all the tofu.
Let it cook in Air fryer for ten mins at 400 °F.
Cook the corn and kale according to your preference.
In four bowls, add the mashed potatoes, corn, and kale in the end top with tofu.
You can add chopped scallions, roasted cashews, and enjoy.

Nutrition: Cal 250 Fat 17 g Protein 21 g Carbs 13 g

122. Vegan Breakfast Sandwich

Prep Time: 10 mins   **Cook Time: 10 mins**
Servings: 4

Ingredients:

Tofu (Egg):
- *Garlic powder: 1 teaspoon*
- *Light soy sauce: 1/4 cup*
- *Turmeric: 1/2 teaspoon*
- *1 block extra firm pressed tofu: cut into 4 round slices*

Breakfast Sandwich:
- *English muffins: four pieces, vegan*
- *Avocado: one cut into slices*
- *Tomato slices*
- *Vegan cheese: 4 slices*
- *Sliced onions*
- *Vegan mayonnaise or vegan butter*

Directions: Let the tofu marinate overnight.
In a deep dish, add the tofu circles with turmeric, soy sauce, and garlic powder. Let it for 10 mins or overnight.
Put the tofu (marinated) in an air fryer. Cook for ten mins at 400 F. shake the basket after 5 mins.
Add vegan butter or vegan mayonnaise to the English muffins. Add vegan cheese, avocado slices, tomato, onions slices, and marinated, cooked tofu. Top with the other half of the English muffin.

Nutrition: Cal 198 Fat 10 g Carbs 12 g Protein 19.9 g

123. Crispy Fat-Free Spanish Potatoes

Prep Time: 10 mins   **Cook Time: 35 mins**
Servings: 3

Ingredients:
- *Small red potatoes: 1 and 1/2 pounds*
- *Liquid from cooked chickpeas or aquafaba: 1 tablespoon*
- *Tomato paste: 1 teaspoon*
- *Sea salt optional: 1 teaspoon*
- *Brown rice flour or any flour (your choice): half tablespoon*
- *Smoked Spanish paprika: 1 teaspoon*
- *Garlic powder: half teaspoon*
- *Sweet smoked paprika: 3/4 tsp.*

Directions: Wash and pat dry the potatoes. Cut the potatoes into small quarters, makes sure they are the same sized. The maximum thickness of potatoes should be one and a half-inch thick.
Boil the potatoes wedges however you like,
Drain the potatoes wedges and add them in a large bowl.
In another bowl, add tomato paste and aquafaba. In the small bowl, mix the remaining ingredients and flour.
Now add the tomato paste mixture to the potatoes, coat all the potatoes wedges gently with light hands. Add the dry mix to the coated potatoes until every potato is covered.
Let the air fryer preheat to 360F for 3 mins. Place the potatoes in the basket and cook for 12 mins.
Shake the basket of air fryer every six mins. Make sure no potatoes get stuck on the bottom.
Let the potatoes be crispy to your liking.
Serve hot with dipping sauce.

Nutrition: Cal 171 Carbs 39 g Protein 5 g

124. Cheese and Veggie Air Fryer Egg Cups

Prep Time: 10 mins
Servings: 4

Cook Time: 20 mins

Ingredients:

- Shredded cheese: 1 cup
- Non-stick cook spray
- Vegetables: 1 cup diced
- Chopped cilantro: 1 Tbsp.
- Half and a half: 4 Tbsp.
- Four large eggs
- Salt and Pepper to taste

Directions: Take four ramekins, grease them with oil.
In a bowl, crack the eggs with half the cheese, cilantro, salt, diced vegetables, half and half, and pepper.
Pour in the ramekins. And put in the air-fryer basket and cook for 12 mins, at 300 F
Then add the cheese to the cups.
Let the air-fryer pre-heat for two mins, at 400 degrees F.
Cook until cheese is lightly browned and melted.

Nutrition: Cal: 195 Carbs: 7 g Protein: 13 g Fat: 12 g

125. Low Carb Air Fryer Baked Eggs

Prep Time: 10 mins
Servings: 4

Cook Time: 15 mins

Ingredients:

- Cooking Spray
- Grated cheese: 1-2 teaspoons
- One large egg
- Frozen or fresh sautéed spinach: 1 tablespoon
- Salt to taste
- Milk: 1 tablespoon, or half & half
- Black pepper to taste

Directions: Take ramekins and spray them with cook spray. Add milk, spinach (if using frozen, thaw it before), egg, cheese.
Add seasoning salt, pepper according to taste, in the ramekins. Stir everything but do not break the yolk.
Let it air fry for 6-12 mins at 330 F. one cup will almost take 5-6 mins. More than one cup will take more time.

Nutrition: Cal: 115 Carbs 1 g Protein 10 g Fat: 7 g

126. Easy Air Fryer Omelet

Prep Time: 10 mins
Servings: 2

Cook Time: 15 mins

Ingredients:

- Breakfast Seasoning: 1 teaspoon
- Two eggs
- A pinch of salt
- Fresh ham
- Milk: 1/4 cup
- Shredded cheese: 1/4 cup
- Diced veggies: green onions, red bell pepper, and mushrooms

Directions: In a bowl, mix the milk and eggs, combine them well. Season with a pinch of salt.
Add chopped vegetables to the egg mixture.
Add the egg mixture to a 6″x3″ baking pan. Make sure it is well greased.
Put the pan in the air fryer basket.
Air fry for 8-10 mins at 350° Fahrenheit.
After 5 mins, add the breakfast seasoning into the eggs and top with shredded cheese.
Take out from the air fryer, and transfer to the plate.
Serve hot with extra green onions and enjoy.

Nutrition: Cal 256 Fat 13 g Protein 15 g Carbs 8 g

127. Breakfast Bombs

Prep Time: 10 mins
Servings: 3

Cook Time: 15 mins

Ingredients:
- Three eggs (large), lightly whisked
- Less-fat cream cheese: two tbsp. Softened
- Chopped chives: 1 tablespoon fresh

- Freshly prepared whole-wheat pizza dough: 1/4 cup or 4 ounces
- Cook spray
- 3 pieces of bacon: center cut

- Freshly prepared whole-wheat pizza dough: 1/4 cup or 4 ounces
- Cook spray

Directions: In a skillet, cook the bacon slices for about ten mins. Crumble the cooked bacon. Add the eggs to the skillet and cook until loose for almost one minute. In another bowl, mix with chives, cheese, and bacon.
Cut the dough into four pieces. Make it into a five-inch circle.
Add 1/4 of egg mixture in the center of dough circle pieces.
Seal the dough seams with water and pinch
Add dough pockets in one single layer in the air fryer. Spray with cook oil
Cook for 5-6 mins, at 350°F or until light golden brown.

Nutrition: Cal 305 Fat 15 g Protein 19 g Carbs 26 g

128. Air Fryer Breakfast Toad-in-the-Hole Tarts

Prep Time: 5 mins
Servings: 4

Cook Time: 25 mins

Ingredients:
- Chopped fresh chives: one tbsp.
- Frozen puff pastry: one sheet, thawed

- Eggs: four large
- Chopped ham: 4 tbsp. (cooked)

- Shredded: 4 tbsp. of Cheddar cheese

Directions: Let the air fryer preheat to 400 F.
Lay puff pastry on a clean surface and slice into four squares.
Add two squares of puff pastry in the air fryer and cook for 8 mins.
Take out from the air fryer and make an indentation in the dough's center and add one tbsp. Of ham and one tbsp. Of cheddar cheese in every hole. Add one egg to it.
Return the basket to the air fryer. Let it cook to your desired doneness, for about six mins or more.
Take out from the basket of the air fryer. Cool for 5 mins.
Top with chives and serve hot.

Nutrition: Cal 154 Fat 7 g Carbs 7 g Protein 10.1 g

129. Air Fried Cheesy Chicken Omelet

Prep Time: 5 mins
Servings: 2

Cook Time: 18 mins

Ingredients:
- Cooked Chicken Breast: half cup (diced) divided
- Four eggs

- Onion powder: 1/4 tsp, divided
- Salt: 1/2 tsp., divided
- Pepper: 1/4 tsp., divided
- Shredded cheese: 2 tbsp. divided

- Garlic powder: 1/4 tsp, divided

Directions: Take two ramekins, grease with olive oil. Add two eggs to each ramekin. Add cheese with seasoning.
Blend to combine. Add 1/4 cup of cooked chicken on top.
Cook for 14-18 mins, in the air fryer at 330 F, or until fully cooked.

Nutrition: Cal 185 Protein 20 g Carbs 10 g Fat 5 g

130. Air Fryer Spicy Chickpeas

Prep Time: 10 Mins
Servings: 4

Cook Time: 12 mins

Ingredients:

- 14 oz can chickpeas, rinsed, drained and pat dry
- 1/2 teaspoon smoked paprika
- 1/4 teaspoon cayenne
- 1/2 teaspoon chili powder
- 1 tablespoon olive oil
- Salt and Pepper

Directions: Add chickpeas, chili powder, cayenne, pepper, paprika, oil, and salt into the bowl and toss well.
Spread chickpeas in the air fryer basket.
Place a baking pan on the oven rack. Set to air fry at 375 degrees F for twelve mins.

Nutrition: Cal 150 Fat 4.7 g Carbs 22.8 g

131. Apple Chips

Prep Time: 10 mins
Servings: 2

Cook time: 15 mins

Ingredients:

- One apple, cored and thinly sliced
- ½ tsp. cinnamon powder
- tbsp. stevia

Directions: Arrange apple slices in your air fryer's basket, add stevia and cinnamon, toss and cook at 390° F for ten mins, turning them halfway.
Transfer to a bowl and serve as a snack.

Nutrition: Cal 90 Fat 0 g Carbs 12 g

132. Air Fryer Walnuts

Prep Time: 10 Mins
Servings: 6

Cook Time: 5 mins

Ingredients:

- 2 cups walnuts
- teaspoon olive oil
- Salt and Pepper

Directions: Add walnuts, oil, pepper, and salt into the bowl and toss well.
Add walnuts to the air fryer basket then place an air fryer basket in baking pan.
Place a baking pan on the oven rack. Set to air fry at 350 degrees F for five mins.

Nutrition: Cal 264 Fat 25.4 g Carbs 4.1 g

133. Avocado Chips

Prep Time: 10 mins
Servings: 3

Cook time: 10 mins

Ingredients:

- One avocado, pitted, peeled and sliced
- Salt and pepper
- ½ cup vegan bread crumbs
- A drizzle of olive oil

Directions: In a bowl, mix bread crumbs with salt and pepper and mix.
Brush avocado slices with the oil, coat them in bread crumbs, place them in your air fryer's basket and cook at the temperature of 390 degrees F for ten mins, shaking halfway. Divide into bowls.

Nutrition: Cal 180 Fat 11 g Carbs 7 g

134. Allspice Chicken Wings

Cook Time: 45 mins

Ingredients:
- ½ tsp celery salt
- ½ tsp bay leaf powder
- ¼ tsp allspice
- 2 pounds chicken wings
- ½ tsp ground black pepper
- ½ tsp paprika
- ¼ tsp dry mustard
- ¼ tsp cayenne pepper

Directions: Grease the air fryer basket and preheat to 340 degrees F. In a bowl, mix celery salt, bay leaf powder, paprika, dry mustard, black pepper, cayenne pepper, and all spice. Coat the wings thoroughly in this mixture.
Arrange the wings in an even layer in the air fryer basket. Cook the chicken until it's no longer pink around the bone, for thirty mins then, increase the temperature to 380 degrees F and cook for six mins more, until crispy on the outside.

Nutrition: Cal 332 Fat 10.1 g Carbs 31.3 g

135. Avocado Rolls

Prep Time: 20 mins
Servings: 5

Cook Time: 25 mins

Ingredients:
- Ten rice paper wrappers
- Three avocados, sliced
- One tomato, diced
- Salt and pepper
- 1 tbsp. olive oil
- 4 tbsp. sriracha
- 1 tbsp. sugar
- 1 tbsp. rice vinegar
- 1 tbsp. sesame oil

Directions: Mash avocados in a bowl.
Toss in the tomatoes, salt and pepper. Mix well.
Arrange the rice paper wrappers. Scoop mixture on top.
Roll and seal the edges with water.
Cook in the air fryer at 350° F for 5 mins.
Mix the rest of the ingredients.

Nutrition: Cal 422 Fat 5.8 g Carbs 38.7 g

136. Baguette Bread

Prep Time: 15 mins
Servings: 8

Cook Time: 20 mins

Ingredients:
- ¾ cup warm water
- cup bread flour
- ½ cup whole-wheat flour
- ½ cup oat flour
- ½ teaspoon demerara sugar
- ¾ teaspoon quick yeast
- 1¼ teaspoons salt

Directions: In a large bowl, place the water and sprinkle with yeast and sugar.
Set aside for five mins or until foamy.
Add the bread flour and salt mix until a stiff dough form.
Put the dough onto a floured surface and with your hands, knead until smooth and elastic.
Now, shape the dough into a ball.
Place the dough into a oiled bowl and turn to coat well.
With a plastic wrap, cover the bowl and place in a warm place for about 1 hour or until doubled in size.
Punch down the dough and form into a long slender loaf.
Place the loaf onto a lightly greased baking sheet and set aside in warm place, uncovered, for about 30 mins.
Select the "Bake" mode. Set the cook time to twenty mins. Set the temperature at 450° F.
Carefully, arrange the dough onto the "Wire Rack" and insert in the oven.
Carefully, invert the bread onto wire rack to cool completely before slicing.
Cut the bread into desired-sized slice.

Nutrition: Cal 114 Fat 0.8 g Carbs 22.8 g

137. Banana Chips

Prep time: 10 mins
Servings: 4

Cook time: 10 mins

Ingredients:
- *Four bananas, peeled and sliced into thin pieces*
- *A drizzle of olive oil*
- *Pepper*

Directions: Put banana slices in your air fryer, drizzle the oil, season with pepper, toss to coat gently and cook at 360° F for ten mins.

Nutrition: Cal 100 Fat 7 g Carbs 20 g

138. Baked Almonds

Prep Time: 10 Mins
Servings: 6

Cook Time: 20 mins

Ingredients:
- *1/2 cups raw almonds*
- *1/2 teaspoon cayenne*
- *1/4 teaspoon onion powder*
- *1/4 teaspoon dried basil*
- *tablespoon butter, melted*
- *1/2 teaspoon garlic powder*
- *1/2 teaspoon cumin*
- *1/2 teaspoon chili powder*
- *1/2 teaspoon sea salt*

Directions: Add almonds and remaining ingredients into the mixing bowl and stir well.
Spread almonds in baking pan.
Set to bake at 350 degrees F for twenty-five mins. After five mins place the baking pan in the preheated oven.

Nutrition: Cal 176 Fat 15.9 g Carbs 5.9 g

139. Basil Crackers

Prep Time: 10 mins
Servings: 6

Cook time: 17 mins

Ingredients:
- *½ tsp. baking powder*
- *Salt and black pepper to the taste*
- *One and ¼ cups whole wheat flour*
- *¼ tsp. basil, dried*
- *One garlic clove, minced*
- *2 tbsp. vegan basil pesto*
- *2 tbsp. olive oil*

Directions: In a prepared bowl, mix flour with salt, pepper, baking powder, garlic, cayenne, basil, pesto and oil, stir until you obtain a dough, spread this on a lined baking sheet that fits your air fryer, introduce in the fryer at 325° F and bake for seventeen mins.
Leave aside to cool down, cut crackers and serve them as a snack.

Nutrition: Cal 170 Fat 20 g Carbs 6 g

140. Banana & Raisin Bread

Prep Time: 15 mins
Servings: 6

Cook Time: 40 mins

Ingredients:
- *1½ cups cake flour*
- *teaspoon baking soda*
- *eggs*
- *½ teaspoon ground cinnamon*
- *½ cup vegetable oil*
- *½ cup sugar*
- *½ teaspoon vanilla extract*
- *three medium bananas, peeled and mashed*
- *½ cup raisins, chopped finely*
- *Salt*

Directions: In a large bowl, mix together cinnamon, flour, baking soda, and salt.

In another bowl, beat well eggs and oil. Add the sugar, vanilla extract, and bananas and beat until well combined.
Add the flour mixture and stir until just combined.
Place the mixture into a lightly greased baking pan and sprinkle with raisins.
With a piece of foil, cover the pan loosely.
Select the "Bake" mode and set the cook time to thirty mins. Set the temperature at 300° F.
Arrange the pan in "Air Fry Basket" and insert in the oven.
After thirty mins of cook, set the temperature to 285° F for ten mins. Place the pan onto a wire rack to cool for ten mins. Carefully, invert the bread onto wire rack to cool completely before slicing.
Cut the bread into desired-sized slices.

Nutrition: Cal 448 Fat 20.2 g Carbs 63.9 g

141. Beets Chips

Prep Time: 10 mins   Cook time: 20 mins
Servings: 4

Ingredients:
- *Four medium beets, peeled and cut into skinny slices*
- *tbsp. chives, chopped*
- *Cook spray*
- *Salt and pepper*

Directions: Arrange beets chips in your air fryer's basket, grease with cook spray, season with salt and black pepper, cook them at 350° F for twenty mins, flipping them halfway, transfer to bowls and serve with chives sprinkled on top as a snack.

Nutrition: Cal 80 Fat 1 g Carbs 6 g

142. Banana & Walnut Bread

Prep Time: 15 mins   **Cook Time:** 25 mins
Servings: 10

Ingredients:
- *1½ cups self-rising flour*
- *2 medium eggs*
- *¼ teaspoon bicarbonate of soda*
- *5 tbsp. + 1 teaspoon butter*
- *2/3 cup plus ½ tablespoon caster sugar*
- *3½ oz. walnuts, chopped*
- *2 cups bananas, peeled and mashed*

Directions: In a bowl, stir together the flour and bicarbonate of soda.
In another bowl, add the butter, and sugar and beat until pale and fluffy.
Add the eggs, one at a time along with a little flour and mix well. Stir in the remaining flour and walnuts. Add the bananas and mix until well combined.
Grease a loaf pan. Place the mixture into the prepared pan.
Select the "Air Fry" mode and set the cook time to ten mins. Set the temperature at 355° F. Press "Start/Pause" button to start.
Arrange the pan in "Air Fry Basket" and insert in the oven.
After ten mins of cook, set the temperature at 338° F for 15 mins. Place the pan onto a wire rack to cool for about 10 mins.
Carefully, invert the bread onto wire rack to cool completely before slicing.
Cut the bread into desired-sized slices.

Nutrition: Cal 270 Fat 12.8 g Carbs 35.5 g

143. Bean Burger

Prep Time: 10 mins   **Cook Time: 25 mins**
Servings: 6

Ingredients:
- *One ¼ cup rolled oats*
- *16 oz. black beans, rinsed and drained*
- *¾ cup of salsa*
- *One ¼ tsp. chilli powder*
- *¼ tsp. chipotle chilli powder*
- *tbsp. soy sauce*
- *½ tsp. garlic powder*

Directions: Pulse the oats inside a food processor until powdery.
Apply all the remaining ingredients and pulse until well combined.
Transfer to a bowl and refrigerate for 15 mins.
Form into burger patties.
Cook in the air fryer at 375 degrees F for 15 mins.

Nutrition: Cal 158 Fat 2 g Carbs 30 g

144. Brown Sugar Banana Bread

Prep Time: 15 mins
Servings: 4

Cook Time: 30 mins

Ingredients:
- 1 egg
- 1 ripe banana, peeled and mashed
- ¼ cup milk
- 2 tablespoons canola oil
- ¾ cup plain flour
- ½ teaspoon baking soda
- 2 tablespoons brown sugar

Directions: Line a very small baking pan with a greased parchment paper.
In a small bowl, add banana and the egg, and beat well.
Add the milk, oil and sugar and beat until well combined.
Add the flour and baking soda and mix until just combined.
Place the mixture into prepared pan.
Select the "Air Fry" mode and set the cook time to 30 mins.
Set the temperature at 320 degrees F.
Arrange the pan in "Air Fry Basket" and insert in the oven.
Place the pan onto a wire rack to cool for about 10 mins.
Carefully, invert the bread onto wire rack to cool completely before slicing.
Cut the bread into desired-sized slices.

Nutrition: Cal 214 Fat 8.7 g Carbs 29.9 g

145. Cabbage Rolls

Prep Time: 10 mins
Servings: 8

Cook time: 25 mins

Ingredients:
- 2 cups cabbage, chopped
- Two yellow onions, chopped
- One carrot, chopped
- ½ red bell pepper, chopped
- 1-inch piece ginger, grated
- Eight garlic cloves, minced
- Salt and pepper
- tsp. coconut aminos
- tbsp. olive oil
- Ten vegan spring roll sheets
- Cook spray
- tbsp. Corn flour mixed with 1 tbsp. water

Directions: Heat a pan with the oil over medium-high heat, add cabbage, onions, carrots, bell pepper, ginger, pepper and amino, garlic, salt, stir, cook for 4 mins take off the heat.
Cut each spring roll sheet and cut it into 4 pieces.
Place 1 tbsp. Veggie mix in one corner, roll and fold edges.
Repeat with the rest of the rolls, place them in your air fryer's basket, grease them with cook oil and cook at 360° F for 10 mins on each side.
Arrange on a plate and then serve as an appetizer.

Nutrition: Cal 150 Fat 3 g Carbs 7 g

146. Butternut Squash with Thyme

Prep Time: 5 mins
Servings: 4

Cook Time: 20 mins

Ingredients:
- 2 cups peeled, butternut squash, cubed
- tbsp olive oil
- ¼ tsp dried thyme
- tbsp finely chopped fresh parsley
- ¼ tsp salt

- *¼ tsp pepper*

Directions: In a bowl, add squash, oil, salt, pepper, and thyme, and toss until squash is well-coated. Place squash in the air fryer and cook for 14 mins at 360 degrees F. When ready, sprinkle with freshly chopped parsley and serve chilled.

Nutrition: Cal 219 Fat 4.3 g Carbs 9.4 g

147. Cauliflower Crackers

Prep Time: 10 mins
Servings: 12

Cook time: 25 mins

Ingredients:
- *One big cauliflower head, florets separated and riced*
- *½ cup cashew cheese, shredded*
- *tbsp. flax meal mixed with 1 tbsp. water*
- *tsp. Italian seasoning*
- *Salt and pepper*

Directions: Spread cauliflower rice on a lined baking sheet that fits your air fryer. Introduce in the fryer and cook at 360 degrees F for 10 mins.
Transfer cauliflower to a bowl, add salt, pepper, cashew cheese, flax meal and Italian seasoning, stir well, spread this into a rectangle pan that fits your air fryer, press well, introduce in the fryer and cook at 360 degrees F for 15 mins more. Cut into medium crackers.

Nutrition: Cal 120 Fat 1 g Carbs 7 g

148. Cheesy Garlic Dip

Prep Time: 10 Mins
Servings: 12

Cook Time: 20 mins

Ingredients:
- *4 garlic cloves, minced*
- *5 oz Asiago cheese, shredded*
- *1 cup mozzarella cheese, shredded*
- *8 oz cream cheese, softened*
- *1 cup sour cream*

Directions: Add all ingredients into the mixing bowl and mix until well combined.
Pour mixture into the baking dish.
Set to bake at 350 degrees F for 25 mins. After 5 mins place the baking dish in the preheated oven.

Nutrition: Cal 157 Fat 14.4 g Carbs 1.7 g

149. Cheese Brussels Sprouts

Prep Time: 10 Mins
Servings: 4

Cook Time: 12 mins

Ingredients:
- *1 lb Brussels sprouts, cut stems and halved*
- *1/4 cup parmesan cheese, grated*
- *1 tablespoon olive oil*
- *1/4 teaspoon paprika*
- *1/4 teaspoon chili powder*
- *1/2 teaspoon garlic powder*
- *Salt and Pepper*

Directions: Stir Brussels sprouts with remaining ingredients except for cheese and place in air fryer basket then place air fryer basket in baking pan.
Place a baking pan on the oven rack. Set to air fry at 350 degrees F for 12 mins.
Top with parmesan cheese.

Nutrition: Cal 100 Fat 5.2 g Carbs 11 g

150. Cheese Onion Dip

Prep Time: 10 Mins　　　　　　　　　　　　　　　　　**Cook Time: 40 mins**
Servings: 8

Ingredients:
- 1 1/2 onions, chopped
- 1/2 teaspoon garlic powder
- 1 1/2 cup Swiss cheese, shredded
- 1 cup mozzarella cheese, shredded
- 1 cup cheddar cheese, shredded
- 1 1/2 cup mayonnaise
- Salt and Pepper

Directions: Add all ingredients into the mixing bowl and mix until well combined.
Pour mixture into the prepared baking dish.
Set to bake at 350 degrees F for 45 mins. After 5 mins place the baking dish in the preheated oven.

Nutrition: Cal 325 Fat 25.7 g Carbs 14 g

151. Cheese Spinach Dip

Prep Time: 10 Mins　　　　　　　　　　　　　　　　　**Cook Time: 20 mins**
Servings: 12

Ingredients:
- 3 oz frozen spinach, defrosted & chopped
- 1 cup sour cream
- 2 cups cheddar cheese, shredded
- 8 oz cream cheese
- 1 teaspoon garlic salt

Directions: Add all ingredients into the mixing bowl and mix well.
Transfer mixture into the baking dish.
Set to bake at 350 degrees F for 25 mins. After 5 mins place the baking dish in the preheated oven.

Nutrition: Cal 185 Fat 16.9 g Carbs 2 g

152. Chickpeas Snack

Prep Time: 10 mins　　　　　　　　　　　　　　　　　**Cook time: 20 mins**
Servings: 4

Ingredients:
- 15 ounces canned chickpeas, drained
- ½ tsp. cumin, ground
- 1 tbsp. olive oil
- 1 tsp. smoked paprika
- Salt and pepper

Directions: In a bowl, mix chickpeas with oil, paprika, cumin, salt and pepper, toss to coat, place them in the fryer's basket, cook at 390° F for 10 mins, and transfer a bowl.

Nutrition: Cal 140 Fat 1 g Carbs 20 g

153. Chocolate Banana Bread

Prep Time: 15 mins　　　　　　　　　　　　　　　　　**Cook Time:** 20 mins
Servings: 8

Ingredients:
- 2 cups flour
- ½ teaspoon baking soda
- 3 eggs
- 1/3 cup butter, softened
- ½ teaspoon baking powder
- ½ teaspoon salt
- ¾ cup sugar
- tablespoon vanilla extract
- cup milk
- ½ cup bananas, peeled and mashed
- cup chocolate chips

Directions: In a bowl, mix together the flour, baking soda, baking powder, and salt.

In another large bowl, add the butter, and sugar and beat until light and fluffy. Add the eggs, and vanilla extract and whisk until well combined. Add the flour mixture and mix until well combined. Add the milk, and mashed bananas and mix well.
Gently, fold in the chocolate chips. Place the mixture into a lightly greased loaf pan.
Select the "Air Fry" mode and set the cook time to 20 mins. Set the temperature at 360 degrees F. Arrange the pan in "Air Fry Basket" and insert in the oven.
Place the pan onto a wire rack to cool for about 10 mins.
Carefully, invert the bread onto wire rack to cool completely before slicing.
Cut the bread into desired-sized slices.

Nutrition: Cal 416 Fat 16.5 g Carbs 59.2 g

154. Cinnamon Banana Bread

Prep Time: 15 mins   **Cook Time:** 20 mins
Servings: 8

Ingredients:
- 1 1/3 cups flour
- 2/3 cup sugar
- 1 teaspoon baking soda
- 1 teaspoon baking powder
- 1 teaspoon ground cinnamon
- 3 bananas, peeled and sliced
- ½ cup milk
- ½ cup olive oil
- 1 teaspoon salt

Directions: In the bowl of a stand mixer, add all the ingredients and mix well.
Grease a loaf pan.
Place the mixture into the prepared pan.
Select the "Air Fry" mode. Set the cook time to 20 mins. Set the temperature at 330 degrees F.
Arrange the pan in "Air Fry Basket" and insert in the oven.
Place the pan onto a wire rack to cool for about 10 mins
Carefully, invert the bread onto wire rack to cool completely before slicing.
Cut the bread into desired-sized slices.

Nutrition: Cal 295 Fat 13.3 g Carbs 44 g

155. Corn Fritters

Prep Time: 15 mins   **Cook Time: 10 mins**
Servings: 4

Ingredients:
- ¼ cup ground cornmeal
- ¼ cup flour
- ¼ tsp. garlic powder
- ¼ tsp. onion powder
- ¼ tsp. paprika
- Salt and pepper
- ½ tsp. baking powder
- ¼ cup parsley, chopped
- One cup corn kernels mixed with 3 tbsp. almond milk
- 2 cups fresh corn kernels
- 4 tbsp. mayonnaise
- 2 tsp. grainy mustard

Directions: Mix the cornmeal, flour, salt, garlic powder, onion powder, pepper, baking powder, paprika and parsley in a bowl.
Put the corn kernels with almond milk in a food processor. Season with salt and pepper. Pulse until well blended.
Add the corn kernels.
Transfer to a bowl and stir into the cornmeal mixture.
Pour a small amount of the batter into the air fryer pan.
Pour another a few centimeters away from the first cake.
Cook in the air fryer set the temperature at 350 degrees for 10 mins or until golden. Flip halfway through.
Serve with mayonnaise mustard dip.

Nutrition: Cal 135 Total Fat 4.6 g Carbs 22.5 g

156. Date & Walnut Bread

Prep Time: 15 mins   **Cook Time:** 35 mins
Servings: 5

Ingredients:
- 1 cup dates, pitted and sliced
- ¾ cup walnuts, chopped
- 1 tablespoon instant coffee powder

- 1 tablespoon hot water
- ½ teaspoon baking powder
- ½ teaspoon baking soda
- 1¼ cups plain flour
- ½ cup condensed milk
- ¼ teaspoon salt
- ½ cup butter, softened
- ½ teaspoon vanilla essence

Directions: In a large bowl, add the dates, butter and top with the hot water. Set aside for about 30 mins.
Dry out well and set aside.
In a small bowl, add the coffee powder and hot water and mix well.
In a large bowl, mix together the flour, baking powder, baking soda and salt.
In another bowl, add the condensed milk and butter and beat until smooth.
Add the flour mixture, coffee mixture and vanilla essence and mix until well combined. Fold in dates and ½ cup of walnut.
Line a baking pan with a lightly greased parchment paper.
Place the mixture into the prepared pan and sprinkle with the remaining walnuts.
Select the "Air Fry" mode and set the cook time to 35 mins. Set the temperature at 320 degrees F. Arrange the pan in "Air Fry Basket" and insert in the oven. Place the pan onto a wire rack to cool for about 10 mins.
Carefully, invert the bread onto wire rack to cool completely before slicing.
Cut the bread into desired-sized slices.

Nutrition: Cal 593 Fat 32.6 g Carbs 69.4 g

157. Date Bread

Prep Time: 15 mins
Servings: 10

Cook Time: 22 mins

Ingredients:
- 2½ cup dates, pitted and chopped
- ¼ cup butter
- 1 egg
- 1½ cups flour
- 1 cup hot water
- ½ cup brown sugar
- 1 teaspoon baking powder
- 1 teaspoon baking soda
- ½ teaspoon salt

Directions: In a large bowl, add the dates, butter and top with the hot water.
Set aside for about 5 mins.
In another bowl, mix together the flour, baking powder, baking soda, brown sugar, and salt.
In the same bowl of dates, mix well the flour mixture, and egg.
Grease a baking pan.
Place the mixture into the prepared pan.
Select the "Air Fry" mode. Set the cook time to 22 mins. Set the temperature at 340 degrees F.
Arrange the pan in "Air Fry Basket" and insert in the oven.
Place the pan onto a wire rack to cool for about 10 mins.
Carefully, invert the bread onto wire rack to cool completely before slicing.
Cut the bread into desired-sized slices.

Nutrition: Cal 269 Fat 5.4 g Carbs 55.1 g

158. Cauliflower Hummus

Prep Time: 10 Mins
Servings: 8

Cook Time: 35 mins

Ingredients:
- 1 cauliflower head, cut into florets
- 3 tablespoon olive oil
- 1/2 teaspoon ground cumin
- 2 tablespoon fresh lemon juice
- 1/3 cup tahini
- 1 teaspoon garlic, chopped
- Pepper
- Salt

Directions: Spread cauliflower florets in baking pan.
Set to bake at 400 degrees F for 40 mins. After 5 mins place the baking dish in the preheated oven.
Transfer roasted cauliflower into the food processor along with remaining ingredients and process until smooth.

Nutrition: Cal 115 Fat 10.7 g Carbs 4.2 g

159. Jalapeno Poppers

Prep Time: 10 Mins
Servings: 10

Cook Time: 7 mins

Ingredients:

- *10 jalapeno peppers, cut in half, remove seeds & membranes*
- *1/2 cup cheddar cheese, shredded*
- *4 oz cream cheese*
- *1/4 teaspoon paprika*
- *1 teaspoon ground cumin*
- *1 teaspoon salt*

Directions: In a bowl, stir together cumin, paprika, cream cheese, cheddar cheese, and salt.
Stuff cream cheese mixture into each jalapeno half.
Place stuffed jalapeno peppers in air fryer basket.
Place a baking pan on the oven rack. Set to air fry at 350 degrees F for 7 mins.

Nutrition: Cal 69 Fat 6.1 g Carbs 1.5 g

160. Cheesy Dip

Prep Time: 10 Mins
Servings: 12

Cook Time: 30 mins

Ingredients:

- *1/2 cup mayonnaise*
- *1 small onion, diced*
- *4 oz cream cheese, cubed*
- *1 1/2 cups mozzarella cheese, shredded*
- *1 1/2 cups cheddar cheese, shredded*

Directions: Add all ingredients into the mixing bowl and mix until well combined.
Pour mixture into the prepared baking dish.
Set to bake at 400 degrees F for 35 mins. After 5 mins place the baking dish in the preheated oven.

Nutrition: Cal 140 Fat 11.9 g Carbs 3.4 g

161. Sweet Potato Fries

Prep Time: 10 Mins
Servings: 2

Cook Time: 16 mins

Ingredients

- *2 sweet potatoes, peeled and cut into fries' shape*
- *tablespoon olive oil*
- *Salt*

Directions: Toss sweet potato fries with oil and salt and place in the air fryer basket then place the air fryer basket in the baking pan.
Place a baking pan on the oven rack. Set to air fry at 375 degrees F for 16 mins.

Nutrition: Cal 178 Fat 7.2 g Carbs 27.9 g

162. Zucchini Chips

Prep Time: 10 mins
Servings: 6

Cook time: 30 mins

Ingredients:

- *Three zucchinis, thinly sliced*
- *Salt and black pepper to the taste*
- *2 tbsp. olive oil*
- *2 tbsp. balsamic vinegar*

Directions: In a bowl, mix oil with vinegar, salt and pepper and whisk well.
Add zucchini slices, toss to coat well. Introduce in your air fryer and cook at 350 degrees F for 30 mins.

Divide zucchini chips into bowls and serve them cold as a snack.

Nutrition: Cal 100 Fat 3 g Carbs 6 g

163. Egg Roll Wrapped with Cabbage and Prawns

Prep Time: 10 mins
Servings: 4

Cook Time: 40 mins

Ingredients:
- 2 tbsp vegetable oil
- 1-inch piece fresh ginger, grated
- tbsp minced garlic
- egg
- carrot, cut into strips
- 8 egg roll wrappers
- ¼ cup chicken broth
- tbsp reduced-sodium soy sauce
- cup shredded Napa cabbage
- tbsp sesame oil
- 8 cooked prawns, minced
- tbsp sugar

Directions: In a skillet over high heat, heat vegetable oil, and cook ginger and garlic for 40 seconds, until fragrant. Stir in carrot and cook for another 2 mins Pour in chicken broth, soy sauce, and sugar and bring to a boil.
Add cabbage and let simmer until softened, for 4 mins Remove skillet from the heat and stir in sesame oil. Let cool for 15 mins Strain cabbage mixture, and fold in minced prawns. Whisk an egg in a small bowl. Fill each egg roll wrapper with prawn mixture, arranging the mixture just below the center of the wrapper.
Fold the bottom part over the filling and tuck under. Fold in both sides and tightly roll up. Use the whisked egg to seal the wrapper. Repeat until all egg rolls are ready. Place the rolls into a greased air fryer basket, spray them with oil and cook for 12 mins at 370 F, turning once halfway through.

Nutrition: Cal 215 Fat 7.9 g Carbs 6.7 g

164. Crab Dip

Prep Time: 10 Mins
Servings: 6

Cook Time: 15 mins

Ingredients:
- 6 oz crab lump meat
- 1 tablespoon mayo
- 1/4 teaspoon salt
- 1/8 teaspoon paprika
- 1 tablespoon green onion, sliced
- 1/4 cup sour cream
- 4 teaspoon bell pepper, diced
- 1 tablespoon butter, softened
- 2 oz cream cheese, softened
- 1 teaspoon parsley, chopped
- 1/4 cup mozzarella cheese, shredded
- 4 teaspoon onion, chopped

Directions: In a bowl, mix together cream cheese, butter, sour cream, and mayonnaise until smooth.
Add remaining ingredients and stir well.
Pour mixture into the greased baking dish.
Set to bake at 350 F for 20 mins. After 5 mins place the baking dish in the preheated oven.

Nutrition: Cal 131 Fat 10.8 g Carbs 8.1 g

165. Pineapple Sticky Ribs

Prep Time: 10 mins
Servings: 4

Cook Time: 20 mins

Ingredients:
- 2 lb. cut spareribs
- 7 oz salad dressing
- 1 (5-oz) can pineapple juice
- 2 cups water
- Garlic salt
- Salt
- Pepper

Directions: Sprinkle the ribs with salt and pepper, and place them in a saucepan. Pour water and cook the ribs for 12 mins on high heat.
Dry out the ribs and arrange them in the fryer; sprinkle with garlic salt. Cook it for 15 mins at 390 F.
Prepare the sauce by combining the salad dressing and the pineapple juice. Serve the ribs drizzled with the sauce.

Nutrition: Cal 316 Fat 3.1 g Carbs 1.9 g

166. Fried Ravioli

Prep Time: 15 mins
Servings: 4

Cook Time: 8 mins

Ingredients:

- ½ cup panko breadcrumbs
- 8 oz. ravioli
- 1 tsp. garlic powder
- 1 tsp. dried oregano
- 1 tsp. dried basil
- 2 tsp. nutritional yeast flakes
- ¼ cup aquafaba liquid
- Cook spray
- ½ cup marinara sauce
- Salt
- Pepper

Directions: Mix the breadcrumbs, salt, pepper, garlic powder, oregano, basil and nutritional yeast flakes on a plate.
In another bowl, pour the aquafaba liquid.
Dip each ravioli into the liquid and then coat it with the breadcrumb mixture.
Put the ravioli in the air fryer.
Spray oil on the ravioli.
Cook at 390° F for 6 mins.
Flip each one and cook for another 2 mins.
Serve with sauce.

Nutrition: Cal 154 Fat 3.8 g Carbs 18.4 g

167. Garlic Cauliflower Florets

Prep Time: 10 Mins
Servings: 4

Cook Time: 20 mins

Ingredients:

- 5 cups cauliflower florets
- 6 garlic cloves, chopped
- 4 tablespoons olive oil
- 1/2 teaspoon cumin powder
- 1/2 teaspoon salt

Directions: Add all ingredients into the large bowl and toss well.
Add cauliflower florets in air fryer basket then place air fryer basket in baking pan.
Place a baking pan on the oven rack. Set to air fry at 400 F for 20 mins.

Nutrition: Cal 159 Fat 14.2 g Carbs 8.2 g

168. Carrot Fries

Prep Time: 10 Mins
Servings: 4

Cook Time: 25 mins

Ingredients:

- 4 medium carrots, peel and cut into fries shape
- 1/2 tablespoon paprika
- 1/2 tablespoon olive oil
- 1/2 teaspoon salt

Directions: Add carrots, paprika, oil, and salt into the mixing bowl and toss well.
Transfer carrot fries in baking pan.
Set to bake at 450 F for 30 mins. After 5 mins place the baking pan in the preheated oven.

Nutrition: Cal 73 Fat 5.4 g Carbs 6.5 g

169. Jalapeno Spinach Dip

Prep Time: 10 Mins
Servings: 6

Cook Time: 30 mins

Ingredients:

- 10 oz frozen spinach, thawed and drained
- 2 teaspoon jalapeno pepper, minced
- 1/2 cup onion, diced
- 1/2 cup cheddar cheese, shredded
- 1/2 cup mozzarella cheese, shredded
- 8 oz cream cheese
- 2 teaspoon garlic, minced

- *1/2 cup Monterey jack cheese, shredded*
- *1/2 teaspoon salt*

Directions: Add all ingredients into the mixing bowl and mix until well combined.
Pour mixture into the 1-quart casserole dish.
Set to bake at 350 F for 35 mins. After 5 mins place the casserole dish in the preheated oven.

Nutrition: Cal 228 Fat 19.8 g Carbs 4.2 g

170. Polenta Biscuits

Prep Time: 10 mins
Servings: 4

Cook time: 25 mins

Ingredients:
- *18 ounces cooked polenta roll, cold*
- *1 tbsp. olive oil*

Directions: Cut polenta into medium slices and brush them with the olive oil.
Place polenta biscuits into your air fryer and cook at 400 degrees F for 25 mins, flipping them after 10 mins.

Nutrition: Cal 120 Fat 0 g Carbs 7 g

171. Potato and Beans Dip

Prep Time: 10 mins
Servings: 10

Cook time: 10 mins

Ingredients:
- *19 ounces canned garbanzo beans, drained*
- *1 cup sweet potatoes, peeled and chopped*
- *¼ cup sesame paste*
- *5 garlic cloves, minced*
- *½ tsp. cumin, ground*
- *1 tbsp. water*
- *1 tbsp. olive oil*
- *1 tbsp. lemon juice*
- *Salt*
- *White pepper*

Directions: Put potatoes in your air fryer's basket, cook them at 360 degrees F for 10 mins, cool them down, peel, put them in your food processor and pulse well.
Add sesame paste, garlic, beans, lemon juice, cumin, water, oil, salt and pepper, pulse again, divide into bowls and serve cold.

Nutrition: Cal 170 Fat 3 g Carbs 12 g

172. Peanut Butter Banana Bread

Prep Time: 15 mins
Servings: 6

Cook Time: 40 mins

Ingredients:
- *1 cup plus 1 tablespoon all-purpose flour*
- *¼ teaspoon baking soda*
- *1 teaspoon baking powder*
- *¼ teaspoon salt*
- *One large egg*
- *1/3 cup granulated sugar*
- *¼ cup canola oil*
- *2 medium ripe bananas, peeled and mashed*
- *¾ cup walnuts, roughly chopped*
- *2 tablespoons creamy peanut butter*
- *2 tablespoons sour cream*
- *1 teaspoon vanilla extract*

Directions: In a bowl and mix the flour, baking powder, baking soda, and salt together.
In another large bowl, add the egg, sugar, oil, peanut butter, sour cream, and vanilla extract and beat until well combined. Add the bananas and beat until well combined. Add the flour mixture and mix.
Gently, fold in the walnuts. Place the mixture into a lightly greased pan.
Select the "Air Fry" mode. Set the temperature at 330 degrees F. Arrange the pan in "Air Fry Basket" and insert in the oven. Place the pan to cool for about 10 mins.
Carefully, invert the bread onto wire rack to cool completely before slicing.
Cut the bread into desired-sized slices.

Nutrition: Cal 384 Fat 23 g Carbs 39.3 g

173. Mushroom Pizza

Prep Time: 15 mins
Servings: 4

Cook Time: 10 mins

Ingredients:
- 4 large Portobello mushrooms, stems and gills removed
- 1 tsp. balsamic vinegar
- 4 tbsp. pasta sauce
- 1 clove garlic, minced
- 3 oz. zucchini, chopped
- 4 olives, sliced
- 2 tbsp. sweet red pepper, diced
- 1 tsp. dried basil
- ½ cups hummus
- Fresh basil, minced
- Salt
- Pepper

Directions: Coat the mushrooms with balsamic vinegar and season with salt and pepper.
Spread pasta sauce inside each mushroom.
Sprinkle with minced garlic.
Preheat your air fryer to 330 degrees F.
Cook mushrooms for 3 mins.
Take the mushrooms out and top with zucchini, olives, and peppers. Season with salt, pepper and basil.
Put them back in the air fryer and cook for another 3 mins.
Serve mushroom pizza with hummus and fresh basil.

Nutrition: Cal 70 Fat 1.56 g Carbs 11 g

174. Crispy Potatoes

Prep Time: 5 mins
Servings: 4

Cook Time: 30 mins

Ingredients:
- 1.5 pounds potatoes, halved
- 3 garlic cloves, grated
- 1 tbsp minced fresh rosemary
- 2 tbsp olive oil
- 1 tsp salt
- ¼ tsp freshly ground pepper

Directions: In a bowl, mix potatoes, garlic, rosemary, olive oil, salt, and pepper, until they are well-coated. Arrange the potatoes in the air fryer and cook on 360 F for 25 mins, shaking twice during the cook. Cook until crispy on the outside and tender on the inside.

Nutrition: Cal 365 Fat 13.2 g Carbs 48.6 g

175. Ranch Potatoes

Prep Time: 10 Mins
Servings: 2

Cook Time: 20 mins

Ingredients:
- 1/2 lb baby potatoes, wash and cut in half
- 1/4 teaspoon parsley
- 1/4 teaspoon paprika
- 1/2 tablespoon olive oil
- 1/4 teaspoon dill
- 1/4 teaspoon garlic powder
- 1/4 teaspoon chives
- 1/4 teaspoon onion powder
- Salt to taste

Directions: Add all ingredients into the bowl and toss well.
Spread potatoes in the air fryer basket then place an air fryer basket in the baking pan.
Place a baking pan on the oven rack. Set to air fry at 400 F for 20 mins.

Nutrition: Cal 99 Fat 3.7 g Carbs 14.8 g

176. Potato Chips

Prep Time: 30 mins
Servings: 4

Cook time: 30 mins

Ingredients:
- 4 potatoes, scrubbed, peeled and cut into thin strips
- A pinch of sea salt
- 2 tsp. rosemary, chopped
- 1 tbsp. olive oil

Directions: In a bowl, mix potato chips with salt and oil, toss to coat, place them in your air fryer's basket and cook at 330° F for 30 mins.
Divide them into bowls, sprinkle rosemary all over.

Nutrition: Cal 200 Fat 4 g Carbs 14 g

177. Rice Balls

Prep Time: 10 mins   **Cook time: 35 mins**
Servings: 6

Ingredients:

- 1 small yellow onion, chopped
- 1 cup Arborio rice
- 1 tbsp. olive oil
- 1 cup veggie stock

- 2 ounces tofu, cubed
- ¼ cup sun-dried tomatoes, chopped
- 1 ½ cups bread crumbs
- Marinara sauce for serving

- A drizzle of olive oil
- Salt
- Pepper

Directions: Heat a pan with 1 tbsp. oil over medium heat, add onion, stir and cook for 5 mins.
Add rice, stock, salt and pepper, stir, and cook on low heat for 20 mins, spread on a baking sheet and leave aside to cool down.
Transfer rice to a bowl, add tomatoes and half of the bread crumbs and stir well.
Shape 12 balls, press a hole in each ball, stuff with tofu cubes, and mound them again.
Dredge them in the rest of the bread crumbs, arrange all balls in your air fryer, drizzle the oil over them and cook at 380 degrees F for 10 mins.
Flip them and cook for 5 mins more.
Arrange them on a plate.

Nutrition: Cal 137 Fat 12 g Carbs 7 g

178. Salsa Cheesy Dip

Prep Time: 10 Mins   **Cook Time: 30 mins**
Servings: 10

Ingredients:

- 16 oz cream cheese, softened
- 3 cups cheddar cheese, shredded

- 1 cup sour cream
- 1/2 cup hot salsa

Directions: In a bowl, mix all ingredients until just combined and pour into the baking dish.
Set to bake at 350 F for 35 mins. After 5 mins place the baking dish in the preheated oven.

Nutrition: Cal 348 Fat 31.9 g Carbs 3.4 g

179. Nuggets with Parmesan Cheese

Prep Time: 5 mins   **Cook Time:** 20 mins
Servings: 4

Ingredients:

- 1 lb. chicken breast, boneless, skinless, cubed
- ½ tsp ground pepper

- ¼ tsp kosher salt
- ¼ tsp seasoned salt
- 5 tbsp plain breadcrumbs
- 2 tbsp panko breadcrumbs

- 2 tbsp grated Parmesan cheese
- 2 tbsp olive oil

Directions: Preheat the air fryer to 380 F and grease. Season the chicken with pepper, kosher salt, and seasoned salt; set aside. In a bowl, pour olive oil. In a separate bowl, add crumb, and Parmesan cheese.
Place the chicken pieces in the oil to coat, then dip into breadcrumb mixture, and transfer to the air fryer. Work in batches if needed. Lightly spray chicken with cook spray.
Cook the chicken for 10 mins, flipping once halfway through. Cook until golden brown on the outside and no more pink on the inside.

Nutrition: Cal 312 Fat 8.9 g Carbs 7 g

180. Sesame Garlic Chicken Wings

Prep Time: 10 mins
Servings: 4

Cook Time: 40 mins

Ingredients:
- *1-pound chicken wings*
- *One cup soy sauce, divided*
- *½ cup brown sugar*
- *½ cup apple cider vinegar*
- *2 tbsp fresh garlic, minced*
- *2 tbsp fresh ginger, minced*
- *2 tbsp cornstarch*
- *1 tsp finely ground black pepper*
- *2 tbsp cold water*
- *1 tsp sesame seeds*

Directions: In a bowl, add chicken wings, and pour in half cup soy sauce. Refrigerate for 20 mins; Dry out and pat dry. Arrange the wings in the air fryer and cook for 30 mins at 380 F, turning once halfway through. Make sure you check them towards the end to avoid overcook.
In a skillet and over medium heat, stir sugar, half cup soy sauce, vinegar, ginger, garlic, and black pepper. Cook until sauce has reduced slightly, about 4 to 6 mins
Dissolve 2 tbsp of cornstarch in cold water, in a bowl, and stir in the slurry into the sauce, until it thickens, for 2 mins Pour the sauce over wings and sprinkle with sesame seeds.

Nutrition: Cal 413 Fat 8.3 g Carbs 7 g

181. Soda Bread

Prep Time: 15 mins
Servings: 10

Cook Time: 30 mins

Ingredients:
- *3 cups whole-wheat flour*
- *1 tablespoon sugar*
- *1 ¼ cup chilled butter, cubed into small pieces*
- *One large egg, beaten*
- *1½ cups buttermilk*
- *2 teaspoon caraway seeds*
- *1 teaspoon baking soda*
- *teaspoon sea salt*

Directions: In a large bowl, mix together the flour, sugar, caraway seeds, baking soda and salt and mix well.
With a pastry cutter, cut in the butter flour until coarse crumbs like mixture is formed.
Make a well in the center of flour mixture. In the well, add the egg, followed by the buttermilk and with a spatula, mix until well combined. With floured hand, shape the dough into a ball.
Place the dough onto a floured surface and lightly need it.
Shape the dough into a 6-inch ball. With a serrated knife, score an X on the top of the dough.
Select the "Air Fry" mode. Set the cook time to 30 mins. Set the temperature at 350 degrees F.
Arrange the dough in lightly greased "Air Fry Basket" and insert in the oven.
Place the pan onto a wire rack to cool for about 10 mins.
Carefully, invert the bread onto wire rack to cool completely before slicing.
Cut the bread into desired-sized slices.

Nutrition: Cal 205 Fat 5.9 g Carbs 31.8 g

182. Sour Cream Banana Bread

Prep Time: 15 mins
Servings: 8

Cook Time: 37 mins

Ingredients:
- *¾ cup all-purpose flour*
- *¼ teaspoon baking soda*
- *2 ripe bananas, peeled and mashed*
- *½ cup granulated sugar*
- *¼ cup sour cream*
- *¼ cup vegetable oil*
- *One large egg*
- *¼ teaspoon salt*
- *½ teaspoon pure vanilla extract*

Directions: In a large bowl, mix together the flour, baking soda and salt.
In another bowl, add the bananas, egg, sugar, sour cream, oil and vanilla and beat until well combined.
Add the flour mixture and continue to mix.
Place the mixture into a lightly greased pan. Select the "Air Fry" mode. Set the cook time to 37 mins. Set the temperature at 310 degrees F. Press "Start/Pause" button to start.
Arrange the pan in "Air Fry Basket" and insert in the oven. Place the pan onto a wire rack to cool for about 10 mins.

Carefully, invert the bread onto wire rack to cool completely before slicing.
Cut the bread into desired-sized slices.

Nutrition: Cal 201 Fat 9.2 g Carbs 28.6 g

183. Spicy Brussels Sprouts

Prep Time: 10 Mins   **Cook Time: 35 mins**
Servings: 6

Ingredients:
- 2 cups Brussels sprouts, halved
- 1/2 teaspoon smoked paprika
- 1/4 teaspoon chili powder
- 1/4 teaspoon garlic powder
- 1/4 cup olive oil
- 1/4 teaspoon salt
- 1/4 teaspoon cayenne pepper

Directions: Add all ingredients into the large bowl and toss well.
Transfer Brussels sprouts on a baking pan.
Set to bake at 400 °F for 40 mins. After 5 mins place the baking pan in the preheated oven.

Nutrition: Cal 86 Fat 8.6 g Carbs 3 g

184. Tortilla Chips

Prep Time: 10 mins   **Cook time: 4 mins**
Servings: 4

Ingredients:
- 8 corn tortillas, each cut into triangles
- Salt and pepper
- 1 tbsp. olive oil

Directions: Brush tortilla chips with the oil, place them in your air fryer's basket and cook for 4 mins at 400 ° F.
Serve them with salt and pepper sprinkled all over.

Nutrition: Cal 530 Fat 1 g Carbs 10 g

185. Spicy Cauliflower Florets

Prep Time: 10 Mins   **Cook Time: 15 mins**
Servings: 4

Ingredients:
- One medium cauliflower head, cut into florets
- 1/2 teaspoon old bay seasoning
- 1/4 teaspoon paprika
- 1/4 teaspoon cayenne
- 1/4 teaspoon chili powder
- 1 tablespoon garlic, minced
- Salt and Pepper
- 3 tablespoon olive oil

Directions: In a bowl, toss cauliflower with remaining ingredients.
Add cauliflower florets in air fryer basket then place air fryer basket in baking pan.
Place a baking pan on the oven rack. Set to air fry at 400 F for 15 mins.

Nutrition: Cal 130 Fat 10.7 g Carbs 8.6 g

186. Sunflower Seed Bread

Prep Time: 15 mins   **Cook Time:** 18 mins
Servings: 6

Ingredients:
- 2/3 cup whole-wheat flour
- 2/3 cup plain flour
- 1/3 cup sunflower seeds
- ½ sachet instant yeast
- 2/3-1 cup lukewarm water
- 1 teaspoon salt

Directions: In a bowl, mix together, sunflower seeds, the flours, yeast, and salt.
Slowly, add in the water, stirring continuously until a soft dough ball form.
Now, move the dough onto a lightly floured surface and knead for about 5 mins using your hands.
Make a ball from the dough and place into a bowl.
With a plastic wrap, cover and place the ball at a warm place for about 30 mins
Grease a cake pan. Coat the top of dough with water and place into the prepared cake pan.
Select the "Air Fry" mode. Set the cook time to 18 mins. Set the temperature at 390 degrees F. Arrange the pan in "Air Fry Basket" and insert in the oven. Place the pan onto a wire rack to cool for about 10 mins. Carefully, invert the bread onto wire rack to cool completely before slicing.
Cut the bread into desired-sized slices.

Nutrition: Cal 132 Fat 1.7 g Carbs 24.4 g

187. Potato Tots

Prep Time: 10 mins   **Cook Time: 12 mins**
Servings: 10

Ingredients:
- 2 cups sweet potato puree
- ½ tsp. cumin
- ½ tsp. coriander
- ½ cup breadcrumbs
- Cook spray
- ½ tsp. salt
- Mayonnaise

Directions: Preheat your air fryer set to 390 degrees F.
Combine all ingredients in a bowl. Form into balls.
Arrange on the air fryer pan. Spray with oil and cook for 6 mins or until golden.
Serve with mayonnaise.

Nutrition: Cal 77 Fat 0.8 g Carbs 15.9 g

188. Cinnamon Chickpeas

Prep Time: 10 Mins   **Cook Time: 12 mins**
Servings: 4

Ingredients:
- 15 oz can chickpeas, rinsed, drained and pat dry
- 1 tablespoon olive oil
- 1/2 teaspoon ground cinnamon
- 1 tablespoon honey
- Salt and Pepper

Directions: Spread chickpeas in the air fryer basket then place an air fryer basket in the baking pan.
Place a baking pan on the oven rack. Set to air fry at 375 degrees F for 12 mins.
In a large bowl, mix cinnamon, honey, oil, pepper, and salt. Add chickpeas and toss well.

Nutrition: Cal 173 Fat 4.7 g Carbs 28.6 g

189. Potato Croquettes

Prep Time: 10 Mins   **Cook Time: 55 mins**
Servings: 6

Ingredients:
- 2 cups cooked quinoa
- 1/4 cup parsley, chopped
- 1/4 cup flour
- 1/4 cup celery, diced
- 2 cups sweet potatoes, mashed
- 2 teaspoon Italian seasoning
- 1 garlic clove, minced
- 1/4 cup scallions, chopped
- Salt and Pepper

Directions: Add all ingredients into the mixing bowl and mix until well combined.
Make 1-inch round croquettes from mixture and place in baking pan.
Set to bake at 375 degrees F for 60 mins. After 5 mins place the baking pan in the preheated oven.

Nutrition: Cal 295 Fat 4.1 g Carbs 55.2 g

190. Veggie Sticks

Prep Time: 10 mins
Servings: 4

Cook time: 30 mins

Ingredients:

- 4 parsnips, cut into thin sticks
- 2 sweet potatoes, cut into sticks
- 4 carrots, cut into sticks
- 2 tbsp. rosemary, chopped
- 2 tbsp. olive oil
- A pinch of garlic powder
- Salt and pepper

Directions: Put parsnips, sweet potatoes and carrots in a bowl, add oil, garlic powder, salt, pepper, rosemary, and toss to coat.
Put sweet potatoes in your preheated air fryer, cook them for 10 mins at 350 degrees F and transfer them to a platter.
Add parsnips to your air fryer, cook for 5 mins and transfer over potato fries.
Add carrots, cook for 15 mins at 350 degrees F, also transfer to the platter.

Nutrition: Cal 140 Fat 0 g Carbs 7 g

191. Potato Wedges

Prep Time: 10 Mins
Servings: 4

Cook Time: 15 mins

Ingredients:

- Two medium potatoes, cut into wedges
- 1/4 teaspoon garlic powder
- 1/2 teaspoon paprika
- 1 1/2 tablespoon olive oil
- 1/8 teaspoon cayenne
- 1 teaspoon sea salt
- 1/4 teaspoon pepper

Directions: Soak potato wedges into the water for 30 mins.
Drain well and pat dry with a paper towel.
In a bowl, toss potato wedges with remaining ingredients.
Place potato wedges in the air fryer basket then place an air fryer basket in the baking pan.
Place a baking pan on the oven rack. Set the air fryer at 400 °F for 15 mins.

Nutrition: Cal 120 Fat 5.4 g Carbs 17.1 g

192. Ricotta Dip

Prep Time: 10 Mins
Servings: 6

Cook Time: 15 mins

Ingredients:

- One cup ricotta cheese, shredded
- 1/4 cup parmesan cheese, grated
- 1/2 cup mozzarella cheese, shredded
- 1 tablespoon rosemary, chopped
- Two garlic cloves, minced
- 2 tablespoon olive oil
- 1 tablespoon lemon juice
- Salt and Pepper

Directions: Add all ingredients into the mixing bowl and mix until well combined.
Pour mixture into the prepared baking dish.
Set to bake at 400 degrees F for 20 mins. After 5 mins place the baking dish in the preheated oven.

Nutrition: Cal 120 Fat 9.3 g Carbs 3.1 g

193. Wontons

Prep Time: 10 mins
Servings: 10

Cook Time: 15 mins

Ingredients:

- Cook spray
- 1/2 cup white onion, grated
- 1/2 cup mushrooms, chopped
- 1/2 cup carrot, grated
- 3/4 cup red pepper, chopped
- 3/4 cup cabbage, grated

- 1 tbsp. chilli sauce
- 1 tsp. garlic powder
- Salt
- 30 wonton wrappers
- Water

Directions: Spray oil in a pan.

Put the pan over medium heat and cook the onion, mushrooms, carrot, red pepper and cabbage until tender.

Stir in the chilli sauce, garlic powder, salt and pepper.

Let it cool for a few mins.

Add a scoop of the mixture on top of the wrappers.

Fold and seal the corners using water.

Cook in the air fryer set the temperature at 320 degrees F for 7 mins or until golden brown.

Nutrition: Cal 290 Fat 1.5 g Carbs 58 g

MAINS

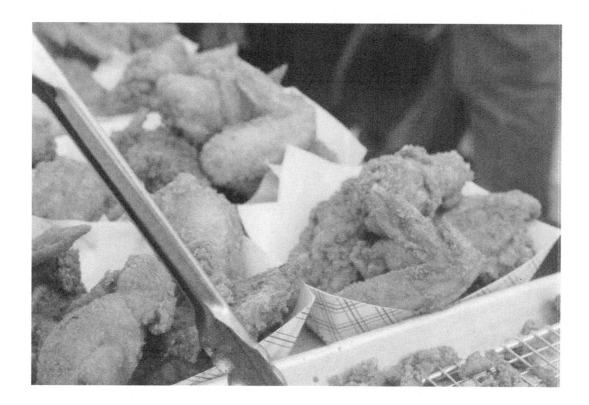

194. Bacon Wrapped Shrimp

Prep Time: 5 Mins
Servings: 4

Cook Time: 5 Mins

Ingredients:
- 1¼ pound tiger shrimp, peeled and deveined
- pound bacon

Directions: Wrap shrimps with a slice of bacon. Refrigerate for about 20 mins. Preheat the Air Fryer to 390 degrees F. Arrange the shrimp in the air fryer basket. Cook for about 5-7 mins.

Nutrition: Cal 202 Fat 7 g Protein 3 g

195. Carrot & Potato Mix

Prep time: 10 mins
Servings: 6

Cook time: 16 mins

Ingredients:
- Two Potatoes
- 3 lb, Carrots
- 1 Yellow onion
- 1 tsp. Dried thyme
- Salt and pepper
- 2 tsp. Curry powder
- 3 tbsp. Coconut milk
- 3 tbsp. Cheese
- 1 tbsp. Parsley

Directions: Cube/chop the parsley, carrots, and onions. Crumble the vegan cheese.
Warm the Air Fryer to reach 365° F. Once it's heated, toss in the veggies, thyme, curry powder, salt, and pepper. Set the timer and air-fry for 16 mins. Stir in the milk and cheese.

Nutrition: Protein: 4 g Carbs: 1 g Fat: 4 g

196. Air Fryer Breaded Pork Chops

Prep Time: 10 mins   **Cook Time: 12 mins Servings: 4**

Ingredients

- *Whole-wheat breadcrumbs: 1 cup*
- *Salt: ¼ teaspoon*
- *Pork chops: 2-4 pieces (center cut and boneless)*
- *Chili powder: half teaspoon*
- *Parmesan cheese: 1 tablespoon*
- *Paprika: 1½ teaspoons*
- *One egg beaten*
- *Onion powder: half teaspoon*
- *Granulated garlic: half teaspoon*
- *Pepper, to taste*

Directions: Let the air fryer preheat to 400 F.
Rub kosher salt on each side of pork chops, let it rest.
Add beaten egg in a big bowl. Add breadcrumbs, garlic, Parmesan cheese, pepper, paprika, chili powder, and onion powder in a bowl and mix well.
Dip pork chop in egg, then in breadcrumb mixture.
Put it in the air fryer and spray with oil.
Let it cook for 12 mins at 400 F. flip it over halfway through. Cook for another six mins.
Serve with a side of salad.

Nutrition: 425 Cal, 20 g Fat, 31 g Protein Carbs 19 g

197. Pork Taquitos in Air Fryer

Prep Time: 10 mins   **Cook Time: 20 mins Servings: 10**

Ingredients

- *Pork tenderloin: 3 cups, cooked & shredded*
- *Cook spray*
- *Shredded mozzarella: 2 and 1/2 cups, fat-free*
- *10 small tortillas*
- *Salsa for dipping*
- *One juice of a lime*

Directions: Let the air fryer preheat to 380 F.
Add lime juice to pork and mix well.
With a damp towel over the tortilla, microwave for ten seconds to soften.
Add pork filling and cheese on top, in a tortilla, roll up the tortilla tightly.
Place tortillas on a greased foil pan.
Spray oil over tortillas. Cook for 7-10 mins or until tortillas is golden brown, flip halfway through.
Serve with fresh salad.

Nutrition: Cal 253 Fat: 18 g Carbs: 10 g Protein: 20 g

198. Air Fryer Tasty Egg Rolls

Prep Time: 10 mins   **Cook Time: 20 mins Servings: 3**

Ingredients

- *Coleslaw mix: half bag*
- *Half onion*
- *Salt: 1/2 teaspoon*
- *Half cups of mushrooms*
- *Lean ground pork: 2 cups*
- *One stalk of celery*
- *Wrappers (egg roll)*

Directions: Put a skillet over medium flame, add onion and lean ground pork and cook for 5-7 mins.
Add mushrooms, coleslaw mixture, salt, and celery to skillet and cook for five mins.
Lay egg roll wrapper flat and add filling (1/3 cup), roll it up, seal with water.
Spray with oil the rolls.
Put in the air fryer for 6-8 mins at 400F, flipping once halfway through.
Serve hot.

Nutrition: Cal 245 Fat: 10 g Carbs: 9 g Protein: 11 g

199. Pork Dumplings in Air Fryer

Prep Time: 30 mins

Cook Time: 20 mins Servings: 6

Ingredients

- 18 dumpling wrappers
- One teaspoon olive oil
- Bok choy: 4 cups (chopped)
- Rice vinegar: 2 tablespoons
- Diced ginger: 1 tablespoon

- Crushed red pepper: 1/4 teaspoon
- Diced garlic: 1 tablespoon
- Lean ground pork: half cup
- Cook spray

- Lite soy sauce: 2 teaspoons
- Honey: half tsp.
- Toasted sesame oil: 1 teaspoon
- Finely chopped scallions

Directions: In a large skillet, heat olive oil, add bok choy, cook for 6 mins, and add garlic, ginger, and cook for one minute. Move on a paper towel and pat dry the excess oil.
In a bowl, add bok choy mixture, crushed red pepper, and lean ground pork and mix well.
Lay a dumpling wrapper on a plate and add one tbsp. of filling in the wrapper's middle. With water, seal the edges and crimp it.
Air spray the air fryer basket, add dumplings in the air fryer basket and cook at 375 F for 12 mins or until browned.
In the meantime, make the sauce: add sesame oil, rice vinegar, scallions, soy sauce, and honey in a bowl. Mix together.
Serve the dumplings with sauce.

Nutrition: Cal 140 Fat 5 g Protein 12 g Carbs 9 g

200. Air Fryer Pork Chop & Broccoli

Prep Time: 20 mins

Cook Time: 20 mins Servings: 2

Ingredients

- Broccoli florets: 2 cups
- Bone-in pork chop: 2 pieces
- Paprika: half tsp.

- Avocado oil: 2 tbsp.
- Garlic powder: half tsp.
- Onion powder: half tsp.

- Two cloves of crushed garlic
- Salt: 1 teaspoon divided

Directions: Let the air fryer preheat to 350 degrees. Spray the basket with cook oil
Add one tbsp. Oil, garlic powder, onion powder, half tsp. of salt, and paprika in a bowl mix well, rub this spice mix to the pork chop's sides
Add pork chops to air fryer basket and let it cook for five mins
In the meantime, add one tsp. oil, garlic, half tsp of salt, and broccoli to a bowl and coat well
Flip the pork chop and add the broccoli, let it cook for five more mins.
Take out from the air fryer and serve.

Nutrition: Cal 483 Fat 20 g Carbs 12 g Protein 23 g

201. Cheesy Pork Chops in Air Fryer

Prep Time: 5 mins

Cook Time: 8 mins Servings: 2

Ingredients

- 4 lean pork chops
- Salt: half tsp.

- Garlic powder: half tsp.
- Shredded cheese: 4 tbsp.

- Chopped cilantro

Directions: Let the air fryer preheat to 350 degrees F.
With cilantro, garlic, and salt, rub the pork chops. Put in the air fryer. Let it cook for four mins. Flip them and cook for two mins more.
Add cheese on top of them and cook for another two mins or until the cheese is melted.
Serve with salad greens.

Nutrition: Cal: 467 Protein: 61 g Fat: 22 g

202. Pork Rind Nachos

Prep time: 5 mins   Cook Time: 5 mins Servings: 2

Ingredients

- 2 tbsp. of pork rinds
- 1/4 cup shredded cooked chicken
- 1/2 cup shredded Monterey jack cheese
- 1/4 cup sliced pickled jalapeños
- 1/4 cup guacamole
- 1/4 cup full-fat sour cream

Directions: Put pork rinds in a baking pan. Fill with grilled chicken and Monterey cheese jack. Place the pan in the basket with the air fryer.
Set the temperature to 370 ° F and set the timer for 5 mins or until the cheese has been melted.
Eat right with jalapeños, guacamole, and sour cream.

Nutrition: Cal 295 Protein: 30.1 g Carbs: 1.8 g Fat: 27.5 g

203. Jamaican Jerk Pork in Air Fryer

Prep Time: 10 mins   Cook Time: 20 mins Servings: 4

Ingredients

- Pork, cut into three-inch pieces
- Jerk paste: ¼ cup

Directions: Rub jerk paste all over the pork pieces.
Let it marinate for four hours, at least, in the refrigerator. Or for more time.
Let the air fryer preheat to 390 F. spray with olive oil
Before putting in the air fryer, let the meat sit for 20 mins at room temperature.
Cook for 20 mins at 390 F in the air fryer, flip halfway through.
Take out from the air fryer let it rest for ten mins before slicing.
Serve with microgreens.

Nutrition: Cal: 234 Protein: 31 g Fat: 9 g Carbs 12 g

204. Pork Tenderloin with Mustard Glazed

Prep Time: 10 mins   Cook Time: 18 mins Servings: 4

Ingredients

- Yellow mustard: ¼ cup
- One pork tenderloin
- Salt: ¼ tsp
- Honey: 3 Tbsp.
- Freshly ground black pepper: ⅛ tsp
- Minced garlic: 1 Tbsp.
- Dried rosemary: 1 tsp
- Italian seasoning: 1 tsp

Directions: With a knife, cut the top of pork tenderloin. Add garlic (minced) in the cuts. Then sprinkle with kosher salt and pepper.
In a bowl, add honey, mustard, rosemary, and Italian seasoning mix until combined. Rub this mustard mix all over pork.
Let it marinate in the refrigerator for at least two hours.
Put pork tenderloin in the air fryer basket. Cook for 18-20 mins at 400 F. with an instant-read thermometer internal temperature of pork should be 145 F
Take out from the air fryer and serve with a side of salad.

Nutrition: Cal: 390 Carbs: 11 g Protein: 59 g Fat: 11 g

205. Balsamic Vinaigrette on Roasted Chicken

Prep Time: 10 mins
Servings: 8

Cook time: 60 mins

Ingredients:
- 1 tbsp chopped fresh parsley
- 1 tsp lemon zest
- 1/2 cup low-salt chicken broth
- One 4-lb whole chicken, cut into pieces
- 2 tbsp olive oil
- Two garlic cloves, chopped
- 2 tbsp fresh lemon juice
- 2 tbsp Dijon mustard
- ¼ cup balsamic vinegar
- Salt
- Freshly ground black pepper

Directions: In a bowl, whisk to blend pepper, garlic, lemon juice, salt, olive oil, mustard, and vinegar.
In a re-sealable bag, combine the above mixture and chicken pieces. Refrigerate and marinate for at least 2 hours to a whole day.
Ensure to turn the bag upside down occasionally.
Grease a baking dish and preheat the oven to 400 °F.
Arrange marinated chicken pieces onto a baking dish and pop into the oven.
Roast chicken for an hour. If chicken is browned and not yet fully cooked, cover with foil and continue cook.
Remove from the oven, and transfer to a serving plate.
Garnish with parsley and drizzle with lemon juice.

Nutrition: Cal 296, Fat 10 g, Carbs 2 g, Protein 47 g

206. Breaded Mushrooms

Prep time: 15 mins
Servings: 2

Cook time: 7 mins

Ingredients:
- ½ pound button mushrooms
- One cup almond meal
- 1 Flax-Egg
- 1 cup almond flour
- 3 ounces cashew cheese
- Salt
- Pepper

Directions: Preheat and set the Air Fryer's temperature to 360 degrees F.
Take a shallow bowl and toss almond meal with cheese into it.
Whisk flax egg in one bowl and spread flour in another.
Wash mushrooms, then pat dry. Coat every mushroom with flour. Dip each of them in the flax egg first, then in breadcrumb.
Spray with cook oil and place back in the Air Fryer. Air fry these mushrooms for 7 mins.
Toss the mushrooms after 3 mins.

Nutrition: Cal: 140 Fat: 9.2 g Carbs: 6.9 g

207. Bang Panko Breaded Fried Shrimp

Prep Time: 5 Mins
Servings: 4

Cook Time: 8 Mins

Ingredients:
- One teaspoon paprika
- Montreal chicken seasoning
- One egg white
- ½ cup almond flour
- ¾ cup panko bread crumbs
- 1 pound raw shrimp (peeled and deveined)

Bang Bang Sauce:
- ¼ cup sweet chili sauce
- 2 tablespoon sriracha sauce
- 1/3 cup plain Greek yogurt

Directions: Ensure your Air Fryer is preheated to 400 degrees. Season all shrimp with seasonings. Add flour to one bowl, egg white in another, and breadcrumbs to a third.
Dip seasoned shrimp in flour, then egg whites, and then breadcrumbs. Spray coated shrimp with olive oil and add to air fryer basket. Set temperature to 400°F, and set time to 4 mins. Cook 4 mins, flip, and cook an additional 4 mins.
To make the sauce, mix together all sauce ingredients until smooth.

Nutrition: Cal 212 Carbs 12 g Fat 1 g

208. Basil Chicken Bites

Prep Time: 10 mins
Serving: 4

Cook Time: 30 mins

Ingredients:
- 1 1/2 lb. chicken breasts, skinless; boneless and cubed
- 1/2 cup chicken stock
- 2 tsp. smoked paprika
- Salt and pepper
- 1/2 tsp. basil; dried

Directions: In a pan that fits the air fryer, combine all the ingredients, toss, introduce the pan in the fryer and cook at 390°F for 25 mins.
Divide between plates and serve for lunch with a side salad.

Nutrition: Cal: 22; Fat: 12 g Carbs: 5 g Protein: 13 g

209. Broccoli Stew

Prep Time: 20 mins
Serving: 4

Cook Time: 15 mins

Ingredients:
- 1 broccoli head, florets separated
- ¼ cup celery; chopped.
- ¾ cup tomato sauce
- 3 tbsp. Chicken stock
- 3 spring onions; chopped.
- Salt and pepper

Directions: In a pan that fits your air fryer, mix all the ingredients, toss, introduce the pan in your fryer and cook at 380°f for 15 mins. Divide into bowls.

Nutrition: Cal 183 Fat 4 g Carbs 4 g

210. Vegan Cauliflower Rice

Prep time: 10 mins
Servings: 3

Cook time: 20 mins

Ingredients:
- 2 carrots, diced
- ½ cup onion, diced
- 2 tbsp. soy sauce
- ½ block firm tofu, crumbled
- 1 tsp. turmeric

For the rice:
- Three cups riced cauliflower
- 2 tbsp. sodium soy sauce, reduced
- ½ cup broccoli, finely chopped
- 1 tbsp. rice vinegar
- ½ cup peas, frozen
- 2 garlic cloves, minced
- 1 and ½ tsp. sesame oil, toasted
- 1 tbsp. ginger, minced
- 1 tbsp. rice vinegar
- ½ cup frozen peas

Directions: Preheat and set the Air Fryer's temperature to 370 degrees F.
Take a large bowl and add tofu alongside remaining tofu ingredients. Stir well to combine.
Set in the Air Fryer to cook for 10 mins.
Take another bowl and add the remaining ingredients. Stir them well.
Transfer into the Air Fryer and cook 10 mins more.

Nutrition: Cal: 153 Fat: 4 g Carbs: 18 g

211. Chicken and Beans

Prep Time: 10 mins
Servings: 6

Cook time: 70 mins

Ingredients:
- 1 lb. chicken breasts, boneless and skinless
- 2 tbsp fresh cilantro, chopped
- 2 cups grated low-fat Monterey Jack cheese
- 2 tsp pure Chile powder
- 2 tsp ground cumin
- One 4-oz can be chopped green chilies

- 1 cup corn kernels
- Two 15-oz cans of white beans drained and rinsed
- 2 garlic cloves
- 1 medium onion, diced
- 2 tbsp extra virgin olive oil
- 3 cups of water
- 1/8 tsp. cayenne pepper

Directions: Slice chicken breasts into 1/2-inch cubes, and with pepper and salt, season it.
On high fire, place a large nonstick fry pan and heat oil.
Sauté chicken pieces for three to four mins or until lightly browned.
Reduce fire to medium and add garlic and onion.
Cook for 5 to 6 mins or until onions is translucent. Add water, spices, chilies, corn, and beans. Bring to a boil.
Once boiling, slow fire to a simmer and continue simmering for an hour, uncovered.
To serve, garnish with a sprinkling of cilantro and a tablespoon of cheese.

Nutrition: Cal 550 Fat 18 g Carbs 51 g Protein 48 g

212. Chicken Pasta Parmesan

Prep Time: 10 mins   **Cook time: 20 mins**
Servings: 1

Ingredients:
- 1/2 cup cooked whole-wheat spaghetti
- 1oz reduced-fat mozzarella cheese, grated
- 2tbsp seasoned dry breadcrumbs
- 4oz skinless chicken breast
- ¼ cup prepared marinara sauce
- 1tbsp olive oil

Directions: On medium-high fire, place an ovenproof skillet and heat oil.
Pan Fry chicken for 3 to 5 mins per side or until cooked through.
Pour marinara sauce, stir and continue cook for 3 mins.
Turn off the fire; add mozzarella and breadcrumbs on top.
Pop into a preheated broiler on high and broil for 10 mins or until breadcrumbs are browned, and mozzarella is melted.
Remove from broiler.

Nutrition: Cal 492, Fat 19 g, Carbs 32 g, Protein 49 g

213. Chinese Chicken Drumsticks

Prep Time: 15 mins   **Cook Time:** 20 mins
Servings: 4

Ingredients:
- 4 (6-ounces) chicken drumsticks
- 1 tablespoon oyster sauce
- 1 teaspoon light soy sauce
- ½ teaspoon sesame oil
- 1 teaspoon Chinese five spice powder
- Salt and ground white pepper, as required
- 1 cup corn flour

Directions: In a bowl, mix together the sauces, oil, five spice powder, salt, and black pepper. Add the chicken drumsticks and coat with the marinade. Refrigerate for at least 30-40 mins.
In a shallow dish, place the corn flour. Remove the chicken from marinade and coat with corn flour.
Set the temperature of Air Fryer to 390 degrees F. Grease an Air Fryer basket. Arrange chicken drumsticks into the prepared Air Fryer basket in a single layer.
Air Fry for about 20 mins. Remove from Air Fryer and transfer the chicken drumsticks onto a serving platter.

Nutrition: Cal 400 Carbs 22.7 g Protein 48.9 g

214. Cilantro-Lime Fried Shrimp

Prep Time: 10 Mins
Servings: 4

Cook Time: 10 Mins

Ingredients:
- 1 pound raw shrimp, peeled and deveined with tails on or off
- ½ cup chopped fresh cilantro
- Juice of 1 lime
- One egg
- ½ cup all-purpose flour
- ¾ cup bread crumbs
- Salt and pepper
- Cook oil
- ½ cup cocktail sauce

Directions: Place the shrimp in a plastic bag and add the cilantro and lime juice. Seal the bag. Shake to combine. Marinate in the refrigerator for 30 mins.
In a small bowl, beat the egg. In another small bowl, place the flour. Place the bread crumbs in a third small bowl, and season with salt and pepper to taste.
Spray the air fryer basket with cook oil.
Remove the shrimp from the plastic bag. Dip each in the flour, then the egg, and then the bread crumbs. Place the shrimp in the Air Fryer Oven. It is okay to stack them. Spray the shrimp with cook oil. Cook for 4 mins.
Open the air fryer and flip the shrimp. I recommend flipping individually instead of shaking to keep the breading intact. Cook for an additional 4 mins, or until crisp. Cool before serving. Serve with cocktail sauce if desired.

Nutrition: Cal 254 Fat 4 g Protein 29 g

215. Cornish Game Hens

Prep Time: 20 mins
Servings: 4

Cook Time: 16 mins

Ingredients:
- ½ cup olive oil
- 1 teaspoon fresh rosemary, chopped
- 1 teaspoon fresh thyme, chopped
- ¼ teaspoon red pepper flakes, crushed
- Salt and ground black pepper
- 2 pounds Cornish game hen, backbone removed and halved
- 1 teaspoon fresh lemon zest, finely grated
- ¼ teaspoon sugar

Directions: In a bowl, mix together oil, herbs, lemon zest, sugar, and spices.
Add the hen portions and generously coat with the marinade.
Cover and refrigerate for about 24 hours.
In a strainer, place the hens and set aside to drain any liquid.
Set the temperature of Air Fryer to 390 degrees F. Grease an Air Fryer basket.
Place hen portions into the prepared Air fryer basket.
Air Fry for about 14-16 mins.
Remove from the Air Fryer and transfer the hen portions onto serving plates.

Nutrition: Cal 523 Carbs 0.8 g Fat 34.1 g

216. Courgettes Casserole

Prep Time: 10 mins
Serving: 4

Cook Time: 25 mins

Ingredients:
- 14 oz. cherry tomatoes; cubed
- 2 spring onions; chopped.
- 3 garlic cloves; minced
- 2 courgettes; sliced
- 2 celery sticks; sliced
- One yellow bell pepper; chopped.
- 1/2 cup mozzarella; shredded
- 1 tbsp. thyme; dried
- 1 tbsp. olive oil
- 1 tsp. smoked paprika

Directions: In a baking dish that fits your air fryer, mix all the ingredients except the cheese and toss.
Sprinkle the cheese on top, introduce the dish in your air fryer and cook at 380°F for 20 mins. Divide between plates.

Nutrition: Cal: 254; Fat: 12 g; Carbs: 4 g

217. Creamy Cauliflower and Broccoli

Prep time: 5 mins
Servings: 6

Cook time: 16 mins

Ingredients:
- 1-pound cauliflower florets
- 1 tbsp. lemon zest, grated
- 1-pound broccoli florets
- ¾ tsp. sea salt flakes
- ½ cup cashew cheese
- ½ tsp. cayenne pepper, smoked
- 2 and ½ tbsp. sesame oil

Directions: Preheat your Air Fryer and set the temperature at 390 degrees F.
Prepare the cauliflower and broccoli using the steaming method.
Drain it and add cayenne pepper, sesame oil, and salt flakes. Cook for 15 mins. Check your vegetables halfway during cook. Stir in the lemon zest and cashew cheese.
Toss to coat well.

Nutrition: Cal: 133 Fat: 9 g Carbs: 7 g

218. Curried Chicken, Chickpeas and Raita Salad

Prep Time: 10 mins
Servings: 5

Cook time: 30 mins

Ingredients:
- 1 cup red grapes halved
- 3-4 cups rotisserie chicken, meat coarsely shredded
- 2 tbsp cilantro
- 1 cup plain yogurt
- Two medium tomatoes, chopped
- 1 tsp ground cumin
- 1 tbsp minced peeled ginger
- 1 tbsp minced garlic
- One medium onion, chopped
- 1 tbsp curry powder
- 2 tbsp vegetable oil

Chickpeas Ingredients:
- ¼ tsp. cayenne
- 1/2 tsp. turmeric
- 1 tsp ground cumin
- one 19-oz can chickpeas, rinsed, drained, and patted dry
- 1 tbsp vegetable oil

Topping and Raita Ingredients:
- 1/2 cup sliced and toasted almonds
- 2 tbsp chopped mint
- 1 cup plain yogurt
- 2 cups cucumber, peeled, cored, and chopped

Directions: To make the chicken salad, place a medium nonstick saucepan and heat oil on a medium-low fire.
Sauté ginger, garlic, and onion for 5 mins or until softened while stirring occasionally.
Add 1 1/2 tsp.: salt, cumin, and curry. Sauté for two mins.
Increase fire to medium-high and add tomatoes. Stirring frequently, cook for 5 mins.
Pour sauce into a bowl, mix in chicken, cilantro, and yogurt. Stir to combine and let it stand to cool to room temperature.
To make the chickpeas, on a nonstick fry pan, heat oil for 3 mins. Add chickpeas and cook for a minute while stirring frequently.
Add ¼ tsp.: salt, cayenne, turmeric, and cumin. Stir to mix well and cook for two mins or until sauce is dried. Transfer to a bowl and let it cool to room temperature.
To make the raita, mix 1/2 tsp.: salt, mint, cucumber, and yogurt. Stir thoroughly to combine and dissolve the salt.
In four 16-oz lidded jars or bowls, to assemble, layer the following: curried chicken, raita, chickpeas, and garnish with almonds.

Nutrition: Cal 403, Fat 16 g, Carbs 42 g

219. Curried Coconut Chicken

Prep Time: 10 mins
Servings: 6

Cook time: 40 mins

Ingredients:
- 4 large tomatoes, sliced
- 1 can make coconut milk (14-oz)
- 6 cloves garlic, crushed then minced
- 1 whole onion, sliced thinly
- 1 tbsp curry
- 1 tbsp. turmeric
- 1 tsp. cinnamon
- 1 tsp. clove powder
- 1 tsp. fenugreek
- 1-inch long ginger around thumb-sized, peeled
- 2 bay leaves
- 2 lbs. boneless and skinless chicken breasts cut into 1-inch cubes

- 2 cups of water
- ¼ of the red bell pepper cut into 1-inch thick strips
- 1/2 tsp. salt
- 1 tsp. pepper
- 2 tbsp olive oil

Directions: In a heavy-bottomed pot, heat oil on the medium-high fire.
Sauté garlic and ginger until garlic is starting to brown, around 1 to 2 mins.
Add curry, turmeric, cinnamon, clove, bay leaf, and fenugreek. Sauté until fragrant, around 3 to 5 mins.
Add tomatoes and onions. Sauté for 5 to ten mins or until tomatoes are wilted, and onions are soft and translucent. If needed, add ¼ cup of water. Add chicken breasts and sauté for 5 mins—season with pepper and salt.
Add remaining water; bring to a boil, then slow fire to medium. While covered, continue cook chicken for at least 15 mins. Add bell pepper and coconut milk. Cook until heated through.
Turn off fire and serve best with brown rice.

Nutrition: Cal 225, Fat 8 g, Carbs 12 g

220. Eggplant Fries

Prep time: 10 mins
Servings: 4

Cook time: 5 mins

Ingredients:
- 1 eggplant, peeled and sliced
- 1 flax-egg
- ½ cup cashew cheese
- 2 tbsp. almond milk
- 2 cups almond meal
- Salt and Black pepper
- Cook spray

Directions: Take a bowl and add flax egg, salt, and pepper to it. Whisk it well.
Take another bowl, mix cheese and panko, then stir.
Dip eggplant fries in the flax egg mixture, coat in panko mix.
Grease the Air Fryer basket using vegan cook spray. Place the eggplant fries in it. Cook for 5 mins at 400 degrees F.

Nutrition: Cal: 162 Fat: 5 g Carbs: 7 g Protein: 6 g

221. Eggplant Bake

Prep Time: 25 mins
Serving: 4

Cook Time: 20 mins

Ingredients:
- 2 eggplants; cubed
- 1/2 lb. Cherry tomatoes; cubed
- 1/2 cup cilantro; chopped.
- 4 garlic cloves; minced
- 1 hot chili pepper; chopped.
- 4 spring onions; chopped.
- Salt and pepper
- 2 tsp. Olive oil

Directions: Grease a baking pan that fits the air fryer with the oil and mix all the pan ingredients.
Put the pan in the preheated air fryer and cook at 380°f for 20 mins, divide into bowls.

Nutrition: Cal: 232; Fat: 12 g; Carbs: 5 g; Protein: 10 g

222. Fennel and Tomato Stew

Prep Time: 10 mins
Serving: 4

Cook Time: 25 mins

Ingredients:
- 2 tbsp. tomato puree
- 2 fennel bulbs; shredded
- 1/2 cup chicken stock
- 1 red bell pepper; chopped.
- 2 garlic cloves; minced
- 2 cups tomatoes; cubed
- 1 tsp. rosemary; dried
- 1 tsp. sweet paprika
- Salt and pepper

Directions: In a pan that fits your air fryer, mix all the ingredients, toss, introduce in the fryer and cook at 380°F for 15 mins.
Divide the stew into bowls.

Nutrition: Cal: 184; Fat: 7 g; Carbs: 3 g; Protein: 8 g

223. Chimichanga

Prep time: 2 mins
Servings: 4

Cook time: 8 mins

Ingredients:
- 1 whole-grain tortilla
- ½ cup vegan refried beans
- ¼ cup grated vegan cheese
- ½ cup fresh salsa
- Two cups romaine lettuce, chopped
- Guacamole
- Chopped cilantro
- Cook oil spray as needed

Directions: Preheat your Air Fryer to 392 degrees F.
Lay tortilla on flat surface and place beans on center, top with cheese and wrap. bottom up over filling, fold insides.
Roll all up and enclose beans inside.
Spray Air Fryer cook basket with oil and place wrap inside the basket, fry for 5 mins, spray on top and cook for 2-3 mins more.
Move to a plate and serve with salsa, lettuce, and guacamole.

Nutrition: Cal: 317 Fat: 6 g Carbs: 55 g Protein: 13 g

224. Garlicky Pork Stew

Prep Time: 30 mins
Serving: 4

Cook Time: 20 mins

Ingredients:
- 3 garlic cloves; minced
- 1 lb. Pork stew meat; cubed
- ¼ cup tomato sauce
- 1cup spinach; torn
- 1/2 tsp. Olive oil

Directions: In a pan that fits your air fryer, mix the pork with the other ingredients except for the spinach, toss, introduce in the fryer and cook at 370°F for 15 mins.
Add the spinach, toss, cook for 10 mins more, divide into bowls.

Nutrition: Cal: 290; Fat: 14 g; Carbs: 5 g; Protein: 13 g

225. Gingered Chicken Drumsticks

Prep Time: 10 mins
Servings: 3

Cook Time: 25 mins

Ingredients:
- ¼ cup full-fat coconut milk
- 2 teaspoons fresh ginger, minced
- 2 teaspoons galangal, minced
- 2 teaspoons ground turmeric
- Salt
- 3 (6-ounces) chicken drumsticks

Directions: In a bowl, mix together the coconut milk, galangal, ginger, and spices. Add the chicken drumsticks and coat with the marinade. Refrigerate to marinate for at least 8 hours.
Set the temperature of Air Fryer to 375 degrees F. Grease an Air Fryer basket. Place chicken drumsticks into the prepared Air Fryer basket in a single layer.
Air Fry for about 20-25 mins. Remove from Air Fryer and transfer the chicken drumsticks onto a serving platter.

Nutrition: Cal 338 Carbs 2.6 g Protein 47.4 g Fat 13.9 g

226. Herbed Roasted Chicken

Prep Time: 15 mins
Servings: 7

Cook Time: 1 hour

Ingredients:
- Three garlic cloves, minced
- 1 (5-pounds) whole chicken
- 1 teaspoon fresh lemon zest, finely grated
- 1 teaspoon dried thyme, crushed
- 1 teaspoon dried oregano, crushed
- 1 teaspoon dried rosemary, crushed
- 1 teaspoon smoked paprika
- 2 tablespoons fresh lemon juice
- 2 tablespoons olive oil
- Salt and ground black pepper

Directions: In a bowl, mix together the garlic, lemon zest, herbs and spices.

Rub the chicken evenly with herb mixture.

Drizzle the chicken with lemon juice and oil. Set aside at the room temperature for about 2 hours.

Set the temperature of Air Fryer to 360 degrees F. Grease an Air Fryer basket.

Place chicken into the prepared Air Fryer basket, breast side down. Air Fry for about 50 mins.

Flip the chicken and Air Fry for about 10 more mins.

Remove from the Air Fryer and place chicken onto a cutting board for about 10 mins before carving.

With a knife, slice the chicken into desired size pieces.

Nutrition: Cal 860 Carbs 1.3 g Protein 71.1 g Fat 50 g

227. Honey Glazed Chicken Drumsticks

Prep Time: 15 mins

Cook Time: 22 mins

Servings: 4

Ingredients:
- ¼ cup Dijon mustard
- 1 tablespoon honey
- ½ tablespoon fresh rosemary, minced
- 1 tablespoon fresh thyme, minced
- 4 (6-ounces) boneless chicken drumsticks
- Salt and ground black pepper
- 2 tablespoons olive oil

Directions: In a bowl, mix well the mustard, honey, oil, herbs, salt, and black pepper. Add the drumsticks and generously coat with the mixture. Cover and refrigerate to marinate overnight.

Set the temperature of Air Fryer to 320 degrees F. Grease an Air Fryer basket. Arrange the chicken drumsticks into the prepared Air Fryer basket in a single layer.

Air Fry for about 12 mins. Now, set the temperature of Air Fryer to 355 degrees F.

Air Fry for 5-10 more mins. Remove from Air Fryer and transfer the chicken drumsticks onto a serving platter.

Nutrition: Cal 377 Carbs 5.9 g Protein 47.6 g Fat 3.6 g

228. Lemon Lentils and Fried Onion

Prep time: 10 mins

Cook time: 30 mins

Servings: 4

Ingredients:
- Four cups of water
- Cook oil spray as needed
- One medium onion, peeled and cut into ¼ inch thick rings
- ½ cup kale stems removed
- Three large garlic cloves, pressed
- 2 tbsp. fresh lemon juice
- 2 tsp. nutritional yeast
- 1 tsp. salt
- 1 tsp. lemon zest
- ¾ tsp. fresh pepper

Directions: Preheat your Air Fryer to 392 degrees F.

Take a large-sized pot and bring lentils to boil over medium-high heat.

Adjust the heat into low and simmer for 30 mins, making sure to stir after every 5 mins.

Once they are cooked, take your Air Fryer basket and spray with cook oil, add onion rings and sprinkle salt.

Fry for 5 mins, shaking basket and fry for 5 mins more.

Remove the basket and spray with oil. Cook for 5 mins more until crispy and browned.

Add kale to the lentils and stir, add sliced greens. Stir in garlic, lemon juice, yeast, salt, pepper, and stir well.

Top with crispy onion rings.

Nutrition: Cal: 220 Fat: 1 g Carbs: 39 g Protein: 15 g

229. Lemony Tuna

Prep Time: 10 Mins

Cook Time: 10 Mins

Servings: 4

Ingredients:
- 2 (6-ounce) cans water packed plain tuna
- 2 teaspoons Dijon mustard
- ½ cup breadcrumbs
- One egg
- Air fryer of hot sauce

- *1 tablespoon fresh lime juice*
- *2 tablespoons fresh parsley, chopped*

- *3 tablespoons canola oil*

- *Salt and freshly ground black pepper*

Directions: Drain most of the liquid from the canned tuna. In a bowl, add the fish, mustard, crumbs, citrus juice, parsley and hot sauce and mix till well combined. Add a little canola oil if it seems too dry. Add egg, salt and stir to combine. Make the patties from tuna mixture. Refrigerate the tuna patties for about 2 hours.
Pour into the Oven rack/basket. Place the Rack on the middle-shelf of the Smart Air Fryer Oven. Set temperature to 355°F, and set time to 12 mins.

Nutrition: Cal 203 Fat 4.7 g Protein 22 g

230. Mexican Stuffed Potatoes

Prep time: 15 mins
Servings: 4

Cook time: 40 mins

Ingredients:
- *4 large potatoes*
- *1 ½ cups cashew cheese*
- *1 cup black beans*

- *2 medium tomatoes, chopped*
- *1 scallion, chopped*
- *1/3 cup cilantro, chopped*

- *1 jalapeno, sliced*
- *1 avocado, diced*
- *Cook oil spray as needed*

Directions: Preheat your Air Fryer to 392 degrees F.
Scrub potatoes and prick with a fork, spray outside with oil.
Transfer to Air Fryer and bake for 30 mins.
Check potatoes at 30 mins mark by poking them. If they are tender, they are ready. If not, cook for 10 mins more.
Once done, warm your cashew cheese and beans in separate pans.
Once potatoes are cooked, cut them across top.
Pry them open with a fork with just enough space to stuff the remaining ingredients.
Top each potato with cashew cheese, beans, tomatoes, scallions, cilantro, jalapeno, and avocado.

Nutrition: Cal: 420 Fat: 5 g Carbs: 80 g Protein: 15 g

231. Okra Casserole

Prep Time: 10 mins
Serving: 4

Cook Time: 20 mins

Ingredients:
- *3 cups okra*
- *2 red bell peppers; cubed*
- *2 tomatoes; chopped.*
- *3 garlic cloves; minced*

- *1/2 cup cheddar; shredded*
- *¼ cup tomato puree*
- *1 tbsp. Cilantro; chopped.*
- *1 tsp. olive oil*

- *2 tsp. coriander, ground*
- *Salt and pepper*

Directions: Grease a heatproof dish that fits your air fryer with the oil add all the ingredients except the cilantro and the cheese, and toss them gently.
Sprinkle the cheese and the cilantro on top, introduce the dish in the fryer and cook at 390°F for 20 mins.
Divide between plates.

Nutrition: Cal: 221; Fat: 7 g; Carbs: 4 g; Protein: 9 g

232. Paprika Cod

Prep Time: 10 mins
Serving: 4

Cook Time: 17 mins

Ingredients:
- *1 lb. cod fillets, boneless, skinless, and cubed*
- *2 cups baby arugula*
- *2 tbsp. Fresh cilantro; minced*

- *1/2 tsp. Sweet paprika*
- *1 spring onion; chopped.*
- *1/2 tsp. oregano, ground*
- *Salt and pepper*

- *A drizzle of olive oil*

Directions: Take a bowl and mix the cod with salt, pepper, paprika, oregano, and the oil, toss, transfer the cubes to your air fryer's basket and cook at 360°F for 12 mins.
In a salad bowl, mix the cod with the remaining ingredients, toss, divide between plates.

Nutrition: Cal: 240; Fat: 11 g; Carbs: 5 g; Protein: 8 g

233. Chicken with Potatoes

Prep Time: 15 mins
Servings: 2

Cook Time: 1 hour

Ingredients:
- 1 (1½-pounds) whole chicken
- 1 tablespoon olive oil
- ½ pound small potatoes
- Salt and ground black pepper

Directions: Set the temperature of Air Fryer to 390 degrees F. Grease an Air Fryer basket.
Season the chicken with salt and pepper. Place chicken into the prepared Air Fryer basket.
Air Fry for about 35-40 mins or until done completely.
Transfer the chicken onto a platter and cover with a piece of foil to keep warm.
In a bowl, add the potatoes, oil, salt, and black pepper and toss to coat well.
Again, set the temperature of Air Fryer to 390 degrees F. Grease an Air Fryer basket. Place potatoes into the prepared Air Fryer basket. Air Fry for about 20 mins or until golden brown.
Remove from the Air Fryer and transfer potatoes into a bowl.
Cut the chicken into desired size pieces using a sharp knife and serve alongside the potatoes.

Nutrition: Cal 431 Fat 16.2 g Carbs 178 g Protein 511 g

234. Roasted Chickpeas

Prep time: 2 mins
Servings: 4

Cook time: 10 mins

Ingredients:
- ¼ tsp. Mango powder, dried
- ½ tsp. Cinnamon powder
- ¼ tsp. cumin powder
- Three cups chickpeas, boiled
- ¼ tsp. Coriander powder, dried
- ½ tsp. chilli powder
- ¼ tsp. rosemary
- 1 tsp. Salt
- 1 tsp. Olive oil

Directions: Preheat and set the air fryer's temperature to 370 degrees F.
Transfer chickpeas with olive oil in your Air Fryer basket.
Cook for 8 mins.
Shake after every 2 mins.
Take a bowl and add chickpeas with all spices and toss to combine.

Nutrition: Cal: 214 Fat: 4.4 g Carbs: 34.27 g Protein: 10.98 g

235. Rosemary Grilled Chicken

Prep Time: 10 mins
Servings: 4

Cook time: 10 mins

Ingredients:
- 1 tablespoon fresh parsley, finely chopped
- 1 tablespoon fresh rosemary, finely chopped
- 1 tablespoon olive oil
- 5 cloves garlic, minced
- 4 pieces of 6-oz chicken breast, boneless and skinless
- 1 teaspoon sea salt

Directions: In a shallow and large bowl, mix salt, parsley, rosemary, olive oil, and garlic. Place chicken breast and marinate in a bowl of herbs for at least an hour or more before grilling.
Grease grill grates and preheat grill to medium-high. Once hot, grill chicken for 4 to 5 mins per side or until juices run a transparent and internal chicken temperature is 168 °F.

Nutrition: Cal 317, Fat 9 g, Carbs 1 g, Protein 53 g

236. Rosemary Russet Potato Chips

Prep time: 10 mins
Servings: 4

Cook time: 60 mins

Ingredients:

- 4 russet potatoes
- 2 tsp. rosemary, chopped
- 1 tbsp. olive oil
- ½ tsp. salt

Directions: Rinse potatoes and scrub to clean.
Peel and cut them in a lengthwise manner similar to thin chips.
Take a bowl and put them into it and soak water for 30 mins.
Take another bowl and toss the chips with olive oil. Transfer them to the cook basket. Cook for 30 mins at 330 ° F.
Toss with salt and rosemary while warm.

Nutrition: Cal: 322 Fat: 3.69 g Carbs: 66 g Protein: 7.5 g

237. Salmon Quiche

Prep Time: 5 Mins
Servings: 4

Cook Time: 12 Mins

Ingredients:

- 5 oz. salmon fillet
- 1/2 tablespoon lemon juice
- 1/2 cup flour
- 1/4 cup butter, melted
- Quiche pan
- 2 eggs and 1 egg yolk
- 3 tbsps. whipped cream
- 1 tsp mustard
- Salt and pepper

Directions: Clean and cut the salmon into small cubes.
Heat the Air Fryer to 375 degrees F.
Pour the lemon juice over the salmon cubes and allow to marinate for an hour.
Combine a tablespoon of water with the butter, flour and yolk in a large bowl. Knead the mixture until smooth.
On a clean surface, use a rolling pin to form a circle of dough. Place this into the quiche pan, using your fingers to adhere the pastry to the edges.
Whisk the cream, mustard and eggs together. Season with salt and pepper. Add the marinated salmon into the bowl and combine.
Pour the content of the bowl into the dough lined quiche pan.
Put the pan in the Air Fryer Oven tray and cook for 25 mins until browned and crispy.

Nutrition: Cal 203 Fat 10 g Protein 19.3 g

238. Spiced Chicken

Prep Time: 15 mins
Servings: 6

Cook Time: 1 hour

Ingredients:

- 1 (5-pounds) whole chicken, necks and giblets removed
- 2 teaspoons dried thyme
- 2 teaspoons paprika
- 1 teaspoon cayenne pepper
- 1 teaspoon ground white pepper
- 1 teaspoon onion powder
- 1 teaspoon garlic powder
- 3 tablespoons oil
- Salt and ground black pepper

Directions: In a bowl, mix together the thyme and spices.
Generously, coat the chicken with oil and then rub it with spice mixture.
Set the temperature of Air Fryer to 350 degrees F. Grease an Air Fryer basket.
Place chicken into the prepared Air Fryer basket, breast side down. Air Fry for about 30 mins.
Flip the chicken and Air Fry for about 30 more mins.
Remove from the Air Fryer and place chicken onto a cutting board for about 10 mins before carving.
Slice the chicken into desired size pieces using a sharp knife.

Nutrition: Cal 871 Carbs 1.7 g Protein 70.6 g Fat 60 g

239. Potato Cauliflower Patties

Prep time: 15 mins   **Cook time: 20 mins**
Servings: 1

Ingredients:

- 1 large sweet potato, peeled and chopped
- 2 cups cauliflower florets
- 2 tbsp. arrowroot powder
- 1 tsp. garlic, minced
- 1 green onion, chopped
- ¼ cup flaxseed, grounded
- 1 cup cilantro, packed
- ¼ tsp. cumin
- 2 tbsp. Ranch seasoning mix
- ¼ cup sunflower seeds
- ½ tsp. chilli powder
- 1 cup cilantro, packed
- Salt and pepper
- Any dipping sauce for serving

Directions: Preheat your Air Fryer and set the temperature at 400 degrees F.
Add sweet potato, cauliflower, onion, garlic, and sizzle into your food processor.
Blend until smooth.
Mould the mixture into patties and place onto a greased baking sheet.
Place into your freezer for 10 mins.
Then transfer into your Air Fryer.
Cook for 20 mins and flip after 10 mins.

Nutrition: Cal: 85 Fat: 2.9 g Carbs: 6 g Protein: 2.7 g

240. Spicy Chicken Legs

Prep Time: 15 mins   **Cook Time:** 25 mins
Servings: 3

Ingredients:

- 3 (8-ounces) chicken legs
- 1 cup buttermilk
- 2 cups white flour
- 1 teaspoon garlic powder
- 1 teaspoon onion powder
- 1 teaspoon ground cumin
- 1 teaspoon paprika
- 1 tablespoon olive oil
- Salt and ground black pepper

Directions: In a bowl, put the chicken legs, and buttermilk. Refrigerate for about 2 hours.
In another bowl, mix together the flour and spices.
Remove the chicken from buttermilk.
Coat the chicken legs with flour mixture, then dip into buttermilk and finally, coat with the flour mixture again.
Set the temperature of Air Fryer to 360 degrees F. Grease an Air Fryer basket.
Arrange chicken legs into the prepared Air Fryer basket and drizzle with the oil
Air Fry for about 20-25 mins.
Remove from the Air Fryer and transfer chicken legs onto a serving platter.

Nutrition: Cal 781 Carbs 69.5 g Protein 55.9 g Fat 7.6 g

241. Tamarind Glazed Potatoes

Prep time: 5 mins   **Cook time: 22 mins**
Servings: 4

Ingredients:

- 5 garnet potatoes, peeled and diced
- 1/3 tsp. white pepper
- 1 tbsp. butter, melted
- 2 tsp. tamarind paste
- ½ tsp. turmeric powder
- 1 ½ tbsp. lime juice
- A pinch of the ground allspice
- A few drops of liquid stevia

Directions: Preheat and set the Air Fryer's temperature to 395 degrees F.
Get a mixing bowl and add all ingredients into it. Mix them until sweet potatoes are well coated. Cook for 12 mins.
Pause the Air Fryer and toss again. Increase the temperature to 390 degrees F.
Cook for 10 mins more.

Nutrition: Cal: 103 Fat: 9.1 g Carbs: 4.9 g

242. Spinach and Olives

Prep Time: 25 mins
Serving: 4

Cook Time: 20 mins

Ingredients:

- 1/2 cup tomato puree
- 4 cups spinach; torn
- 2 cups black olives pitted and halved
- 3 celery stalks; chopped.
- 1 red bell pepper; chopped.
- 2 tomatoes; chopped.
- Salt

Directions: In a pan that fits your air fryer, mix all the ingredients except the spinach, toss, introduce the pan to the air fryer and cook at 370°f for 15 mins.
Add the spinach, toss, cook for 5 - 6 mins more, divide into bowls and serve.

Nutrition: Cal: 193; Fat: 6 g; Carbs: 4 g

243. The Cheesy Sandwich (Vegan)

Prep time: 3 mins
Servings: 4

Cook time: 12 mins

Ingredients:

- 2 slices sprouted whole grain bread
- 1 tsp. vegan margarine
- 2 slices of vegan cheese
- 1 tsp. mellow white miso
- One medium-large garlic clove, minced
- 2 tbsp. fermented vegetables, kimchi or sauerkraut
- Romaine lettuce

Directions: Preheat your Air Fryer to 392 degrees F.
Spread outside of bread with Vegan margarine, place sliced cheese inside and close sandwich back up.
Transfer Sandwich to Air Fryer and cook 6 mins, flip and cook for 6 mins more.
Transfer to plate and spread miso and garlic clove inside one of the slices, top with fermented veggies and lettuce.
Close sandwich and cut in half.

Nutrition: Cal: 288 Fat: 13 g Carbs: 34 g

244. Spinach and Shrimp

Prep Time: 10 mins
Serving: 4

Cook Time: 20 mins

Ingredients:

- 2 cups baby spinach
- 15 oz. shrimp; peeled and deveined
- ¼ cup veggie stock
- 2 tomatoes; cubed
- 4 spring onions; chopped.
- 1 tbsp. garlic; minced
- 2 tbsp. Cilantro; chopped.
- 1 tbsp. Lemon juice
- 1/2 tsp. cumin, ground
- Salt and black pepper

Directions: In a pan that fits your air fryer, mix all the ingredients except the cilantro, toss, introduce in the air fryer and cook at 360°F for 15 mins.
Add the cilantro, stir, and divide into bowls.

Nutrition: Cal: 201; Fat: 8 g; Carbs: 4 g

245. Chicken Drumsticks

Prep Time: 15 mins
Servings: 4

Cook Time: 20 mins

Ingredients:

- 4 (6-ounces) chicken drumsticks
- 1 garlic clove, crushed
- 1 tablespoon mustard
- 2 teaspoons brown sugar
- 1 teaspoon cayenne pepper
- 1 teaspoon red chili powder
- 1 tablespoon vegetable oil
- Salt

Directions: In a bowl, mix together garlic, mustard, brown sugar, oil, and spices Rub the chicken drumsticks with marinade and refrigerate to marinate for about 20-30 mins.

Set the temperature of Air Fryer to 390 degrees F. Grease an Air Fryer basket. Arrange drumsticks into the prepared Air Fryer basket in a single layer.

Air Fry for about 10 mins and then 10 more mins at 300 degrees F. Remove from Air Fryer and transfer the chicken drumsticks onto a serving platter.

Nutrition: Cal 341 Carbs 3.3 g Fat 14.1 g

246. Tandoori Chicken Legs

Prep Time: 15 mins

Cook Time: 20 mins

Servings: 4

Ingredients:

- Four chicken legs
- 3 tablespoons lemon juice
- 3 teaspoons ginger paste
- 3 teaspoons garlic paste
- 4 tablespoons hung curd*
- 2 tablespoons tandoori masala powder
- 2 teaspoons red chili powder
- 1 teaspoon garam masala powder
- 1 teaspoon ground cumin
- 1 teaspoon ground coriander
- 1 teaspoon ground turmeric
- Pinch of orange food color
- Salt and pepper

Directions: In a bowl, mix well chicken legs, lemon juice, ginger paste, garlic paste, and salt.

Set aside for about 15 mins.

Meanwhile, in another bowl, mix together the curd, spices, and food color. Add the chicken legs into bowl and generously coat with the spice mixture. Cover the bowl of chicken and refrigerate for at least 10-12 hours.

Set the temperature of air fryer to 445 degrees F. Line an air fryer basket with a piece of foil.

Arrange chicken legs into the prepared air fryer basket. Air fry for about 18-20 mins.

Remove from air fryer and transfer the chicken legs onto serving plates.

Nutrition: Cal 356 Carbs 3.7 g Fat 13.9 g

247. Bean Dish

Prep time: 5 mins

Cook time: 8 mins

Servings: 4

Ingredients:

- 1 can (15 ounces) pinto beans, drained
- ¼ cup tomato sauce
- 2 tbsp. nutritional yeast
- Two large garlic cloves, minced
- ½ tsp. dried oregano
- ½ tsp. cumin
- 1/8 tsp. ground pepper
- Cook oil spray as needed
- ¼ tsp. salt

Directions: Preheat your Air Fryer to 392 degrees F.

Take a medium bowl and add beans, tomato sauce, yeast, garlic, oregano, cumin, salt, pepper and mix well.

Take your baking pan and add oil, pour bean mixture.

Transfer to Air Fryer and bake for 4 mins until cooked thoroughly with a slightly golden crust on top.

Nutrition: Cal: 284 Fat: 4 g Carbs: 47 g

248. Thyme Eggplant and Beans

Prep Time: 25 mins

Cook Time: 20 mins

Serving: 6

Ingredients:

- 1 lb. Green beans; trimmed and halved
- 2 eggplants; cubed
- 1 red bell pepper; chopped.
- 1 cup veggie stock
- 1 red chili pepper
- 1 tbsp. Olive oil
- 1/2 tsp. Thyme; dried
- Salt

Directions: In a pan that fits your air fryer, mix all the ingredients, toss, introduce the pan in the machine and cook at 350°f for 20 mins.

Nutrition: Cal: 180; Fat: 3 g; Carbs: 5 g

249. Tomato and Avocado

Prep Time: 5 mins   **Cook Time: 8 mins**
Serving: 4

Ingredients:
- *1/2 lb. cherry tomatoes; halved*
- *2 avocados, pitted; peeled, and cubed*
- *1 ¼ cup lettuce; torn*
- *1/3 cup coconut cream*
- *A pinch of salt and pepper*
- *Cook spray*

Directions: Grease the air fryer with cook spray, combine the tomatoes with avocados, salt, pepper, and the cream, and cook at 350°F for 5 mins, shaking once.
In a salad bowl, mix the lettuce with the tomatoes and avocado mix, toss.

Nutrition: Cal: 226; Fat: 12 g; Carbs: 4 g

250. Paneer Pizza

Prep time: 5 mins   **Cook time: 9 mins**
Servings: 4

Ingredients:
- *1 flour tortilla sprouted*
- *¼ cup pizza sauce*
- *½ cup cheese*
- *Cook oil spray*

Directions: Preheat your Air Fryer 347 Degrees F.
Spray your Air Fryer cook basket with oil, add tortilla to your Air Fryer basket and pour the sauce in the center.
Evenly distribute cheese on top.
Bake for 9 mins.

Nutrition: Cal: 210 Fat: 6 g Carbs: 33 g

251. Tomato and Beef Sauce

Prep Time: 25 mins   **Cook Time: 20 mins**
Serving: 4

Ingredients:
- *1 lb. Lean beef meat; cubed and browned*
- *16 oz. Tomato sauce*
- *2 garlic cloves; minced*
- *Salt and pepper*
- *Cook spray*

Directions: Preheat the air fryer at 400°f, add the pan inside, grease it with cook spray, add the meat and all the other ingredients, toss and cook for 20 mins.

Nutrition: Cal: 270; Fat: 15 g; Carbs: 6 g

252. Tomatoes and Cabbage Stew

Prep Time: 10 mins
Serving: 4

Cook Time: 25 mins

Ingredients:
- 14 oz. Canned tomatoes; chopped.
- 1 green cabbage head; shredded
- 4 oz. chicken stock
- 2 tbsp. Dill; chopped.
- 1 tbsp. sweet paprika
- Salt and pepper

Directions:
In a pan that fits your air fryer, mix the cabbage with the tomatoes and all the other ingredients except the dill, toss, introduce the pan in the fryer and cook at 380°F for 20 mins.
Divide into bowls and serve with dill sprinkled on top.

Nutrition: Cal: 200; Fat: 8 g; Carbs: 4 g

253. Turkey and Bok Choy

Prep Time: 25 mins
Serving: 4

Cook Time: 20 mins

Ingredients:
- One turkey breast, boneless, skinless, and cubed
- Two cups bok choy; torn and steamed
- 1 tbsp. Balsamic vinegar
- 1/2 tsp. Sweet paprika
- Salt and pepper
- 2 tsp. Olive oil

Directions: Take a bowl and mix the turkey with the oil, paprika, salt, and pepper, toss, transfer them to your air fryer's basket and cook at 350°F for 20 mins.
In a salad, mix the turkey with all the other ingredients and toss.

Nutrition: Cal: 250; Fat: 13 g; Carbs: 6 g

254. Vegan Taquito

Prep time: 15 mins
Servings: 4

Cook time: 15 mins

Ingredients:
- 8 corn tortillas
- 1 (15 ounces) can vegan refried beans
- 1 cup shredded vegan cheese
- Guacamole
- Cashew cheese
- Vegan sour cream
- Fresh salsa
- Cook oil spray

Directions: Preheat your Air Fryer to 392 degrees F.
Warm your tortilla and run them underwater for a second, transfer to Air Fryer cook basket and cook for 1 minute.
Remove to the flat surface and place equal amounts of beans at the center of each tortilla, top with vegan cheese.
Roll tortilla sides up over filling, place seam side down in Air Fryer.
Spray oil on top and cook for 7 mins until golden brown.

Nutrition: Cal: 420 Fat: 5 g Carbs: 80 g

255. Turkey and Broccoli Stew

Prep Time: 10 mins
Serving: 4

Cook Time: 30 mins

Ingredients:
- turkey breast, skinless; boneless, and cubed
- broccoli head, florets separated
- cup tomato sauce
- tbsp. Parsley, chopped.
- Salt and pepper
- tbsp. olive oil

Directions: In a baking dish that fits your air fryer, mix the turkey with the rest of the ingredients except the parsley, toss, introduce the plate in the fryer, bake at 380°F for 25 mins.
Divide into bowls and sprinkle the parsley on top.

Nutrition: Cal: 250; Fat: 11 g; Carbs: 6 g

256. Turkey and Mushroom Stew

Prep Time: 10 mins
Serving: 4

Cook Time: 30 mins

Ingredients:
- 1 turkey breast, skinless, boneless; cubed and browned
- 1/2 lb. brown mushrooms; sliced
- ¼ cup tomato sauce
- 1 tbsp. Parsley, chopped.
- Salt and pepper

Directions: In a pan that fits your air fryer, mix the turkey with the mushrooms, salt, pepper, and tomato sauce toss, introduce to the fryer and cook at 350°F for 25 mins.
Divide into bowls and serve with parsley sprinkled on top.

Nutrition: Cal: 220; Fat: 12 g; Carbs: 5 g

257. Turkey and Quinoa Stuffed Peppers

Prep Time: 15 mins
Servings: 6

Cook time: 35 mins

Ingredients:
- 3 large red bell peppers
- 2 tsp chopped fresh rosemary
- 2 tbsp chopped fresh parsley
- 3 tbsp chopped pecans, toasted
- 1/2 cup chicken stock
- 1/2 lb. fully cooked smoked turkey sausage, diced
- 2 cups of water
- 2 tbsp. extra virgin olive oil
- 1 cup uncooked quinoa
- 1/2 tsp. salt

Directions: On high fire, place a large saucepan and add salt, water, and quinoa. Bring to a boil.
Once boiling, reduce fire to a simmer, cover, and cook until all water is absorbed, around 15 mins.
Uncover quinoa, turn off the fire, and let it stand for another 5 mins.
Add rosemary, parsley, pecans, olive oil, chicken stock, and turkey sausage into quinoa pan. Mix well.
Slice peppers lengthwise in half and discards membranes and seeds. In another boiling pot of water, add peppers, boil for 5 mins, drain and discard water.
Grease a 13 x 9 baking dish and preheat oven to 350 °F.
Place boiled bell pepper onto a prepared baking dish, evenly fill with the quinoa mixture, and pop into the oven.
Bake for 15 mins.

Nutrition: Cal 253, Fat 13 g, Carbs 21 g, Protein 14 g

258. Chicken and Asparagus

Prep Time: 25 mins
Serving: 4

Cook Time: 20 mins

Ingredients:

- *Four chicken breasts, skinless; boneless and halved*
- *One bunch asparagus; trimmed and halved*
- *1 tbsp. Sweet paprika*
- *Salt and pepper*
- *1 tbsp. Olive oil*

Directions:

Take a bowl and mix all the ingredients, toss, put them in your air fryer's basket and cook at 390°F for 20 mins.

Nutrition: Cal: 230; Fat: 11 g; Carbs: 5 g; Protein: 12 g

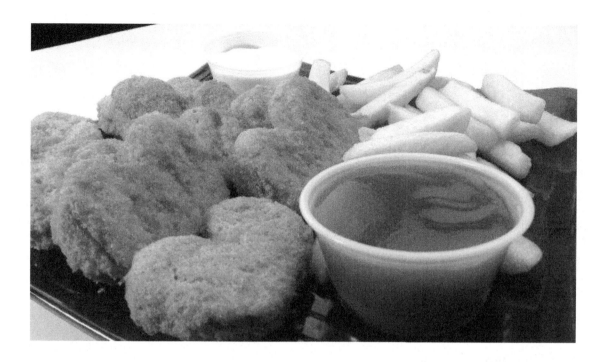

259. Air-Fried Lemon and Olive Chicken

Prep Time: 10 mins
Servings: 4

Cook Time: 15 mins

Ingredients:

- *Four Boneless Skinless Chicken Breasts*
- *½ teaspoon organic cumin*
- *½ cup butter, melted*
- *One lemon 1/2 juiced, 1/2 thinly sliced*
- *1 cup chicken bone-broth*
- *1 can pitted green olives*
- *½ cup red onions, sliced*
- *1 teaspoon sea salt*
- *¼ teaspoon pepper*

Directions:
Season the chicken breasts with sea salt, cumin, and black pepper.
Preheat your air fryer toast oven to 370 degrees and brush the chicken breasts with the melted butter.
Cook in the pan of your air fryer oven for about 5 mins until evenly browned.
Add all remaining ingredients and cook at 320 degrees for 10 mins.

Nutrition: Cal: 310 kcal Carbs: 10.2 g Fat: 9.4 g Protein: 21.8 g

260. Breaded Chicken Tenderloins

Prep Time: 10 mins
Servings: 4

Cook Time:12 mins

Ingredients

- *Eight chicken tenderloins*
- *Olive oil: 2 tablespoons*
- *One egg whisked*
- *1/4 cup breadcrumb*

Directions: Let the air fryer heat to 370°F.
In a big bowl, add oil and breadcrumbs, mix well until forms a crumbly mixture.
Dip chicken tenderloin in whisked egg and coat in breadcrumbs mixture.
Place the chicken in the air fryer and cook for 12 mins or more. Take out from the air fryer and serve with your favorite green salad.

Nutrition: per serving: Cal 206, Protein 20 g, Carbs 17 g Fat 10 g

261. Parmesan Chicken Meatballs

Prep Time: 10 mins
Servings: 20

Ingredients

- *Pork rinds: half cup, ground*
- *Ground chicken: 4 cups*
- *Parmesan cheese: half cup grated*
- *Kosher salt: 1 tsp.*
- *Garlic powder: 1/2 tsp.*
- *One egg beaten*
- *Paprika: 1/2 tsp.*
- *Pepper: half tsp.*

Breading

- *Whole wheat breadcrumbs: half cup ground*

Directions: Let the Air Fryer pre-heat to 400°F.
Add cheese, chicken, egg, pepper, half cup of pork rinds, garlic, salt, and paprika in a big mixing ball. Mix well into a dough, make into 1and half-inch balls.
Coat the meatballs in whole wheat bread crumbs.
Spray the oil in the air fry basket and add meatballs in one even layer.
Let it cook for 12 mins at 400°F, flipping once halfway through.
Serve with salad greens.

Nutrition: Cal 240, Fat 10 g, Carbs 12.1 g, Protein 19.9 g

262. Lemon Rosemary Chicken

Prep Time: 30 mins
Servings: 2

Cook Time:20 mins

Ingredients
For marinade

- *Chicken: 2 and ½ cups*
- *Ginger: 1 tsp, minced*
- *Olive oil: 1/2 tbsp.*
- *Soy sauce: 1 tbsp.*

For the sauce

- *Half lemon*
- *Honey: 3 tbsp.*
- *Oyster sauce: 1 tbsp.*
- *Fresh rosemary: half cup, chopped*

Directions: In a big mixing bowl, add the marinade ingredients with chicken, and mix well.
Keep in the refrigerator for at least half an hour.
Let the oven preheat to 400 °F for three mins.
Place the marinated chicken in the air fryer in a single layer. And cook for 6 mins.
Meanwhile, add all the sauces ingredients in a bowl and mix well except for lemon wedges.
Brush the sauce generously over half-baked chicken add lemon juice on top.
Cook for another 13 mins. flip the chicken halfway through. Let the chicken evenly brown.
Serve right away and enjoy.

Nutrition: Cal 308, Protein 25 g, Carbs 7 g, Fat 12 g

263. Air Fryer Chicken & Broccoli

Prep Time: 10 mins
Servings: 4

Cook Time:15 mins

Ingredients

- *Olive oil: 2 Tablespoons*
- *Chicken breast: 4 cups, bone and skinless (cut into cubes)*
- *Half medium onion, roughly sliced*
- *Low sodium soy sauce: 1 Tbsp.*
- *Garlic powder: half teaspoon*
- *Rice vinegar: 2 teaspoons*
- *Broccoli: 1-2 cups, cut into florets*
- *Hot sauce: 2 teaspoons*
- *Fresh minced ginger: 1 Tbsp.*
- *Sesame seed oil: 1 teaspoon*
- *Salt & black pepper, to taste*

Directions: In a bowl, add chicken breast, onion, and broccoli. Combine them well.

In another bowl, add ginger, oil, sesame oil, rice vinegar, hot sauce, garlic powder, and soy sauce mix it well. Then add the broccoli, chicken, and onions to marinade.

Coat well the chicken with sauces. And let it rest in the refrigerator for 15 mins.

Place chicken mix in one even layer in air fryer basket and cook for 16-20 mins, at 380 F. halfway through, toss the basket gently and cook the chicken evenly. Add five mins more, if required.

Add salt and pepper, if needed.

Serve hot with lemon wedges.

Nutrition: Cal 191, Fat 7 g, Carbs 4 g, Protein 25 g

264. Air Fried Maple Chicken Thighs

Prep Time: 10 mins
Servings: 4

Cook Time:25 mins

Ingredients
- *One egg*
- *Buttermilk: 1 cup*

- *Maple syrup: half cup*
- *Chicken thighs: 4 pieces*

- *Granulated garlic: 1 tsp.*

Dry Mix
- *Granulated garlic: half tsp.*
- *All-purpose flour: half cup*
- *Salt: one tbsp.*
- *Sweet paprika: one tsp.*

- *Smoked paprika: half tsp.*
- *Tapioca flour: ¼ cup*
- *Cayenne pepper: ¼ teaspoon*
- *Granulated onion: one tsp.*

- *Black pepper: ¼ teaspoon*
- *Honey powder: half tsp.*

Directions: In a ziploc bag, add egg, one tsp. of granulated garlic, buttermilk, and maple syrup, add in the chicken thighs and let it marinate for one hour or more in the refrigerator.

In a mixing bowl, add sweet paprika, tapioca flour, granulated onion, half tsp. of granulated garlic, flour, cayenne pepper, salt, pepper, honey powder, and smoked paprika mix it well.

Let the air fry preheat to 380 F.

Coat the marinated chicken thighs in the dry spice mix, shake the excess off.

Put the chicken skin side down in the air fryer.

Let it cook for 12 mins. Flip thighs halfway through and cook for 13 mins more.

Serve with salad greens.

Nutrition: 415.4 Cal, Protein 23.3 g, Carbs 20.8 g, Fat 13.4 g

265. Mushroom Oatmeal

Prep time: 10 min
Servings: 4

Cook time: 20 mins

Ingredients
- *One small yellow onion, chopped*
- *1 cup steel-cut oats*
- *1 Garlic cloves, minced*
- *2 Tablespoons butter*

- *½ cup of water*
- *One and a half cup of canned chicken stock*
- *Thyme springs, chopped*
- *2 Tablespoons extra virgin olive oil*

- *½ cup gouda cheese, grated*
- *1 cup mushroom, sliced*
- *Salt and black pepper to taste*

Directions: Heat a pan over medium heat, which suits your air fryer with the butter, add onions and garlic, stir and cook for 4 mins.

Add oats, sugar, salt, pepper, stock, and thyme, stir, place in the air fryer and cook for 16 mins at 360 degrees F.

In the meantime, prepare a skillet over medium heat with the olive oil, add mushrooms, cook them for 3 mins, add oatmeal and cheese, whisk, divide into bowls and serve for breakfast.

Nutrition: Cal 284, Fat 8 g, Carbs 20 g, Protein 17 g

266. Bell Peppers Frittata

Prep time: 10 min
Servings: 4

Cook time: 20 mins

Ingredients

- 2 Tablespoons olive oil
- 2 cups chicken sausage, casings removed and chopped
- One sweet onion, chopped

- 1 red bell pepper, chopped
- 1 orange bell pepper, chopped
- 1 green bell pepper, chopped
- Salt and black pepper to taste

- 8 eggs, whisked
- ½ cup mozzarella cheese, shredded
- 2 teaspoons oregano, chopped

Directions: Add 1 spoonful of oil to the air fryer, add bacon, heat to 320 degrees F, and brown for 1 minute.
Remove remaining butter, onion, red bell pepper, orange and white, mix and simmer for another 2 mins.
Stir and cook for 15 mins, add oregano, salt, pepper, and eggs.
Add mozzarella, leave frittata aside for a couple of mins, divide and serve between plates.

Nutrition: per serving: cal 212, fat 4g, fiber 6g, carbs 8g, protein 12g

267. Southwest Chicken in Air Fryer

Prep Time: 20 mins
Servings: 4

Cook Time:30 mins

Ingredients

- Avocado oil: one tbsp.
- Four cups of boneless, skinless, chicken breast
- Chili powder: half tsp.

- Salt to taste
- Cumin: half tsp.
- Onion powder: 1/4 tsp.
- Lime juice: two tbsp.

- Garlic powder: 1/4 tsp

Directions: In a ziploc bag, add chicken, oil, and lime juice.
Add all spices in a bowl and rub all over the chicken in the ziploc bag.
Let it marinate in the fridge for ten mins or more.
Take chicken out from the ziploc bag and put it in the air fryer.
Cook for 25 mins at 400 F, flipping chicken halfway through until internal temperature reaches 165 degrees.

Nutrition: Cal: 165, Carbs: 1 g, Protein: 24 g, Fat: 6 g

268. No-Breading Chicken Breast in Air Fryer

Prep Time: 10 mins
Servings: 2

Cook Time: 20 mins

Ingredients

- Olive oil spray
- Chicken breasts: 4 (boneless)
- Onion powder: 3/4 teaspoon

- Salt: ¼ cup
- Smoked paprika: half tsp.
- 1/8 tsp. of cayenne pepper

- Garlic powder: 3/4 teaspoon
- Dried parsley: half tsp.

Directions: In a large bowl, add six cups of warm water, add salt (1/4 cup) and mix to dissolve.
Put chicken breasts in the warm salted water and let it refrigerate for almost 2 hours.
Remove from water and pat dry.
In a bowl, add all spices with ¾ tsp. of salt. Spray the oil all over the chicken and rub the spice mix all over the chicken.
Let the air fryer heat at 380F.
Put the chicken in the air fryer and cook for ten mins. Flip halfway through and serve with salad green.

Nutrition: Cal: 208, Carbs: 1 g, Protein: 39 g, Fat: 4.5 g

269. Lemon Pepper Chicken Breast

Prep Time: 3 mins
Servings: 2

Cook Time:15 mins

Ingredients
- Two Lemons rind, juice, and zest
- One Chicken Breast
- Minced Garlic: 1 Tsp
- Black Peppercorns: 2 tbsp.
- Chicken Seasoning: 1 Tbsp.
- Salt & pepper, to taste

Directions: Let the air fryer preheat to 370°F.
In a large aluminum foil, add all the seasonings along with lemon rind.
Add salt and pepper to chicken and rub the seasonings all over chicken breast.
Put the chicken in aluminum foil. And fold it tightly.
Flatten the chicken inside foil with a rolling pin.
Put it in the air fryer and cook for 15 mins.

Nutrition: Cal: 140, Carbs: 24 g, Protein: 13 g, Fat: 2 g

270. Herb-Marinated Chicken Thighs

Prep Time: 30 mins
Servings: 4

Cook Time:10 mins

Ingredients
- Chicken thighs: 8 skin-on, bone-in,
- Lemon juice: 2 Tablespoon
- Onion powder: half teaspoon
- Garlic powder: 2 teaspoon
- Spike Seasoning: 1 teaspoon.
- Olive oil: 1/4 cup
- Dried basil: 1 teaspoon
- Dried oregano: half teaspoon.
- Black Pepper: 1/4 tsp.

Directions: In a bowl, add dried oregano, olive oil, lemon juice, dried sage, garlic powder, Spike Seasoning, onion powder, dried basil, black pepper.
In a ziploc bag, add the spice blend and the chicken and mix well.
Marinate the chicken in the refrigerator for at least six hours or more.
Preheat the air fryer to 360 °F.
Put the chicken in the air fryer basket, cook for six-eight mins, flip the chicken, and cook for six mins more.
Take out from the air fryer and serve with microgreens.

Nutrition: per serving: Cal 100|Fat: 9g| Carbs 1g|Protein 4g

271. Air Fried Chicken Fajitas

Prep Time: 10 mins
Servings: 6

Cook Time:20 mins

Ingredients
- Chicken breasts: 4 cups, cut into thin strips
- Bell peppers, sliced
- Salt: half tsp.
- Cumin: 1 tsp.
- Garlic powder: 1/4 tsp
- Chili powder: half tsp.
- Lime juice: 1 tbsp.

Directions: In a bowl, add seasonings, chicken and lime juice, and mix well. Then add sliced peppers and coat well.
Spray the air fryer with olive oil.
Put the chicken and peppers in, and cook for 15 mins at 400 F. flip halfway through.
Serve with wedges of lemons and enjoy.

Nutrition: Cal 140, Protein 22 g, Carbs 6 g, Fat 5 g

272. Air Fried Blackened Chicken Breast

Prep Time: 10 mins
Servings: 2

Cook Time: 20 mins

Ingredients

- Paprika: 2 teaspoons
- Ground thyme: 1 teaspoon
- Cumin: 1 teaspoon
- Cayenne pepper: half tsp.
- Onion powder: half tsp.
- Black Pepper: half tsp.
- Salt: ¼ teaspoon
- Vegetable oil: 2 teaspoons
- Pieces of chicken breast halves (without bones and skin)

Directions: In a mixing bowl, add onion powder, salt, cumin, paprika, black pepper, thyme, and cayenne pepper. Mix it well.
Drizzle oil over chicken and rub. Dip each piece of chicken in blackening spice blend on both sides.
Let it rest for five mins while the air fryer is preheating.
Preheat it for five mins at 360F.
Put the chicken in the air fryer and let it cook for ten mins. Flip and then cook for another ten mins.
After, let it sit for five mins, then slice and serve with the side of greens.

Nutrition: 432.1 Cal, Protein 79.4 g, Carbs 3.2 g, Fat 9.5 g

273. Chicken with Mixed Vegetables

Prep Time: 20 mins
Servings: 2

Cook Time: 20 mins

Ingredients

- 1/2 onion diced
- Chicken breast: 4 cups, cubed pieces
- Half zucchini chopped
- Italian seasoning: 1 tablespoon
- Bell pepper chopped: 1/2 cup
- Clove of garlic pressed
- Broccoli florets: 1/2 cup
- Olive oil: 2 tablespoons
- Half teaspoon of chili powder, garlic powder, pepper, salt,

Directions: Let the air fryer heat to 400 F and dice the vegetables
In a bowl, add the seasoning, oil and add vegetables, chicken and toss well
Place chicken and vegetables in the air fryer, and cook for ten mins, toss half way through, cook in batches.
Make sure the veggies are charred and the chicken is cooked through.

Nutrition: Cal: 230, Carbs: 8 g, Protein: 26 g, Fat: 10 g

274. Garlic Parmesan Chicken Tenders

Prep Time: 5 mins
Servings: 4

Cook Time: 12 mins

Ingredients

- One egg
- Eight raw chicken tenders
- Water: 2 tablespoons
- Olive oil

To coat

- Panko breadcrumbs: 1 cup
- Half tsp of salt
- Black Pepper: 1/4 teaspoon
- Garlic powder: 1 teaspoon
- Onion powder: 1/2 teaspoon
- Parmesan cheese: 1/4 cup
- Any dipping Sauce

Directions: Add all the coating ingredients in a big bowl.
In another bowl, mix water and egg.
Dip the chicken in the egg mix, then in the coating mix.
Put the tenders in the air fry basket in a single layer.
Spray with the olive oil light
Cook at 400 degrees for 12 mins. Flip the chicken halfway through.
Serve with salad greens and enjoy.

Nutrition: Cal: 220, Carbs: 13 g, Protein: 27 g, Fat: 6 g

275. Chicken Thighs Smothered Style

Prep Time: 30 mins   Cook Time:30 mins
Servings: 4

Ingredients
- *8-ounce of chicken thighs*
- *1 tsp paprika*
- *One pinch salt*
- *Mushrooms: half cup*
- *Onions, roughly sliced*

Directions: Let the air fryer preheat to 400F.
Chicken thighs season with paprika, salt, and pepper on both sides.
Place the thighs in the air fryer and cook for 20 mins.
Meanwhile, sauté the mushroom and onion.
Take out the thighs from the air fryer serve with sautéed mushrooms and onions.
And serve with chopped scallions and on the side of salad greens.

Nutrition: Cal 466.3, Fat: 32 g, Carbs: 2.4 g, Protein: 40.5 g

276. Lemon-Garlic Chicken

Prep Time: 2 hours' mins   Cook Time: 35 mins
Servings: 4

Ingredients
- *Lemon juice ¼ cup*
- *1 Tbsp. olive oil*
- *1 tsp mustard*
- *Cloves of garlic*
- *¼ tsp salt*
- *⅛ tsp black pepper*
- *Chicken thighs*
- *Lemon wedges*

Directions: In a bowl, whisk together the lemon juice, olive oil, mustard Dijon, garlic, salt, and pepper.
Place the chicken thighs in a ziploc bag. Spill marinade over chicken & seal bag, ensuring all chicken parts are covered. Cool for at least 2 hours.
Preheat a frying pan to 360 F.
Remove the chicken with towels from the marinade, & pat dry.
Place pieces of chicken in the air fryer basket, if necessary, cook them in batches.
Fry till chicken is no longer pink on the bone & the juices run smoothly, 22 to 24 min. Upon serving, press a lemon slice across each piece.

Nutrition: Cal 258, Fat: 18.6 g, Carbs: 3.6 g, Protein: 19.4 g

277. Buttermilk Chicken in Air-Fryer

Prep Time: 30 mins   Cook Time:20 mins
Servings: 6

Ingredients
- *Chicken thighs: 4 cups skin-on, bone-in*

Marinade
- *Buttermilk: 2 cups*
- *Black pepper: 2 tsp.*
- *Cayenne pepper: 1 tsp.*
- *Salt: 2 tsp.*

Seasoned Flour
- *Baking powder: 1 tbsp.*
- *All-purpose flour: 2 cups*
- *Paprika powder: 1 tbsp.*
- *Salt: 1 tsp.*
- *Garlic powder: 1 tbsp.*

Directions: Let the air fry heat at 370°F.
With a paper towel, pat dry the chicken thighs.
In a mixing bowl, add paprika, black pepper, salt mix well, then add chicken pieces. Add buttermilk and coat the chicken well. Let it marinate for at least 6 hours.
In another bowl, add baking powder, salt, flour, pepper, and paprika. Put one by one of the chicken pieces and coat in the seasoning mix.

Spray oil on chicken pieces and place breaded chicken skin side up in air fryer basket in one layer, cook for 8 mins, then flip the chicken pieces' cook for another ten mins
Take out from the air fryer and serve right away.

Nutrition: Cal 210, Fat 18 g, Protein 22 g, Carbs 12 g

278. Orange Chicken Wings

Prep Time: 5 mins
Servings: 2

Cook Time: 14 mins

Ingredients
- *Honey: 1 tbsp.*
- *Chicken Wings, Six pieces*
- *One orange zest and juice*
- *Worcestershire Sauce: 1.5 tbsp.*
- *Black pepper to taste*
- *Herbs (sage, rosemary, oregano, parsley, basil, thyme, and mint)*

Directions: Wash and pat dry the chicken wings.
In a bowl, add chicken wings, pour zest and orange juice.
Add the rest of the ingredients and rub on chicken wings. Let it marinate for at least half an hour.
Let the Air fryer preheat at 370°F.
In an aluminum foil, wrap the marinated wings and put them in an air fryer, and cook for 20 mins.
After 20 mins, remove aluminum foil and brush the sauce over wings and cook for 15 mins more. Then again, brush the sauce and cook for another ten mins.
Take out from the air fryer and serve hot.

Nutrition: Cal 271, Protein 29 g, Carbs 20 g, Fat 15 g

279. Air Fryer Brown Rice Chicken Fried

Prep Time: 10 mins
Servings: 2

Cook Time: 20 mins

Ingredients
- *Olive Oil Cook Spray*
- *Chicken Breast: 1 Cup, Diced & Cooked &*
- *White Onion: 1/4 cup chopped*
- *Celery: 1/4 Cup chopped*
- *Cooked brown rice: 4 Cups*
- *Carrots: 1/4 cup chopped*

Directions: Place foil on the air fryer basket, make sure to leave room for air to flow, roll up on the sides.
Spray with olive oil, the foil. Mix all ingredients.
On top of the foil, add all ingredients in the air fryer basket. Give an olive oil spray on the mixture. Cook for five mins at 390F.
Open the air fryer and give a toss to the mixture. Cook for five more mins at 390F.
Take out from air fryer and serve hot.

Nutrition: Cal 350, Fat: 6 g, Carbs 20 g, Protein 22 g

280. Chicken Cheesy Quesadilla in Air Fryer

Prep Time: 4 mins
Servings: 2

Cook Time: 7 mins

Ingredients
- *Precooked chicken: one cup, diced*
- *Tortillas: 2 pieces*
- *Low-fat cheese: one cup (shredded)*

Directions: Spray oil the air basket and place one tortilla in it. Add cooked chicken and cheese on top.
Add the second tortilla on top. Put a metal rack on top. Cook for 6 mins at 370 degrees, flip it halfway through so cook evenly.
Slice and serve with dipping sauce.

Nutrition: Cal: 171, Carbs: 8 g, Protein: 15 g, Fat: 8 g

281. Delicious Chicken Pie

Prep Time: 10 mins
Servings: 2

Cook Time: 30 mins

Ingredients

- Puff pastry: 2 sheets
- Chicken thighs: 2 pieces, cut into cubes
- One small onion, chopped
- Small potatoes: 2, chopped
- Mushrooms: 1/4 cup
- Light soya sauce
- One carrot, chopped
- Black pepper to taste
- Worcestershire sauce: to taste
- Salt to taste
- Italian mixed dried herbs
- Garlic powder: a pinch
- Plain flour: 2 tbsp.
- Milk, as required
- Melted butter

Directions: In a mixing bowl, add light soya sauce and pepper add the chicken cubes, and coat well.
In a pan over medium heat, sauté potatoes, carrot, and onion. Add some water, if required, to cook the vegetables.
Add the chicken cubes and mushrooms and cook them too.
Stir in black pepper, salt, Worcestershire sauce, garlic powder, and dried herbs.
When the chicken is cooked through, add some of the flour and mix well.
Add in the milk and let the vegetables simmer until tender.
Place one piece of puff pastry in the baking tray of the air fryer, poke holes with a fork.
Add on top the cooked chicken filling and eggs and puff pastry on top with holes. Cut the excess pastry off. Glaze with oil spray or melted butter.
Air fry at 180 F for six mins, or until it becomes golden brown.
Serve right away and enjoy.

Nutrition: Cal 224, Protein 20 g, Fat 18 g, Carbs 17 g

282. Chicken Bites in Air Fryer

Prep Time: 10 mins
Servings: 3

Cook Time: 10 mins

Ingredients

- Chicken breast: 2 cups
- Kosher salt& pepper to taste
- Smashed potatoes: one cup
- Scallions: ¼ cup
- One Egg beat
- Whole wheat breadcrumbs: 1 cup

Directions: Boil the chicken until soft.
Shred the chicken with the help of a fork.
Add the smashed potatoes, scallions to the shredded chicken. Season with kosher salt and pepper.
Coat with egg and then in bread crumbs.
Put in the air fryer, and cook for 8 mins at 380F. Or until golden brown.
Serve warm.

Nutrition: Cal: 234, Protein 25 g, Carbs 15 g, Fat 9 g

283. Popcorn Chicken in Air Fryer

Prep Time: 10 mins
Servings: 4

Cook Time:20 mins

Ingredients
For Marinade

- 8 cups, chicken tenders, cut into bite-size pieces
- Freshly ground black pepper: 1/2 tsp
- Almond milk: 2 cups
- Salt: 1 tsp
- paprika: 1/2 tsp

Dry Mix

- Salt: 3 tsp
- Flour: 3 cups
- Paprika: 2 tsp
- Oil spray
- Freshly ground black pepper: 2 tsp

Directions: In a bowl, add all marinade ingredients and chicken. Mix well, and put it in a ziploc bag and refrigerator for two hours for the minimum, or six hours.

In a large bowl, add all the dry ingredients.

Coat the marinated chicken to the dry mix. Into the marinade again, then for the second time in the dry mixture.

Spray the air fryer basket with olive oil and place the breaded chicken pieces in one single layer. Spray oil over the chicken pieces too.

Cook at 370 degrees for 10 mins, tossing halfway through.

Serve immediately with salad greens or dipping sauce.

Nutrition: Cal 340, Protein 20 g, Carbs 14 g, Fat 10 g

284. Turkey Fajitas Platter in Air Fryer

Prep Time: 5 mins   **Cook Time:20 mins**
Servings: 2

Ingredients

- *Cooked Turkey Breast: 1/4 cup*
- *Six Tortilla Wraps*
- *One Avocado*
- *One Yellow Pepper*
- *One Red Pepper*
- *Half Red Onion*
- *Soft Cheese: 5 Tbsp.*
- *Mexican Seasoning: 2 Tbsp.*
- *Cumin: 1 Tsp*
- *Kosher salt& Pepper*
- *Cajun Spice: 3 Tbsp.*
- *Fresh Coriander*

Directions: Chop up the avocado and slice the vegetables.

Dice up turkey breast into small bite-size pieces.

In a bowl, add onions, turkey, soft cheese, and peppers along with seasonings. Mix it well.

Place it in foil and the air fryer.

Cook for 20 mins at 200 F.

Nutrition: Cal: 379, Carbs: 84 g, Protein: 30 g, Fat: 39 g

285. Turkey Juicy Breast Tenderloin

Prep Time: 5 mins   **Cook Time:25 mins**
Servings: 3

Ingredients

- *Turkey breast tenderloin: one-piece*
- *Thyme: half tsp.*
- *Sage: half tsp.*
- *Paprika: half tsp.*
- *Pink salt: half tsp.*
- *Freshly ground black pepper: half tsp.*

Directions: Let the air fryer preheat to 350 F.

In a bowl, mix all the spices and herbs, rub it all over the turkey.

Spray oil on the air fryer basket. Put the turkey in the air fryer and let it cook at 350 F for 25 mins, flip halfway through.

Serve with your favorite salad.

Nutrition: Cal: 162, Carbs: 1 g, Protein: 13 g, Fat: 1 g

286. Turkey Breast with Mustard Maple Glaze

Prep Time: 10 mins   **Cook Time:55 mins**
Servings: 6

Ingredients

- *Whole turkey breast: 5 pounds*
- *Olive oil: 2 tsp.*
- *Maple syrup: 1/4 cup*
- *Dried sage: half tsp.*
- *Smoked paprika: half tsp.*
- *Dried thyme: one tsp.*
- *Salt: one tsp.*
- *Freshly ground black pepper: half tsp.*
- *Dijon mustard: 2 tbsp.*

Directions: Let the air fryer preheat to 350 F.

Rub the olive oil over the turkey breast.

In a bowl, mix salt, sage, pepper, thyme, and paprika. Mix well and coat turkey in this spice rub.

Place the turkey in an air fryer, cook for 25 mins at 350ºF. Flip the turkey over and cook for another 12 mins. Flip again and cook for another ten mins. With an instant-read thermometer, the internal temperature should reach 165ºF.

In the meantime, in a saucepan, mix mustard, maple syrup, and with one tsp. of butter.

Brush this glaze all over the turkey when cooked.
Cook again for five mins. Slice and Serve with fresh salad.

Nutrition: Cal 379, Fat: 23 g, Carbs: 21 g, Protein: 52 g

287. Zucchini Turkey Burgers

Prep Time: 10 mins
Servings: 5

Cook Time:10 mins

Ingredients
- Gluten-free breadcrumbs: 1/4 cup (seasoned)
- Grated zucchini: 1 cup
- Red onion: 1 tbsp. (grated)
- Lean ground turkey: 4 cups
- One clove of minced garlic
- 1 tsp of kosher salt and fresh pepper

Directions: In a bowl, add zucchini (moisture removed with a paper towel), ground turkey, garlic, salt, onion, pepper, breadcrumbs. Mix well.
With your hands make five patties. But not too thick.
Let the air fryer preheat to 375 F.
Put in an air fryer in a single layer and cook for 7 mins or more. Until cooked through and browned.
Place in buns with ketchup and lettuce and enjoy.

Nutrition: Cal: 161, Carbs: 4.5 g, Protein: 18 g, Fat: 7 g

288. No-breaded Turkey Breast

Prep Time: 5 mins
Servings: 10

Cook Time:55 mins

Ingredients
- Turkey breast: 4 pounds, ribs removed, bone with skin
- Olive oil: 1 tablespoon
- Salt: 2 teaspoons
- Dry turkey seasoning (without salt): half tsp.

Directions: Rub half tbsp of olive oil over turkey breast. Sprinkle salt, turkey seasoning on both sides of turkey breast with half tbsp of olive oil.
Let the air fryer preheat at 350 F. put turkey skin side down in air fryer and cook for 20 mins until the turkey's temperature reaches 160 F for half an hour to 40 mins.
Let it sit for ten mins before slicing. Serve with fresh salad.

Nutrition: Cal: 226, Protein: 32.5 g, Fat: 10 g, Carbs 22 g

289. Almond Flour Coco-Milk Battered Chicken

Prep Time: 5 mins
Serving: 4

Cook Time: 30 mins

Ingredients:
- 4 small chicken thighs
- ¼ cup of coconut milk
- 1/2 cup almond flour
- 1 1/2 tablespoon old bay Cajun seasoning
- 1 egg, beaten
- Salt and pepper

Directions: Preheat the air fryer oven for 5 mins.
Mix the egg and coconut milk in a bowl.
Soak the chicken thighs in the beaten egg mixture.
In a mixing bowl, combine Cajun seasoning, almond flour, salt, and pepper.
Dredge the chicken thighs in the almond flour mixture. Place in the air fryer basket.
Cook for 30 mins at 350°F.

Nutrition: Cal: 590 Fat: 38 g Carbs: 3.2 g Protein: 32.5 g

290. Almond-Crusted Chicken

Prep Time: 20 mins
Servings: 2

Cook Time: 25 mins

Ingredients:
- 2x 6-oz. boneless skinless chicken breasts
- ¼ cup slivered almonds
- 1 tbsp. full-fat mayonnaise
- 2 tbsp. Dijon mustard

Directions: Pulse the almonds in a food processor until they are finely chopped. Spread the almonds on a plate and set aside. Cut each chicken breast in half lengthwise.
Mix the mayonnaise and mustard and then spread evenly on top of the chicken slices.
Place the chicken into the chopped almonds plate to coat thoroughly, laying each coated slice into the basket of your fryer.
Cook for 25 mins at 350°F until golden. Test the temperature, making sure the chicken has reached 165°F.

291. Bacon Chicken Lasagna

Prep Time: 10 Mins
Servings: 8

Cook Time: 25 mins

Ingredients:
- 12 lasagna noodles, cooked
- 3 cups chicken, cooked and shredded
- 2 1/2 cups mozzarella cheese, grated
- 3/4 lb bacon, cooked and crumbled
- 16 oz cream cheese
- 1/2 cup sun-dried tomatoes, chopped
- 14 oz artichoke hearts, drained and chopped
- 1/2 cup parmesan cheese, grated
- 3 tablespoon ranch dressing
- 1 1/4 cups milk

Directions: Spray a 9*13-inch baking dish with cook spray and set aside.
Insert wire rack in rack position 6. Select bake, set temperature 350 F, timer for 25 mins. Press start to preheat the oven.
In a bowl, mix together chicken, tomatoes, artichokes, parmesan cheese, 1 cup mozzarella cheese, and bacon.
In a separate bowl, mix together ranch dressing, milk, and cream cheese.
Pour half milk mixture over the chicken and stir well. Pour half milk mixture in the baking dish.
Place 3 lasagna noodles in the baking dish then place 1/3 chicken mixture and half cup mozzarella cheese. Repeat layers twice.
Bake for 25 mins.

Nutrition: Cal 851 Fat 44.3 g Carbs 60 g Protein 53.1 g

292. Baked Chicken & Potatoes

Prep Time: 10 Mins
Servings: 5

Cook Time: 60 mins

Ingredients:
- 5 chicken thighs
- 1 lemon juice
- 1/2 cup olive oil
- 1 tbsp fresh rosemary, chopped
- 1 tsp. dried oregano
- 2 lbs. potatoes, cut into chunks
- 4 garlic cloves, minced
- Salt and Pepper

Directions: Select bake, set temperature 375 F, timer for 60 mins. Press start to preheat the oven.
In a large mixing bowl, add chicken and remaining ingredients and mix well.
Place chicken in the baking dish and spread potatoes around the chicken.
Bake chicken for 60 mins.

Nutrition: Cal 333 Fat 21.6 g Carbs 30.1 g Protein 7.3 g

293. Basil Pesto Chicken

Prep Time: 10 Mins
Servings: 4

Cook Time: 40 mins

Ingredients:

- Four chicken breasts, skinless, boneless, and cut in half
- 1/2 cup basil pesto
- 1 cup mozzarella cheese, shredded
- Three tomatoes, sliced

Directions: Line a roasting pan with aluminum foil and spray with cook spray. Set aside.
Select bake, set temperature 390 F, timer for 35 mins. Press start to preheat the oven.
In a bowl, mix together pesto and chicken until well coated.
Place chicken on roasting pan and bake for 35 mins.
Remove from oven and top with cheese and tomatoes.
Bake for 5 mins more.

Nutrition: Cal 315 Fat 12.3 g Carbs 3.9 g Protein 45.1 g

294. Basil-Garlic Breaded Chicken Bake

Prep Time: 5 mins
Serving: 2

Cook Time: 30 mins

Ingredients:
- 2 boneless skinless chicken breast halves (4 ounces each)
- 1 tablespoon butter, melted
- 1 large tomato, seeded and chopped
- 2 garlic cloves, minced
- 1 1/2 tablespoons minced fresh basil
- 1/4 cup all-purpose flour
- 1/4 cup egg substitute
- 1/4 cup grated Parmesan cheese
- 1/4 cup dry bread crumbs
- 1/4 teaspoon pepper
- 1/2 teaspoon salt
- 1/2 tablespoon olive oil

Directions: In a shallow bowl, whisk OK egg substitute and place flour in a separate bowl—dip chicken in flour, then egg, and then flour. In a small bowl, whisk OK butter, bread crumbs, and cheese. Sprinkle over chicken.
Lightly grease the baking pan of the air fryer with cook spray. Place chicken on the bottom of the pan. Cover with foil.
For 20 mins, cook at 390°F.
Meanwhile, in a bowl, whisk well-remaining ingredient.
Remove foil from the pan and then pour over chicken the remaining Ingredients.
Cook for 8 mins.

Nutrition: Cal: 311; Fat: 11 g; Protein: 31 g; Carbs: 22 g

295. BBQ Chicken Wings

Prep Time: 10 Mins
Servings: 8

Cook Time: 55 mins

Ingredients:
- 32 chicken wings
- 1 1/2 cups BBQ sauce
- Salt and pepper
- 1/4 cup olive oil

Directions: Line baking sheet with parchment paper and set aside.
Select bake, set temperature 375 F, timer for 55 mins. Press start to preheat the oven.
In a mixing bowl, toss chicken wings with olive oil, pepper, and salt.
Arrange chicken wings on a baking sheet and bake for 50 mins.
Toss chicken wings with BBQ sauce and bake for 5 mins more.

Nutrition: Cal 173 Fat 8.3 g Carbs 17 g Protein 7.4 g

296. BBQ Spicy Chicken Wings

Prep Time: 10 Mins
Servings: 6

Cook Time: 45 mins

Ingredients:

- 3 lbs. chicken wings
- 2 tbsp olive oil
- 1/2 cup BBQ spice rub

Directions: Select bake, set temperature 390 F, timer for 45 mins. Press start to preheat the oven.
Brush chicken wings with olive oil and place in a large mixing bowl.
Add BBQ spice over chicken wings and toss until well coated.
Arrange chicken wings on rack in a single layer and bake for 45 mins.

Nutrition: Cal 483 Fat 22.2 g Carbs 1.5 g Protein 65.8 g

297. Baked Chicken

Prep Time: 5 mins
Servings: 6

Cook time: 45 mins

Ingredients:

- 1/2 cup butter
- 1tsp. pepper
- 3tbsp. garlic, minced
- 1whole chicken

Directions: Pre-heat your fryer at 350°F.
Allow the butter to soften at room temperature, then mix well in a small bowl with the pepper and garlic.
Massage the butter into the chicken. Any remaining butter can go inside the chicken.
Cook the chicken in the fryer for half an hour. Flip, then cook on the other side for another thirty mins.
Test the temperature of the chicken by sticking a meat thermometer into the fat of the thigh to make sure it has reached 165°F.
Take care when removing the chicken from the fryer. Let sit for ten mins before you carve it.

298. Buffalo Chicken Wings

Prep Time: 5 mins
Serving: 8

Cook Time: 30 mins

Ingredients:

- 1-2 tbsp. brown sugar
- 1 tbsp. Worcestershire sauce
- 1/2 C. butter
- 1/2 C. cayenne pepper sauce
- 4 pounds of chicken wings
- 1 tsp. salt

Directions: Whisk brown sugar, salt, Worcestershire sauce, butter, and hot sauce together and set aside.
Dry wings and put to the air fryer basket.
Set temperature to 380°F, and set time to 25 mins. Cook was tossing halfway through.
When the timer sounds, shake wings, bump up the temperature to 400 degrees, and cook another 5 mins.
Take out wings and place them into a bowl. Add sauce and toss well.
Serve alongside celery sticks.

Nutrition: Cal: 402; Fat: 16 g; Protein: 17 g

299. Buffalo Chicken Tenders

Prep Time: 15 mins
Servings: 2

Cook Time: 10 mins

Ingredients:

- One egg
- 1 cup mozzarella cheese, shredded
- ¼ cup feta cheese
- ¼ cup buffalo sauce
- 1 cup cooked chicken, shredded

Directions: Combine all ingredients (except feta). Line the basket of your fryer with a suitably-sized piece of parchment paper. Lay the mixture into the fryer and press it into a circle about half an inch thick. Crumble the feta cheese over it. Cook for 8 mins at 400°F. Turn the fryer off and allow the chicken to rest inside before removing it with care. Cut the mixture into slices.

300. Caribbean Chicken

Prep Time: 10 Mins   **Cook Time: 10 mins**
Servings: 8

Ingredients:

- 3 lbs chicken thigh, skinless and boneless
- 1 tablespoon cayenne
- 1 tablespoon cinnamon
- 1 tablespoon coriander powder
- 3 tablespoon coconut oil, melted
- 1/2 teaspoon ground nutmeg
- 1/2 teaspoon ground ginger
- Salt and Pepper

Directions: Select air fry, set temperature 390 F, timer for 10 mins. Press start to preheat the oven.
In a bowl, mix together all ingredients except chicken.
Rub bowl mixture all over the chicken.
Place chicken into the air fryer basket and air fry for 10 mins.

Nutrition: Cal 373 Fat 17.9 g Carbs 1.2 g Protein 49.3 g

301. Carne Asada Tacos

Prep Time: 5 mins   **Cook Time: 14 mins**
Serving: 4

Ingredients:

- 1/3 cup olive oil
- 11/2 pounds (680 g) flank steak
- 1/3 cup freshly squeezed lime juice
- 1/2 cup chopped fresh cilantro
- 4 teaspoons minced garlic
- 1 teaspoon ground cumin
- 1 teaspoon chili powder
- Salt and freshly ground black pepper

Directions: Brush the fry basket with olive oil.
Put the flank steak in a large mixing bowl—season with salt and pepper.
Add the lime juice, cilantro, garlic, cumin, and chili powder and toss to coat the steak.
For the best flavor, let the steak marinate in the refrigerator for about 1 hour.
Preheat the air fryer oven to 400°F.
Put the steak in the fry basket. Insert the fry basket at mid position. Select Air Fry, Convection, and set time to 7 mins. Flip the steak. Air fry for 7 mins more or until an internal temperature reaches at least 145°F.
Let the steak rest for about 5 mins and then cut into strips to serve.

302. Cheddar Turkey Bites

Prep Time: 5 mins   **Cook Time: 20 mins**
Servings: 4

Ingredients:

- One big turkey breast, skinless; boneless, and cubed
- 1/4 cup cheddar cheese, grated
- 1/4 tsp. garlic powder
- Salt and pepper
- 1 tbsp. Olive oil

Directions: Rub the turkey cubes with the oil, season with salt, pepper, garlic powder, and dredge in cheddar cheese.
Put the turkey bits in your air fryer's basket and cook at 380°F for 20 mins. Divide between plates and serve with a side salad.

Nutrition: Cal: 240 Fat: 11 g Carbs: 5 g

303. Chicken Lasagna

Prep Time: 10 Mins
Servings: 9

Cook Time: 45 mins

Ingredients:
- Eight lasagna noodles, cooked and drained
- 3 cups chicken, cooked and diced
- 1/2 cup onion, chopped
- 1/2 cup green bell pepper, chopped
- 1/2 cup parmesan cheese, grated
- 1/2 Teaspoon dried basil
- 2 cups processed cheese, shredded
- 16 oz cottage cheese
- 6 oz can mushroom, drained and sliced
- 10 oz can cream of chicken soup
- 1/4 cup pimento peppers, chopped
- 3/4 cup milk
- 3 tablespoon butter

Directions: Select bake, set temperature 350 F, timer for 45 mins. Press start to preheat the oven.
Melt butter in a saucepan. Add bell pepper, onion and sauté.
Stir in soup, pimento, basil, processed cheese, milk, and mushrooms.
Place 1/2 noodles in a baking dish then layer with 1/2 cream sauce, half cottage cheese, half chicken, and half parmesan cheese.
Repeat layers.
Bake for 45 mins.

Nutrition: Cal 449 Fat 16.8 g Carbs 38.8 g Protein 35 g

304. Cheesy Meatloaf

Prep Time: 10 Mins
Servings: 8

Cook Time: 35 mins

Ingredients:
- 2 lbs. ground turkey
- 1 teaspoon garlic powder
- 1 teaspoon garlic, minced
- One egg
- 1 tablespoon onion, minced
- 1 cup cheddar cheese, shredded
- 2 oz BBQ sauce, sugar-free
- 1 teaspoon ground mustard
- 1 teaspoon chili powder
- 1 teaspoon salt

Directions:
Spray 9*13-inch casserole dish with cook spray and set aside.
Select bake, set temperature 390 F, timer for 35 mins. Press start to preheat the oven.
In a large bowl, mix all ingredients then transfer into the casserole dish.
Bake for 30-35 mins.

Nutrition: Cal 302 Fat 17.9 g Carbs 3.6 g Protein 35.5 g

305. Chicken Breasts & Spiced Tomatoes

Prep Time: 5 mins
Servings: 4

Cook time: 15 mins

Ingredients:
- lb. boneless chicken breast
- 1 cup butter
- 1 cup tomatoes, diced
- 1 1/2 tsp. paprika
- 1 tsp. pumpkin pie spices
- Salt and pepper

Directions: Preheat your fryer at 375°F.
Cut the chicken into relatively thick slices and put them in the fryer. Sprinkle with salt and pepper to taste. Cook for fifteen mins.
In the meantime, melt the butter in a saucepan, before adding the tomatoes, paprika, and pumpkin pie spices. Leave simmering while the chicken finishes cook.
When the chicken is cooked through, place it on a dish and pour the tomato mixture over.

306. Chicken Casserole

Prep Time: 10 Mins
Servings: 8

Cook Time: 40 mins

Ingredients:
- 2 lbs. cooked chicken, shredded
- 6 oz cream cheese, softened
- 4 oz butter, melted
- 5 oz Swiss cheese
- 1 oz fresh lemon juice
- 6 oz ham, cut into small pieces
- 1 tablespoon Dijon mustard
- 1/2 teaspoon salt

Directions: Select bake, set temperature 350 F, timer for 40 mins. Press start to preheat the oven.
Arrange chicken in the baking dish and top with ham pieces.
Add butter, lemon juice, mustard, cream cheese, and salt into the blender and blend until a thick sauce.
Spread sauce on top of chicken in the baking dish.
Arrange Swiss cheese slices on top of the sauce and bake for 40 mins.

Nutrition: Cal 451 Fat 29.2 g Carbs 2.5 g Protein 43 g

307. Cheesy Chicken Rice

Prep Time: 10 Mins
Servings: 4

Cook Time: 25 mins

Ingredients:
- 1 cup chicken breast, cooked and shredded
- 2 tablespoon all-purpose flour
- 2 cup cooked brown rice
- 1 tablespoon garlic, minced
- 2 tablespoon butter
- 1 cup cheddar cheese, shredded
- 1 cup chicken stock
- 1/2 tablespoon fresh thyme, chopped
- 1/1 teaspoon salt
- 1/2 teaspoon pepper

Directions: Spray a baking dish with cook spray and set aside.
Select bake, set temperature 350 F, timer for 25 mins. Press start to preheat the oven.
Melt butter in a saucepan over medium-high heat. Add garlic and cook for 1 minute. Add thyme, pepper, salt, and flour stir well.
Pour chicken stock into the pan and whisk constantly. Whisk until thick then add cheese and stir until melted.
Add chicken and cooked rice stir well to combine. Transfer pan mixture into the baking dish and bake for 25 mins.

Nutrition: Cal 559 Fat 18.5 g Carbs 77 g Protein 20.3 g

308. Chicken Coconut Meatballs

Prep Time: 10 Mins
Servings: 4

Cook Time: 10 mins

Ingredients:
- 1 lb ground chicken
- 1 tablespoon soy sauce
- 1 tablespoon hoisin sauce
- 1/2 cup fresh cilantro, chopped
- 2 green onions, chopped
- 1/4 cup shredded coconut
- 1 teaspoon sriracha
- Salt and Pepper
- 1 teaspoon sesame oil

Directions:
Select air fry, set temperature 350 F, timer for 10 mins. Press start to preheat the oven.
Add all ingredients into the large bowl and mix.
Make small balls and place them into the air fryer basket and air fry for 10 mins.

Nutrition: Cal 258 Fat 11.4 g Carbs 3.7 g Protein 33.5 g

309. Chicken Fajitas

Prep Time: 10 mins
Serving: 4

Cook Time: 20 mins

Ingredients:

- 4 boneless, skinless chicken breasts, sliced
- 1 small red onion, sliced
- 2 avocados, peeled and chopped
- 2 red bell peppers, sliced
- 1/2 cup spicy ranch salad dressing, divided
- 1/2 teaspoon dried oregano
- 8 corn tortillas
- 2 cups torn butter lettuce

Directions: Place the chicken, onion, and pepper in the air fryer basket. Drizzle with one tablespoon of the salad dressing and add the oregano. Toss to combine.
Place the Rack on the middle-shelf of the Air fryer oven. Set temperature to 165°F, and set time to 14 mins. Grill for 10 to 14 mins or until the chicken is 165°F on a food thermometer. Transfer the chicken and vegetables to a bowl and toss with the remaining dressing. Serve the chicken mixture with the tortillas, lettuce, and avocados and let everyone make their creations.

Nutrition: Cal: 783; Fat: 38 g; Protein: 72 g

310. Chicken Fillets, Brie & Ham

Prep Time: 5 mins
Serving: 4

Cook Time: 15 mins

Ingredients:

- 2 Large Chicken Fillets
- Freshly Ground Black Pepper
- 4 Small Slices of Brie (Or your cheese of choice)
- 1 Tbsp. Freshly Chopped Chives
- 4 Slices Cured Ham

Directions: Slice the fillets into four and make incisions as you would for a hamburger bun. Leave a little "hinge" uncut at the back. Season the inside and pop some brie and chives in there. Close them, and wrap them each in a slice of ham. Brush with oil and pop them into the basket.
Heat your fryer to 350° F. Pour into the Oven rack/basket. Place the Rack on the middle-shelf of the Air fryer oven. Set temperature to 400°F, and time to 15 mins. Roast the little parcels until they look tasty (15 min).

311. Chicken Kabab

Prep Time: 10 Mins
Servings: 3

Cook Time: 6 mins

Ingredients:

- 1 lb ground chicken
- 1/4 cup almond flour
- Two green onion, chopped
- One egg, lightly beaten
- 1/3 cup fresh parsley, chopped
- Two garlic cloves
- 4 oz onion, chopped
- 1/4 teaspoon turmeric powder
- 1 tablespoon fresh lemon juice
- 1/2 teaspoon pepper

Directions: Select air fry, set temperature 400 F, timer for 6 mins. Press start to preheat the oven.
Add all ingredients into the food processor and mix until well combined.
Transfer chicken mixture to the bowl and place it in the refrigerator for 30 mins.
Divide mixture into the 6 equal portions and roll around the soaked wooden skewers.
Place kabab into the air fryer basket air fry for 6 mins.

Nutrition: Cal 391 Fat 17.3 g Carbs 7.9 g Protein 48.6 g

312. Chicken Meatballs

Prep Time: 10 Mins
Servings: 4

Cook Time: 15 mins

Ingredients:
- 1 lb ground chicken
- 1 teaspoon cumin
- Three garlic cloves, minced
- 2 tablespoon soy sauce
- 1/4 cup breadcrumbs
- 1/2 cup parmesan cheese, grated
- One egg, lightly beaten
- Salt and Pepper

Directions: Line baking sheet with parchment paper and set aside.
Select bake, set temperature 390 F, timer for 15 mins. Press start to preheat the oven.
Add all ingredients into the mixing bowl and process until well combined.
Make small balls from the meat mixture and arrange on a baking sheet.
Bake meatballs for 15 mins.

Nutrition: Cal 304 Fat 12.4 g Carbs 6.9 g Protein 39.4 g

313. Chicken Mushrooms Bake

Prep Time: 10 Mins
Servings: 4

Cook Time: 30 mins

Ingredients:
- 2 lbs. chicken breasts, halved
- 8 oz mushrooms, sliced
- 1/2 cup mayonnaise
- 1/3 cup sun-dried tomatoes
- 1 teaspoon salt

Directions: Grease baking dish with butter and set aside.
Select bake, set temperature 390 F, timer for 30 mins. Press start to preheat the oven.
Place chicken into the baking dish and top with sun-dried tomatoes, mushrooms, mayonnaise, and salt. Mix well.
Bake for 30 mins.

Nutrition: Cal 560 Fat 26.8 g Carbs 9.5 g Protein 67.8 g

314. Chicken Paillard

Prep Time: 10 Mins
Servings: 8

Cook Time: 25 mins

Ingredients:
- Four chicken breasts, skinless and boneless
- 1/2 cup olives, diced
- One small onion, sliced
- One fennel bulb, sliced
- 28 oz can tomatoes, diced
- 1/4 cup pine nuts
- 2 tablespoon olive oil
- 1/4 cup fresh basil, chopped
- 1/4 cup fresh parsley, chopped
- Salt and Pepper

Directions:
Select bake, set temperature 390 F, timer for 25 mins. Press start to preheat the oven.
Arrange chicken in baking dish and season with pepper and salt and drizzle with oil.
In a bowl, mix together olives, tomatoes, pine nuts, onion, fennel, pepper, and salt.
Pour olive mixture over chicken and bake for 25 mins.
Garnish with basil and parsley.

Nutrition: Cal 242 Fat 12.8 g Carbs 9.3 g Protein 23.2 g

315. Chicken Parmesan

Prep Time: 5 mins
Servings: 4

Cook Time: 25 mins

Ingredients:
- 2 (6-oz.) boneless, skinless chicken breasts
- 1 oz. Pork rinds, crushed
- 1 cup low-carb, no-sugar-added pasta sauce
- 1 cup shredded mozzarella cheese, divided.
- 4 tbsp. Full-fat mayonnaise, divided.
- 1/2 tsp. Garlic powder.
- ¼ tsp. Dried oregano.
- 1/2 cup grated Parmesan cheese, divided.
- 1/2 tsp. Dried parsley.

Directions: Slice each chicken breast in half lengthwise and lb. out to 3/4-inch thickness. Sprinkle with garlic powder, oregano, and parsley.
Spread 1 tbsp. Mayo on top of each piece of chicken and then sprinkle ¼ cup mozzarella on each piece.
In a small bowl, mix the pork rinds and Parmesan. Sprinkle the mixture on top of mozzarella.
Pour sauce into a 6-inch round baking pan and place chicken on top. Place pan into the air fryer basket. Set the temperature to 320°F and set the timer for 25 mins.
The cheese will be browned, and the internal temperature will be at least 165°F when fully cooked.

Nutrition: Cal: 393 Protein: 34.2 g Fat: 22.8 g Carbs: 6.8 g

316. Chicken Pizza Crust

Prep Time: 10 mins
Servings: 4

Cook Time: 25 mins

Ingredients:
- 1 lb. ground chicken thigh meat
- ¼ cup grated Parmesan cheese
- 1/2 cup shredded mozzarella

Directions: Take a large bowl, mix all ingredients. Separate into four even parts.
Cut out four, 6-inch circles of parchment and press each part of the chicken mixture out onto one of the processes. Place into the air fryer basket, working in batches as needed.
Set the temperature to 375°F and the timer for 25 mins. Flip the crust halfway through the cook time.
Once fully cooked, you may top it with cheese and your favorite toppings and cook five additional mins. Or you may place crust into refrigerator or freezer and top when ready to eat.

Nutrition: Cal: 230 Protein: 24.7 g Fat: 12.8 g Carbs: 1.2 g

317. Chicken Pizza Crusts

Prep Time: 15 mins
Servings: 2

Cook Time: 30 mins

Ingredients:
- 1 lb. ground chicken
- 1/2 cup mozzarella, shredded
- ¼ cup parmesan cheese, grated

Directions: In a large bowl, combine all the ingredients and then spread the mixture out, dividing it into four equal-size parts.
Cut a sheet of parchment paper into four circles, roughly six inches in diameter, and put some of the chicken mixtures onto the center of each piece, flattening the mix to fill out the ring.
Cook either one or two circles at a time at 375°F for 25 mins. Halfway through, turn the crust over to cook on the other side. Keep each batch warm.
Once all the crusts are cooked, top with cheese and the toppings of your choice. If desired, cook the topped crusts for an additional five mins.

318. Chicken Pram

Prep Time: 10 mins
Servings: 4

Cook time: 35 mins

Ingredients:
- 4 chicken breast halves, skinless & boneless
- 1/2 cup flour
- 2 eggs
- 2/3 cup panko breadcrumbs
- 2/3 cup Italian seasoned breadcrumbs
- 1/3 + ¼ cup parmesan cheese, divided
- 2 tbsp. fresh parsley, chopped
- Nonstick cook spray
- 24 oz. marinara sauce
- 1 cup mozzarella cheese, grated
- 1/2 tsp. salt
- ¼ tsp. pepper

Directions: Place the baking pan in position 2 of the oven. Lightly spray the fryer basket with cook spray.
Place flour in a shallow dish.
In a separate shallow dish, beat the eggs.
In a third shallow dish, combine both breadcrumbs, 1/3 cup parmesan cheese, two tablespoons parsley, salt, and pepper.
Place chicken between two sheets of plastic wrap and pound to 1/2-inch thick.
Dip chicken first in flour, then eggs, and breadcrumb mixture to coat. Place in the basket and then put the basket on the baking pan.
Set oven to air fry on 375°F for 10 mins. Turn chicken over halfway through cook time.
Remove chicken and baking pan from the oven. Set range to bake on 425°F for 30 mins.
Pour 1 1/2 cups marinara in the bottom of an 8x11-inch baking dish. Place chicken over the sauce and add another two tablespoons marinara to tops of chicken. Top the chicken with mozzarella and parmesan cheese once oven preheats for 5 mins, place the dish in the oven and bake 20-25 mins until bubbly and cheese is golden brown.

Nutrition: Cal: 529 Fat: 13 g Carbs: 52 g Protein: 51 g

319. Chicken Stir-Fry

Prep Time: 10 mins
Servings: 2

Cook Time: 20 mins

Ingredients:
- 1 (6-oz.) chicken breast; cut into 1-inch cubes
- 1/2 medium red bell pepper; seeded and chopped
- 1/2 medium zucchini; chopped
- ¼ medium red onion; peeled and sliced
- 1/2 tsp. Garlic powder
- 1 tsp. Dried oregano
- ¼ tsp. dried thyme
- 1 tbsp. Coconut oil

Directions: Place all ingredients into a mixing bowl and stir until the coconut oil covers the meat and vegetables. Pour the contents of the bowl into the basket of the Air Fryer.
Adjust the temperature to 375°F and set the timer for 15 mins. Shake the fryer basket halfway through the cooking time to redistribute the food.

Nutrition: Cal: 186 Protein: 20.4 g Fat: 8 g Carbs: 5.6 g

320. Chicken with Oregano Chimichurri

Prep Time: 5 mins
Servings: 4

Cook Time: 12 mins

Ingredients:
- 700 g chicken breast, cut into 4 pieces
- 1 teaspoon finely grated orange zest
- 1 teaspoon dried oregano
- One small garlic clove, grated
- 2 teaspoon vinegar (red wine, cider, or white wine)
- 1 tablespoon fresh orange juice
- 1/2 cup chopped fresh flat-leaf parsley leaves
- Sea salt and pepper
- 1/4 cup and 2 teaspoons extra virgin olive oil
- 4 cups arugula
- Two bulbs fennel, shaved
- 2 tablespoons whole-grain mustard

Directions: To make chimichurri: In a medium bowl, combine orange zest, oregano, and garlic. Mix in vinegar, orange juice, and parsley and then slowly whisk in ¼ cup of olive oil until emulsified. Season with sea salt and pepper.

Sprinkle the chicken with pepper and salt, and set your air fryer toast oven to 350 degrees F.

Brush the chicken steaks with the remaining olive oil and cook for about 6 mins per side or until evenly browned. Take out from the fryer and let rest for at least 10 mins.

Toss the cooked chicken, greens, and fennel with mustard in a medium bowl; season with salt and pepper.

Serve steak with chimichurri and salad.

Nutrition: Cal: 312 Carbs: 12.8 g Fat: 33.6 g Protein: 29 g

321. Chimichurri Turkey

Prep Time: 20 mins　　　　　　　　　　　　　　　　　　　　　　　　**Cook Time: 50 mins**
Servings: 4

Ingredients:
- 1 lb. Turkey breast
- 1/2 cup chimichurri sauce
- 1/2 cup butter
- ¼ cup parmesan cheese, grated
- ¼ tsp. garlic powder

Directions: Massage the chimichurri sauce over turkey breast, refrigerate in an airtight container for at least a half-hour.

Meanwhile, prepare the herbed butter. Mix the butter, parmesan, and garlic powder, using a hand mixer if you like (this will make it extra creamy)

Preheat your fryer at 350°F and place a wire rack inside. Remove the turkey from the refrigerator and let it to return to room temperature for about 20 mins while the fryer warms.

Place the turkey in the fryer and allow it to cool for 20 mins. Flip and cook on the other side for another 20 mins.

Take care when removing the turkey from the fryer. Place it on a serving dish with the herbed butter.

322. Collard Wraps with Satay Dipping Sauce

Prep Time: 10 mins　　　　　　　　　　　　　　　　　　　　　　　　**Cook Time: 16 mins**
Servings: 6

Ingredients:
- Wraps 4 large collard leaves, stems removed
- Six (200g) grilled chicken breasts, diced
- One medium avocado, sliced
- 1/2 cucumber, thinly sliced
- One cup diced mango
- Six large strawberries, thinly sliced
- 24 mint leaves
- Dipping Sauce
- 2 tablespoons almond butter
- 2 tablespoons coconut cream
- 1 bird eye chili, finely chopped
- 2 tablespoons unsweetened applesauce
- ¼ cup fresh lime juice
- 1 teaspoon sesame oil
- 1 tablespoon apple cider vinegar
- 1 tablespoon tahini
- 1 clove garlic, crushed
- 1 tablespoon grated fresh ginger
- 1/8 teaspoon of sea salt

Directions:

For the chicken breasts:
Start by setting your air fryer to 350 degrees F. Lightly coat the air fryer's basket with oil.

Season the briskets with salt and pepper and place on the prepared basket and fry for 8 mins on each side.

Once done, remove from the air fryer oven and place on a platter to cool slightly then dice.

For the wraps:
Divide the vegetables and diced chicken breasts equally between the four large collard leaves; fold bottom edges over the filling. Then, both sides and roll very tightly to the end of the leaves; secure with toothpicks and cut each in half.

For the sauce:
Combine all the sauce ingredients in a blender and blend until very smooth. Divide among bowls and serve with the wraps.

Nutrition: Cal: 389, Carbs: 11.7 g, Fat: 38.2 g, Protein: 26 g

323. Creamy Chicken Wings

Prep Time: 5 mins
Servings: 4

Cook Time: 30 mins

Ingredients:
- 2 lb. chicken wings
- ¼ cup parmesan, grated
- 1/2 cup heavy cream
- Three garlic cloves; minced
- 3 tbsp. Butter; melted
- 1/2 tsp. Oregano; dried
- 1/2 tsp. basil; dried
- Salt and black pepper to taste.

Directions: In a dish suitable for your air fryer, mix the chicken wings with all the ingredients except the parmesan cheese and toss.
Place the dish in your air fryer and cook at 380°F for 30 mins. Sprinkle on the cheese, set the mixture aside for 10 mins, divide between plates.

Nutrition: Cal: 270 Fat: 12 g Carbs: 6 g Protein: 17 g

324. Crisp Chicken with Mustard Vinaigrette

Prep Time: 15 mins
Servings: 1

Cook Time: 10 mins

Ingredients:

Salad:
- 250 g chicken breast
- One cup shaved Brussels sprouts
- Two cups baby spinach
- Two cups mixed greens
- 1/2 avocado sliced
- Segments of one orange
- 1 teaspoon raw pumpkin seeds
- 1 teaspoon toasted almonds
- 1 teaspoon hemp seeds

Dressing:
- 1/2 shallot, chopped
- One garlic clove, chopped
- 2 teaspoons balsamic vinegar
- 1 teaspoon olive oil
- 1/2 cup fresh orange juice
- 1 teaspoon Dijon mustard
- 1 teaspoon raw honey
- Fresh ground pepper

Directions: In a blender, blend all dressing ingredients until very smooth; set aside.
Set your air fryer to 350 degrees and brush the basket of the oven with oil.
Place the chicken breast on the basket and cook for 10 mins, 5 mins per side.
Remove from the air fryer and transfer to a plate. Allow to rest for 5 mins and then cut into pieces.
Combine all salad ingredients in a bowl; drizzle with dressing and toss to coat well.

Nutrition: Cal: 457, Carbs: 13.6 g, Fat: 37 g, Protein: 31.8 g

325. Crispy Chicken Thighs

Prep Time: 20 mins
Servings: 2

Cook Time: 30 mins

Ingredients:
- 1 lb. chicken thighs
- Two cups roasted pecans
- One cup water
- One cup almond flour
- Salt and pepper

Directions: Preheat the fryer to 400°F.
Season the chicken with salt and pepper and set aside.
Grind the toasted pecans in a food processor until a flour-like consistency is achieved.
Fill one plate with the water, another with the almond flour and a third with the pecans.
Coat the thighs with the almond flour. Mix the remaining flour with the processed pecans.
Dip the thighs in the water and then press into the almond and pecan mix, ensuring the chicken is completely covered.
Cook the chicken in the fryer for twenty-two mins, with an extra five mins, added if you would like the chicken a darker-brown color. Check the temperature has reached 165°F before serving.

326. Crispy Honey Garlic Chicken Wings

Prep Time: 10 mins
Serving: 8

Cook Time: 25 mins

Ingredients:

- 16 chicken wings
- 1/8 C. water
- 1/2 tsp. salt
- 4 tbsp. minced garlic
- ¼ C. butter
- ¼ C. raw honey
- ¾ C. almond flour
- Extra-Virgin Olive Oil

Directions: Rinse off and dry the chicken wings well.
Spray the basket with extra-virgin olive oil.
Coat chicken wings with flour and add coated attachments to the air fryer.
Pour into the Oven basket. Place the basket on the middle shelf of the Air fryer oven. Set temperature to 380°F, and set time to 25 mins. Cook was shaking every 5 mins.
When the timer goes off, cook 5-10 mins at 400 degrees until skin is crispy and dry.
While the chicken is cook, melt the butter in a saucepan and add the garlic. Sauté garlic 5 mins. Add salt and honey, simmer for 20 mins. Add a bit of water after 15 mins to make the sauce doesn't harden.
Remove the wings from the air fryer and coat in sauce.

Nutrition: Cal: 435; Fat: 19 g; Protein: 31 g

327. Crunchy Almond and Salad with Roasted Chicken

Prep Time: 10 mins
Servings: 1

Cook Time: 20 mins

Ingredients:

- Roasted Chicken
- 100g chicken thighs
- Salad
- 1 teaspoon olive oil
- 100g Lacinato kale, sliced into thin strips
- 1/4 cup roasted almonds
- Pinch of salt and pepper
- 1 teaspoon apple cider vinegar
- 1/2 teaspoon extra-virgin olive oil
- 1 tablespoon rosemary
- 1 tablespoon cup sage

Directions:
Place kale in a bowl with olive oil; massage oil until kale is tender; sprinkle with salt and pepper and toss with toasted almonds.
Preheat your air fryer to 360°F.
Sprinkle chicken with salt and pepper; add vinegar and oil and season with rosemary and sage.
Roast in the basket for about 20 mins, turning chicken halfway through cook.
Serve chicken with kale and almond salad.

Nutrition: Cal: 293, Carbs: 10 g, Fat: 16.4 g, Protein: 14 g

328. Curried Coconut Chicken

Prep Time: 5 mins
Servings: 4

Cook Time: 30 mins

Ingredients:

- 1.5 kg chicken - breasts, thighs, or a combo
- One can full-fat coconut milk
- ¼ cup lemon juice
- 1 tbsp. curry powder
- 1 tsp. turmeric
- 1/2-1 tsp. lemon zest
- 1/2 tsp. salt

Directions: Mix the coconut milk, lemon juice, and spices in a bowl.
Pour some onto the pan of your air fryer and then add the chicken pieces.
Pour the rest over the chicken.
Cook at 370 degrees F for 15-20 mins.

Test chicken for doneness by cutting open and looking at the center, if you see any pink, cook for 5-10 mins.
Use 2 forks to shred the chicken.
Add lemon zest and serve with steamed rice or roasted vegetables.

Nutrition: Cal: 411, Carbs: 9.1 g, Fat: 11.9 g, Protein: 19.2 g

329. Fennel Chicken

Prep Time: 5mins   Cook time: 15 mins
Servings: 4

Ingredients:
- *1 1/2 lb. chicken thighs*
- *11/2 cup coconut milk*
- *2 tbsp. garam masala*
- *¾ tbsp. coconut oil, melted*

Directions: Combine the coconut oil and garam masala in a bowl. Pour the mixture over the chicken thighs and let marinate for half an hour.
Preheat your fryer at 375°F. Cook the chicken for 15 mins.
Add the coconut milk, giving it a good stir, then cook for another 10 mins.
Remove the chicken and place on a serving dish.

330. Greek Chicken Meatballs

Prep Time: 10 mins   Cook Time: 15 mins
Servings: 2

Ingredients:
- *1 lb. ground chicken*
- *1 tsp. Greek seasoning*
- *1/2 oz. finely ground pork rinds*
- *1/3 cup feta, crumbled*
- *1/3 cup frozen spinach, drained and thawed*
- *Tzatziki*

Directions: Place all ingredients in a large bowl, and combine with your hands. Take equal-sized portions of this mixture and roll each into a 2-inch ball. Place the balls in your fryer.
Cook the meatballs at 350°F for 12 mins, in several batches, if necessary.
Once they are golden, make sure they have reached an ideal temperature of 165°F and remove from the air fryer. Keep each batch warm. Serve with Tzatziki.

331. Honey Chicken Breasts

Prep Time: 15 mins   Cook Time: 20 mins
Serving: 4

Ingredients:
- *2 chicken breasts, rinsed and halved*
- *1 tablespoon melted butter*
- *1/2 teaspoon ground pepper*
- *3/4 teaspoon sea salt*
- *1 teaspoon paprika*
- *1 teaspoon dried rosemary*
- *2 tablespoons dry white wine*
- *1 tablespoon honey*

Directions: First, pat the chicken breasts dry. Lightly coat them with the butter. Next, add the remaining ingredients.
Transfer to the air fryer basket; cook about 15 mins at 330 degrees F.

Nutrition: Cal: 189; Fat: 14 g; Protein: 11 g

332. Chicken Drumsticks with Garlic & Thyme

Prep Time: 10 mins
Servings: 4

Cook Time: 20 mins

Ingredients:

- 11/2 red onions, diced
- Eight cloves of garlic
- Eight chicken drumsticks
- ¼ teaspoon chili powder

- 2 tablespoons thyme leaves
- Zest of ¼ lemon
- 1 tbsp. extra-virgin olive oil
- 2/3 cup diced tinned tomatoes

- 2 tbsp. sweet balsamic vinegar
- 11/2 teaspoons salt
- 1/2 teaspoon pepper

Directions: Set air fryer to 370 degrees F and add the olive oil, onions, and 1/2 tsp of salt to the pan of your air fryer. Cook for two mins until golden.
Add chicken drumsticks and sprinkle with the rest of the salt, pepper, and chili, then add the thyme, garlic cloves, and lemon zest; add the balsamic vinegar and tomatoes and distribute the mixture between the drumsticks.
Cook for about twenty mins.
Serve the creamy chicken over rice, pasta, or potatoes.

Nutrition: Cal: 329 Carbs: 13.3 g Fat: 0.4 g Protein: 20.8 g

333. Chicken Thighs

Prep Time: 20 mins
Servings: 2

Cook Time: 35 mins

Ingredients:

- Four skin-on bone-in chicken thighs
- 2 tbsp. unsalted butter, melted

- 3 tsp. herbs
- 1/2 tsp. Garlic powder

- ¼ tsp. onion powder

Directions: Using a brush, coat the chicken thighs with the butter. Combine the herbs with the onion powder and garlic powder, then massage into the chicken thighs. Place the thighs in the air fryer.
Cook at 380°F for twenty mins, turning the chicken halfway through to cook on the other side.
When the thighs have achieved a golden color, check the temperature with a meat thermometer. Once they reach 165°F, remove from the air fryer.

334. Korean Chicken Wings

Prep Time: 5 mins
Serving: 8

Cook Time: 10 mins

Ingredients

Wings:

- 2 pounds of chicken wings

- 1 tsp. pepper

- 1 tsp. salt

Sauce:

- 2 packets Splenda
- 1 tbsp. minced garlic
- 1 tbsp. minced ginger

- 1 tbsp. sesame oil
- 1 tsp. agave nectar
- 1 tbsp. mayonnaise

- 2 tbsp. gochujang

Finishing:

- ¼ C. chopped green onions

- 2 tsp. sesame seeds

Directions: Ensure air fryer is preheated to 400 degrees.
Line a small pan with aluminum foil, place a rack onto the pan, and then place in the air fryer.
Season wings with salt and pepper and put them on the grill.
Set the temperature to 160°F, set the time to twenty mins, and fry twenty mins, turning at 10 mins.
While the chicken is air frying, mix all the sauce components together.
Once a thermometer says the chicken has reached 160 degrees, pull out the wings and a bowl.
Pour half of the sauce mixture on top of the wings, mixing well to coat.

Return the coated wings to the air fryer for five mins.
Remove and sprinkle with green onions and sesame seeds.

Nutrition: Cal: 356 Fat: 26 g Protein: 23 g

335. Lemon Pepper Chicken Legs

Prep Time: 20 mins
Servings: 2

Cook Time: 30 mins

Ingredients:
- 8 chicken legs
- 1/2 tsp. garlic powder
- 2 tsp. baking powder
- 1 tbsp. salted butter, melted
- 1 tbsp. lemon-pepper seasoning

Directions: In a bowl, combine the baking powder and garlic powder, and then use this mixture to coat the chicken legs. Place the chicken in the Air Fryer basket.
Cook the chicken legs at 375°F for 25 mins. Halfway through cook, turn them over and let them to cook on the other side.
When the chicken is golden brown, test with a thermometer to make sure it has reached an ideal temperature of 165°F. Remove from the air fryer.
Stir the melted butter and lemon-pepper seasoning, and toss with the chicken legs until the chicken is coated.

336. Lemon Pepper Drumsticks

Prep Time: 5 mins
Servings: 8

Cook Time: 25 mins

Ingredients:
- 8 chicken drumsticks
- 4 tbsp. Salted butter; melted
- 2 tsp. Baking powder
- 1/2 tsp. Garlic powder
- 1 tbsp. lemon-pepper seasoning

Directions: Sprinkle the baking powder and the garlic powder over drumsticks and rub into the skin of the chicken-place the drumsticks in the basket of the air fryer.
Adjust the temperature to 375°F and the time at twenty-five mins.
Use tongs to turn drumsticks halfway through the cook time. When the skin is golden brown, and the internal temperature is at least 165°F, remove from the air fryer.
Take a large bowl, mix butter, and lemon pepper seasoning. Add drumsticks to the bowl and stir until coated.

Nutrition: Cal: 532 Carbs: 1.2 g Protein: 48.3 g Fat: 32.3

337. Mustard Turkey Bites

Prep Time: 5 mins
Servings: 4

Cook Time: 20 mins

Ingredients:
- 1 big turkey breast, skinless; boneless, and cubed
- 4 garlic cloves; minced
- 1 tbsp. mustard
- 1 1/2 tbsp. extra-virgin olive oil
- Salt and pepper

Directions: In a bowl, mix the chicken with the garlic and the other ingredients and toss.
Put the turkey in the basket of your air fryer, cook at 360°F for twenty mins, divide among plates and serve with a side salad.

Nutrition: Cal: 240 Carbs: 6 g Fat: 12 g Protein: 15 g

338. Nutmeg Chicken Thighs

Prep Time: 15 mins   Cook Time: 20 mins
Servings: 4

Ingredients:
- 2 lb. chicken thighs
- 1/2 tsp. nutmeg, ground
- A pinch of salt and pepper
- 2 tbsp. Olive oil

Directions: Season the chicken thighs with pepper and salt, and rub with the rest of the ingredients.
Place chicken thighs in the basket of the air fryer, cook at 360°F for fifteen mins on each side, divide among plates.

Nutrition: Cal: 271 Carbs: 6 g Fat: 12 g Protein: 13 g

339. Chicken Parmesan

Prep Time: 5 mins   Cook Time: 225 mins
Serving: 2

Ingredients:
- 2 sizeable white meat chicken breasts, approximately 5-6 ounces
- One cup of breadcrumbs (Panko brand works well)
- 2 medium-sized eggs
- 1 tablespoon of dried oregano
- One cup of marinara sauce
- 2 slices of provolone cheese
- 1 tablespoon of parmesan
- Pinch of salt and pepper

Directions: Cover the air fryer's basket with a foil liner, leaving the edges uncovered to allow air to circulate through the basket.
Preheat the air fryer to 350 degrees.
In a bowl, beat the eggs until, the yolks and whites are fully combined, and set aside.
In a separate bowl, combine the breadcrumbs, salt, oregano and pepper, and set aside.
One by one, dip the raw chicken breasts into the bowl with the dry ingredients, coating both sides, dipping into the bowl with wet ingredients, and then dropping back into the dry ingredients.
Lay the coated chicken breasts on the foil covering the air fryer basket in a single flat layer.
Set the air fryer timer for ten mins.
The air fryer will turn off, and the chicken should be halfway cooked and the breaded coating should begin to brown.
Turn each piece of chicken over to ensure complete frying.
Set the air fryer to 320 degrees for another ten mins.
While the chicken is cook, pour half the marinara sauce into a 7-inch heatproof skillet.
After fifteen mins, when the air fryer shuts off, remove the fried chicken breasts with tongs and set in the marinara-covered pan.
Pour the rest of the sauce over the fried chicken, then place the provolone slices on top both and spread the parmesan cheese all over the pan.
Reset the air fryer to 350 degrees F for 5 mins.
After 5 mins, when the air fryer shuts off, remove the dish from the air fryer using tongs or oven mitts. The chicken will be perfectly crisped and the cheese melted and lightly toasted.

340. Fried Chicken Roast Served with Fruit Compote

Prep Time: 15 mins   Cook Time: 50 mins
Servings: 12

Ingredients:
- One full chicken, dissected
- 2 tablespoons olive oil
- 2 tablespoons chopped garlic
- 12 dried apricots, sliced
- 16 dried figs, coarsely chopped
- 1 tablespoon chopped fresh thyme
- 1 tablespoon chopped fresh rosemary
- Fruit Compote
- One apple, diced
- 1/2 cup red grapes, halved, seeds removed
- 1/2 cup chopped red onion
- 1/2 cup cider vinegar
- 1/2 cup dry white wine
- 2 teaspoons liquid stevia
- 2 1/2 teaspoon salt
- 1 1/2 teaspoon pepper

Directions: In a small bowl, mix together thyme, garlic, rosemary, salt, and pepper and rub the mixture over the pork.
Light your air fryer and set it to 320°F, place the chicken on the basket and cook for ten mins.

Increase the temperature and cook for another ten mins, turning the chicken pieces once. Increase the temperature once more time to 400° F and cook for five mins to get a crispy finish.
Make Fruit Compote: In a saucepan, combine all ingredients and cook over medium heat, stirring, for about twenty-five mins. Once the chicken is cooked, serve with a spoon of fruit compote

Nutrition: Cal: 511 kcal, Carbs: 15 g, Fat: 36.8 g, Protein: 31.5 g

341. Roasted Chicken

Prep Time: 10mins
Servings: 4

Cook time: 25 mins

Ingredients:
- 6 lb. whole chicken
- 1 tbsp. minced garlic
- One white onion, peeled and halved
- 3 tbsp. butter
- 1 tsp. olive oil

Directions: Pre-heat the fryer at 360°F.
Massage the chicken with oil and the minced garlic.
Place the peeled and halved onion, as well as the butter, inside of the chicken.
Cook the chicken in the fryer for 75 mins.
Take care when removing the chicken from the fryer, then carve.

342. Spiced Chicken Breasts

Prep Time: 15 mins
Servings: 4

Cook Time: 10 mins

Ingredients:
- 4 chicken breasts, skinless and boneless
- 1 tbsp. parsley; chopped
- 1 tsp. smoked paprika
- 1 tsp. garlic powder
- 1 tsp. chili powder
- A pinch of salt and pepper
- A drizzle of olive oil

Directions: Season chicken with salt and pepper and rub it with oil and all other ingredients except the parsley.
Put the chicken breasts in the basket of the air fryer and cook at 350°F for ten mins on each side.
Divide among plates and sprinkle with parsley.

Nutrition: Cal: 222 Carbs: 6 g Fat: 11 g Protein: 12 g

343. Spiced Duck Legs

Prep Time: 5 mins
Servings: 4

Cook Time: 25 mins

Ingredients:
- 2 garlic cloves; minced
- 2 tsp. five-spice
- 1 tsp. hot chili powder
- A pinch of salt and pepper
- 2 tbsp. extra-virgin olive oil

Directions: Take a bowl and mix the duck legs with all the other ingredients and rub them in well.
Put the duck legs in the basket of your air fryer and cook at 380°F for twenty-five mins, flipping them halfway.
Divide between plates.

Nutrition: Cal: 287 Carbs: 6 g Fat: 12 g Protein: 17 g

344. Stir-Fried Chicken with Water Chestnuts

Prep Time: 10 mins
Servings: 4

Cook Time: 15 mins

Ingredients:
- Four small chicken breasts, sliced
- One small cabbage, chopped
- Three garlic cloves, chopped
- 1 teaspoon Chinese five-spice powder
- 1 cup dried plums
- 2 tablespoons sesame oil
- ¼ cup wheat-free tamari
- 1 cup water chestnuts
- Toasted sesame seeds

Directions: Start by preheating your air fryer at 370 degrees F.
Heat sesame oil in fryer pan over medium heat; mix all the ingredients, except sesame seeds, and transfer to the air fryer.
Cook until cabbage and chicken are tender for 15-20 mins.
Serve warm sprinkled with toasted sesame seeds.

Nutrition: Cal: 404 kcal, Carbs: 11.3 g, Fat: 29 g, Protein: 22 g

345. Strawberry Turkey

Prep Time: 15 mins
Servings: 2

Cook Time: 25 mins

Ingredients:
- 2 lb. turkey breast
- 1 tbsp. olive oil
- 1 cup fresh strawberries
- Salt and pepper

Directions: Preheat your fryer to 375°F.
Massage the turkey breast with oil before seasoning with a generous amount of salt and pepper.
Cook the turkey in the fryer for 15 mins. Turn the turkey and cook for another 15 mins.
Blend the strawberries in a food processor until smooth.
Pile the strawberries on the top of the turkey and cook for another 7 mins.

346. Sweet and Sour Chicken

Prep Time: 20 mins
Serving: 6

Cook Time: 25 mins

Ingredients:
- Three Chicken Breasts, cubed
- 1/2 Cup Flour
- 1/2 Cup Cornstarch
- Two Red Peppers, sliced
- One Onion, chopped
- Two Carrots, julienned
- 2 Tbsps. Cornstarch
- 1/3 Cup Vinegar
- 2/3 Cup Water
- 3/4 Cup Sugar
- 1/4 cup Soy sauce
- 1 Tbsp. Ketchup

Directions: Preheat the air fryer oven to 375 degrees.
Combine flour, cornstarch, and chicken in an airtight container and shake to combine.
Remove chicken from container and shake off excess flour.
Add the chicken to the tray of the Air Fryer and cook for twenty mins.
In a saucepan, whisk together water, vinegar, soy sauce, sugar, and ketchup. Bring to a boil over medium heat, reduce heat, then simmer for two mins.
After chicken has cooked for twenty mins, add vegetables and sauce mixture to the air fryer and cook for an additional five mins.

347. Teriyaki Chicken Wings

Prep Time: 15 mins
Servings: 2

Cook Time: 30 mins

Ingredients:
- 2 lb. chicken wings
- ¼ tsp. ground ginger
- 2 tsp. minced garlic

- *1/2 cup sugar-free teriyaki sauce*
- *2 tsp. baking powder*

Directions: In a small bowl, combine the garlic, ginger, and teriyaki sauce. Place the chicken wings in a separate, larger bowl and pour the mixture over them. Stir to coat until chicken is well covered.
Refrigerate for at least an hour.
Remove the marinated wings from the fridge and add the baking powder, stirring again to coat. Then place the chicken in the basket of air fryer.
Cook for twenty-five mins at 400 degrees F, shaking the basket intermittently throughout the cook time.
When the wings are 165 degrees F and golden brown, remove from the fryer, and serve immediately.

348. Teriyaki Duck Legs

Prep Time: 15 mins   **Cook time: 2 hours**
Servings: 6

Ingredients:
- *3 lbs. duck legs*
- *1/2 cup teriyaki sauce*
- *2 tbsp. malt vinegar*
- *2 tbsp. soy sauce*

Directions: Place duck legs, skin side up, in a baking dish.
In a small bowl, whisk together remaining ingredients and pour around duck legs. The liquid should reach the skin level. If not, add water until it does.
Set the convection oven at 300 degrees F for 60 mins. After 5 mins, place the ducks in the range and cook 90 mins. Remove duck from the oven. Pour the cook liquid into a small saucepan, skim off the fat and reserve. Bring sauce to a boil and cook until reduced, about 10 mins, stirring occasionally.
Place the duck legs in the fryer basket and brush with reserved fat and sauce. Place the basket in the oven and set to cook at 400°F for 10 mins. Turn the duck halfway through cook and brush with fat and sauce again.

Nutrition: Cal: 608 Fat: 20 g Carbs: 6 g Protein: 101 g

349. Turkey Turnovers

Prep Time: 10 mins   **Cook time: 10 mins**
Servings: 8

Ingredients:
- *2 cups turkey, cooked & chopped*
- *1 cup cheddar cheese, grated*
- *1 cup broccoli, cooked & chopped*
- *2 cans of refrigerated crescent rolls*
- *1/2 cup mayo*
- *1/2 tsp. salt*
- *¼ tsp. pepper*

Directions: In a large bowl, combine all ingredients, except rolls, mix well.
Separate each can of rolls into 4 squares, press holes to seal.
Put a spoon of turkey mixture into the center of each square. Fold in diagonally and seal edges.
Set oven to bake at 375°F for 15 mins.
Brush the tops of the pies with more mayo. After oven has preheated for 5 mins, place turnovers on baking sheet and cook 10-12 mins or until golden brown.

Nutrition: Cal: 309 Fat: 21 g Carbs: 15 g Protein: 15 g

350. Crispy & Spicy Chicken Thighs

Prep Time: 15 mins   **Cook Time: 35 mins**
Servings: 4

Ingredients
- *500g chicken thighs*
- *1 teaspoon red pepper flakes*
- *1 teaspoon sweet paprika*
- *1 teaspoon freshly ground black pepper*
- *1 tablespoon garlic powder*
- *1-2 tablespoons coconut oil*
- *1 teaspoon dried oregano*
- *1 teaspoon curry powder*

Directions: Start by preheating your air fryer to 370° F and prepare the fryer basket by lining it with parchment paper.
Combine all the spices in a bowl and set aside.

Now arrange the thighs on the prepared basket with the skin side down (remember first to pat the skin dry with kitchen towels). Sprinkle the top side of the chicken thighs with half the seasoning mix, turn them over and sprinkle the bottom side with the remaining seasoning mix.

Bake for about 30 mins until the chicken thighs are cooked through and the skin is crispy.

Turn once halfway through cook.

To make the skin crispier, increase the heat to 400° F, and bake for an additional five mins.

Nutrition: Cal: 281, Carbs: 3 g, Fat: 13 g, Protein: 36.8 g

351. Zingy & Nutty Chicken Wings

Prep Time: 5 mins   **Cook Time: 18 mins**
Serving: 4

Ingredients:
- 1 tablespoon fish sauce
- 1 tablespoon fresh lemon juice
- 1 teaspoon sugar
- 12 chicken middle wings, cut into half
- 2 fresh lemongrass stalks, chopped finely
- ¼ cup unsalted cashews, crushed

Directions: In a bowl, mix sugar, fish sauce, and lime juice.

Add wings and coat generously with mixture. Refrigerate to marinate for about 1-2 hours.

Preheat the air fryer oven to 355° F.

In the air fryer oven, place lemongrass stalks—Cook for about 2-3 mins. Remove the cashew mixture from the oven and transfer it to a bowl. Now, set the air fryer to 390° F.

Place the chicken wings into. Cook for about 13-15 mins further.

Transfer the wings into serving plates. Sprinkle with cashew mixture.

352. Lemongrass Chicken

Prep time: 10 mins   **Cook time: 20 mins**
Servings: 5

Ingredients:
- Four garlic cloves, peeled and crushed
- 2 tablespoons fish sauce
- One bunch lemongrass, bottom removed and trimmed
- 1-inch piece ginger root, peeled and chopped
- 3 tablespoons coconut aminos
- One cup coconut milk
- 1 teaspoon Chinese five spice powder
- Ten chicken drumsticks
- 1 teaspoon butter
- One yellow onion, peeled and chopped
- 1 tablespoon lime juice
- ¼ cup cilantro, diced
- Salt and pepper

Directions: In a food processor, blend the lemongrass with garlic, ginger, amines, fish sauce and the five-spice powder and mix well. Add the coconut milk and pulse again.

Add the onion, stir and cook for five mins. Add the chicken, salt and pepper, mix and cook for one minute. Add the coconut milk and lemongrass mixture, stir, cover, and cook for fifteen mins.

Add more salt and pepper and lemon juice, stir, divide among plates and serve with coriander sprinkled on top.

Nutrition: Cal: 400, Fat: 18 g, Carbs: 6 g, Proteins: 20 g

353. Salsa Chicken

Prep time: 10 mins   **Cook time: 25 mins**
Servings: 5

Ingredients:
- ¾ teaspoon cumin
- 1 pound chicken breast, skinless and boneless
- 1 cup chunky salsa
- Dried oregano
- Salt and pepper

Directions: Add salt and pepper to the chicken to taste and add to the oven.
Add the oregano, cumin and sauce, stir, cover, and cook for 25 mins.
Transfer the chicken with the sauce to a bowl, cut the meat into pieces with a fork and serve with tortillas on the side.

Nutrition: Cal: 125, Fat: 3 g, Carbs: 3 g, Protein: 22 g

354. Sweet Chicken

Prep time: 10 mins
Servings: 4

Cook time: 10 mins

Ingredients:
- ½ cup fish sauce
- One cup lime juice
- 2 pounds chicken thighs, boneless and skinless
- 2 tablespoons coconut nectar
- 2 teaspoons cilantro, diced
- ¼ cup olive oil
- 1 teaspoon ginger, grated
- 1 teaspoon fresh mint, chopped

Directions: In a bowl, toss the lemon juice with the fish sauce, ginger, mint and cilantro, olive oil, coconut nectar, and beat well.
Pour over the chicken and cook for ten mins.

Nutrition: Cal: 300, Fat: 5 g, Carbs: 23 g, Protein: 32 g

355. Chicken with Vegetables

Prep Time: 10 Mins
Servings: 4

Cook Time: 50 mins

Ingredients:
- Eight chicken thighs, skinless and boneless
- Ten oz roasted red peppers, sliced
- Two cups cherry tomatoes
- 1 1/2 lbs potatoes, cut into chunks
- 4 tablespoon extra-virgin olive oil
- 1 teaspoon dried oregano
- Five garlic cloves, crushed
- 1/4 cup capers, drained
- Salt and Pepper

Directions: Select bake, set temperature 390 degrees F, timer for 50 mins. Press start to preheat the oven.
Season chicken with salt and pepper.
Heat 2 tbsp of oil in a skillet over medium-high heat. Add chicken and sear until brown on both sides.
Place chicken in a baking dish. Stir in potatoes, oregano, red peppers, garlic, capers, and tomatoes. Drizzle with olive oil.
Bake for 50 mins.

Nutrition: Cal 837, Fat 36.3 g, Carbs 36.7 g, Protein 89.3 g

356. Chicken Zucchini Casserole

Prep Time: 10 Mins
Servings: 8

Cook Time: 40 mins

Ingredients:
- 2 1/2 lbs. chicken breasts, boneless and cubed
- Five zucchini, cut into cubes
- Twelve oz roasted red peppers, drained and chopped
- 1 teaspoon xanthan gum
- 1 tablespoon tomato paste
- 5.5 oz coconut cream
- Ten garlic cloves
- 2/3 cup mayo
- 1 teaspoon salt

Directions: Select bake, set temperature 390 degrees F, timer for 35 mins. Press start to preheat the oven.
Add chicken and zucchini to the casserole dish. Cover pan with aluminum foil. Bake for 35 mins.
Meanwhile, in a bowl, stir together the remaining ingredients.
Pour the mixture bowl over chicken and zucchini and bake for five mins.

Nutrition: Cal 429, Fat 22 g, Carbs 14.6 g, Protein 43.9 g

357. Chinese Chicken Wings

Prep Time: 10 Mins
Servings: 2

Cook Time: 30 mins

Ingredients:
- *Four chicken wings*
- *1 tablespoon Chinese spice*
- *1 teaspoon mixed spice*
- *1 tablespoon soy sauce*
- *Salt and Pepper*

Directions: Select air fry, set temperature 350 degrees F, timer for 30 mins. Press start to preheat the oven.
Add chicken wings into the bowl. Add remaining ingredients and mix well.
Transfer chicken wings into the basket of the air fryer and fry for fifteen mins.

Nutrition: Cal 429 Fat 17.3 g Carbs 2.1 g Protein 62.4 g

358. Delicious Curried Chicken

Prep Time: 10 Mins
Servings: 4

Cook Time: 40 mins

Ingredients:
- *Four chicken breasts, skinless and boneless*
- *4 tsp. curry powder*
- *1/3 cup butter*
- *1/3 cup honey*
- *1/4 cup mustard*

Directions: Select bake, set temperature 375 degrees F, timer for forty mins. Press start to preheat the oven.
Add honey and butter in a saucepan and heat over low heat until butter is melted.
Remove saucepan from heat and mix in curry powder and mustard.
Arrange chicken in a casserole dish and pour butter mixture over chicken and bake for forty mins.

Nutrition: Cal 552, Fat 29.3 g, Carbs 27.9 g, Protein 45.2 g

359. Cheesy Parmesan Chicken

Prep Time: 10 Mins
Servings: 4

Cook Time: 35 mins

Ingredients:
- *Four chicken breasts*
- *1 cup breadcrumbs*
- *1 cup parmesan cheese, shredded*
- *1/4 cup olive oil*
- *Salt and Pepper*

Directions: Select bake, set temperature 350 degrees F, timer for 35 mins. Press start to preheat the oven.
Season chicken with salt, pepper and olive oil.
In a shallow dish, mix together parmesan and bread crumbs. Coat the chicken with parmesan and breadcrumb mixture and place in the baking dish.
Bake chicken for 35 mins.

Nutrition: Cal 564, Fat 29.7 g, Carbs 20.3 g, Protein 53.1 g

360. Honey Mustard Sauce Chicken

Prep Time: 10 Mins
Servings: 6

Cook Time: 40 mins

Ingredients:
- *Six chicken thighs, bone-in & skin-on*
- *1/4 cup yellow mustard*
- *1/2 cup honey*

- *Salt and Pepper*

Directions: Select bake, set temperature 350 degrees F, timer for 30 mins. Press start to preheat the oven.
Season chicken with salt and pepper and place in baking dish.
Mix honey and yellow mustard and pour over chicken and bake for 30 mins.
Spoon honey mustard mixture over chicken and bake chicken for another ten mins.

Nutrition: Cal 119, Fat 1.4 g, Carbs 23.9 g, Protein 4.5 g

361. Mexican Chicken Lasagna

Prep Time: 10 Mins   **Cook Time: 15 mins**
Servings: 15

Ingredients:
- *Four tortillas*
- *1 1/2 lbs chicken breast, cooked and shredded*
- *2 teaspoon ground cumin*
- *2 tablespoon chili powder*
- *One cup of salsa*
- *3/4 cup sour cream*
- *Two cup cheese, shredded*
- *1 teaspoon dry onion, minced*

Directions: Select bake, set temperature 390 degrees F, timer for fifteen mins. Press start to preheat the oven.
Mix chicken, dried onion, salsa, cumin, chili powder, and sour cream.
Spray baking sheet with cook spray.
Spread half of chicken mixture in baking dish then place two tortillas on top.
Sprinkle 1/2 cheese over the tortillas then repeat the layers.
Bake for fifteen mins.

Nutrition: Cal 160, Fat 9 g, Carbs 5.3 g, Protein 14.5 g

362. Fajita Chicken

Prep Time: 10 Mins   **Cook Time: 15 mins**
Servings: 4

Ingredients:
- *Four chicken breasts, make horizontal cuts on each piece*
- *2 tablespoon fajita seasoning*
- *One onion, sliced*
- *One bell pepper, sliced*
- *2 tablespoon extra-virgin olive oil*

Directions: Select air fry, set temperature 380 degrees F, timer for fifteen mins. Press start to preheat the oven.
Rub oil and seasoning over the chicken breast.
Place chicken in the basket of the air fryer and top with bell peppers and onion.
Cook for fifteen mins.

Nutrition: Cal 374, Fat 17.9 g, Carbs 8 g, Protein 42.8 g

363. Garlicky Chicken Wings

Prep Time: 10 Mins   **Cook Time: 20 mins**
Servings: 4

Ingredients:
- *Twelve chicken wings*
- *1 tablespoon chili powder*
- *1/2 tablespoon baking powder*
- *1 teaspoon granulated garlic*
- *1/2 teaspoon sea salt*

Directions: Select air fry, set temperature 410 degrees F, timer for twenty mins. Press start to preheat the oven.
Add chicken wings into a bowl and stir with remaining ingredients.
Transfer chicken wings in the basket and air fry for 20 mins.

Nutrition: Cal 580, Fat 22.6 g, Carbs 2.4 g, Protein 87.1 g

364. Herb Garlic Meatballs

Prep Time: 10 Mins
Servings: 6

Cook Time: 25 mins

Ingredients:
- 2 lbs. ground chicken
- teaspoon dry parsley
- One onion, diced
- Two cups bread crumbs
- 1/2 cup milk
- Two eggs, lightly beaten
- Four garlic cloves, minced
- Salt and Pepper

Directions: Line baking sheet with parchment paper and set aside.
Select bake, set temperature 390 degrees F, timer for twenty-five mins. Press start.
Add all ingredients into the mixing bowl and stir until well combined.
Make 1-inch balls from meat mixture and arrange on a baking sheet. Bake meatballs for twenty-five mins.

Nutrition: Cal 471 Fat 15 g Carbs 29.4 g Protein 51.4 g

365. Hot Chicken Wings

Prep Time: 10 Mins
Servings: 4

Cook Time: 25 mins

Ingredients:
- Two lbs chicken wings
- 1/2 teaspoon Tabasco
- 6 tablespoon butter, melted
- twelve oz hot sauce
- 1/2 teaspoon Worcestershire sauce

Directions: Select air fry, set temperature 380 degrees F, timer for fifty-five mins. Press start.
Add chicken wings into the basket and cook for twenty-five mins.
Meanwhile, in a bowl, stir together Worcestershire sauce, hot sauce, and butter. Set aside.
Add cooked chicken wings into the sauce bowl and stir.

Nutrition: Cal 594 Fat 34.4 g Carbs 1.6 g Protein 66.2 g

366. Italian Turkey

Prep Time: 10 Mins
Servings: 4

Cook Time: 45 mins

Ingredients:
- 1 1/2 lbs. turkey breast tenderloin
- 1 tsp. Italian seasoning
- 1/2 tbsp extra-virgin olive oil
- 1/2 tsp. salt
- 1/4 tsp. pepper

Directions: Select bake, set temperature 390 degrees F, timer for 45 mins.
Brush turkey tenderloin with oil and rub with Italian seasoning, salt and pepper.
Place turkey in a baking dish and bake for 40-45 mins or until internal temperature reaches 165 degrees F.

Nutrition: Cal 200 Fat 4.3 g Carbs 0.2 g Protein 42.2 g

367. Juicy Baked Chicken Wings

Prep Time: 10 Mins
Servings: 5

Cook Time: 50 mins

Ingredients:
- 3 lbs. chicken wings
- Four garlic cloves, minced
- One cup honey
- 2 tbsp BBQ sauce
- 1/2 cup soy sauce
- 2 tbsp olive oil
- Salt and Pepper

Directions: Line the baking sheet with aluminum foil and set aside.

Select bake, set temperature 350 degrees F, timer for fifty mins. Press start to preheat the oven.
Season chicken wings with pepper and salt and arrange on a baking sheet in a single layer.
In a bowl, mix together BBQ sauce, soy sauce, honey, garlic, and olive oil and pour over chicken wings.
Bake the chicken wings for fifty mins.

Nutrition: Cal 798 Fat 25.8 g Carbs 60.9 g Protein 80.7 g

368. Juicy Garlic Chicken

Prep Time: 10 Mins
Servings: 6

Cook Time: 40 mins

Ingredients:
- 2 lbs chicken thighs, skinless and boneless
- 2 tablespoon fresh parsley, chopped
- Lemon juice
- Eight garlic cloves, sliced
- 2 tablespoon olive oil
- Salt and Pepper

Directions: Select bake, set temperature 390 degrees F, timer for forty mins.
Place chicken on roasting pan and season with salt and pepper.
Sprinkle garlic and parsley, lemon juice and olive oil on the top of the chicken.
Bake for forty mins.

Nutrition: Cal 336 Fat 16 g Carbs 1.6 g Protein 44.1 g

369. Pepper Lemon Chicken Breasts

Prep Time: 10 Mins
Servings: 4

Cook Time: 30 mins

Ingredients:
- Four chicken breasts, skinless and boneless
- 1/2 teaspoon paprika
- 1 teaspoon lemon pepper seasoning
- Four teaspoon lemon juice
- Four teaspoon butter, sliced
- 1 teaspoon garlic powder
- Salt and Peppe

Directions: Select bake, set temperature 350 degrees F, timer for thirty mins. Dress chicken with salt and pepper and place in the baking dish.
Pour lemon juice over chicken. Stir together garlic powder, paprika, and lemon pepper seasoning and drizzle over chicken.
Add butter slices on top of the chicken and cook for thirty mins.

Nutrition: Cal 323 Fat 14.8 g Carbs 2.5 g Protein 42.8 g

370. Pepper Lemon Baked Chicken Legs

Prep Time: 10 Mins
Servings: 6

Cook Time: 30 mins

Ingredients:
- 2 1/2 lbs. chicken legs
- 1 1/2 tablespoon lemon pepper spice
- 2 teaspoon extra-virgin olive oil
- 2 tablespoon lemon juice
- 1/2 teaspoon garlic powder

Directions: Add chicken legs to the zip-lock bag.
Add the remaining ingredients over chicken. Seal the bag and shake and place in the refrigerator for one hour.
Select bake, set temperature 390 degrees F, timer for thirty mins.
Place marinated chicken legs on a rack over a baking sheet and bake for thirty mins.

Nutrition: Cal 374 Fat 15.6 g Carbs 0.3 g Protein 54.8 g

371. Pepper Lemon Chicken

Prep Time: 10 Mins   **Cook Time: 35 mins**
Servings: 4

Ingredients:

- *Four chicken thighs*
- *1 tablespoon lemon pepper seasoning*
- *2 tablespoon lemon juice*
- *1/2 teaspoon Italian seasoning*
- *1/2 teaspoon onion powder*
- *2 tablespoon extra-virgin olive oil*
- *1/2 teaspoon paprika*
- *1 teaspoon garlic powder*
- *1 teaspoon salt*

Directions: Select bake, set temperature 390 degrees F, timer for thirty-five mins.
Add chicken in a bowl.
Stir lemon juice and olive oil and pour over chicken.
Mix paprika, onion powder, garlic powder, Italian seasoning, lemon pepper seasoning, salt and rub all over the chicken.
Dispose chicken on a roasting pan and bake for thirty-five mins.

Nutrition: Cal 338 Fat 17.7 g Carbs 2.2 g Protein 40.9 g

372. Lemon Rosemary Chicken

Prep Time: 10 Mins   **Cook Time: 25 mins**
Servings: 2

Ingredients:

- *Two chicken breasts, boneless and skinless*
- *One garlic clove, minced*
- *Twelve oz small potatoes, halved*
- *One spring rosemary, chopped*
- *1 tablespoon rosemary leaves*
- *1/2 tablespoon olive oil*
- *1 teaspoon red chili flakes*
- *Lemon juice*
- *Salt*

Directions: Select bake, set temperature 390 degrees F, timer for twenty-five mins. Press start to preheat the oven.
Add potatoes to boiling water and cook for ten mins. Drain and set aside.
In a bowl, place the chicken and add rosemary, chili, garlic, lemon juice, rosemary, and oil.
In a skillet, place the chicken over medium-high heat for five mins.
Transfer the chicken to a baking dish and add potatoes.
Place sheet in the oven and roast for twenty-five mins.

Nutrition: Cal 446 Fat 15.5 g Carbs 29.2 g Protein 46 g

373. Old Bay Chicken

Prep Time: 10 Mins   **Cook Time: 45 mins**
Servings: 4

Ingredients:

- *Three lbs chicken wings*
- *1 tablespoon old bay seasoning*
- *2 teaspoons xanthan gum*
- *Lemon juice*
- *1/2 cup butter, melted*

Directions: Select air fry, set temperature 360 degrees F, timer for forty-five mins.
Add chicken wings, old bay seasoning, and xanthan gum to a bowl and toss well.
Transfer chicken wings to the basket and air fry for forty-five mins.
In a bowl stir lemon juice and melted butter.
Add cooked chicken wings to the butter lemon mixture.

Nutrition: Cal 853 Fat 48.2 g Carbs 4.1 g Protein 99 g

374. Olive Tomato Chicken

Prep Time: 10 Mins
Servings: 4

Cook Time: 22 mins

Ingredients:
- Four chicken breast, boneless and halves
- Fifteen olives, pitted and halved
- Two cups cherry tomatoes
- 3 tablespoon extra-virgin olive oil
- 3 tablespoon capers, rinsed and drained
- Salt and Pepper

Directions: Select bake, set temperature 390 degrees F, timer for twenty mins.
In a bowl, mix tomatoes, olives, capers with 2 tablespoons of olive oil. Set aside.
Season chicken with salt and pepper.
Heat the remaining oil in a skillet over high heat.
Place the chicken in the pan and cook for four mins.
Transfer chicken to the pan, top with tomato mixture and bake for twenty mins.

Nutrition: Cal 241 Fat 15 g Carbs 4.9 g Protein 22.3 g

375. Parmesan Chicken & Vegetables

Prep Time: 10 Mins
Servings: 4

Cook Time: 30 mins

Ingredients:
- Four chicken breasts, skinless and boneless
- 1/2 teaspoon garlic powder
- 1/2 cup Parmesan cheese, grated
- One zucchini, sliced
- 1/2 cup Italian seasoned bread crumbs
- Four tablespoon butter, melted
- 1/2 lb baby potatoes cut into fourths
- One yellow squash, sliced
- 2 tablespoon extra-virgin olive oil
- Salt and Pepper

Directions: Spray a baking sheet with cook spray and set aside.
Select bake, set temperature 350 F, timer for thirty mins. Press Start to preheat the oven.
Place melted butter in a shallow dish.
In another dish mix together parmesan cheese, bread crumbs, and garlic powder.
Season chicken with salt and pepper then dip into the melted butter and coat with cheese mixture.
Place coated chicken in an ovenproof dish.
In a bowl, add potatoes, zucchini, yellow squash, and olive oil and mix.
Add vegetables to the baking dish around the chicken and bake for thirty mins.

Nutrition: Cal 579 Fat 32.7 g Carbs 20.4 g Protein 50.2 g

376. Parmesan Pesto Chicken

Prep Time: 10 Mins
Servings: 4

Cook Time: 25 mins

Ingredients:
- Four chicken breasts, skinless & boneless
- 1/2 cup parmesan cheese, shredded
- 1/2 cup pesto
- Salt and Pepper

Directions: Select bake, set temperature 390 degrees F, timer for twenty-five mins. Press Start to preheat the oven.
Season chicken with salt and pepper and place into the baking dish.
Take pesto on top of the chicken and sprinkle with cheese.
Bake chicken for twenty-five mins.

Nutrition: Cal 449 Fat 26.2 g Carbs 2.4 g Protein 48.9 g

377. Baked Chicken Breasts

Prep Time: 10 Mins
Servings: 4

Cook Time: 30 mins

Ingredients:
- Four chicken breasts, bone-in & skin-on
- 1/4 tsp. pepper
- 1 tsp. olive oil
- 1/2 tsp. kosher salt

Directions: Insert wire rack in rack position 6. Select bake, set temperature 375 F, timer for 30 mins. Press start to preheat the oven.
Season chicken with olive oil, pepper and salt.
Place chicken on roasting pan and bake for 30 mins.

Nutrition: Cal 288 Fat 12 g Carbs 0.1 g Protein 42.3 g

378. Pumpkin Chicken Lasagna

Prep Time: 10 Mins
Servings: 5

Cook Time: 35 mins

Ingredients:
- Nine lasagna noodles
- One lb chicken, boneless and chopped
- One cup milk
- Fourteen oz can cream of pumpkin soup
- One teaspoon olive oil
- 1 1/2 cups mozzarella, shredded
- Sixteen oz pasta sauce

Directions: Select bake, set temperature 390 degrees F, timer for thirty-five mins.
In a bowl, combine soup and milk. Set aside.
Heat oil in a saucepan over medium heat.
Add chicken in a saucepan and sauté until cooked.
Stir in pasta sauce and simmer for fifteen mins.
Spread 1/3 sauce in the baking dish then place three noodles and top with 1/3 of the sauce. Repeat layers twice. Sprinkle the noodles with cheese.
Bake for thirty-five mins.

Nutrition: Cal 597 Fat 10.9 g Carbs 77.6 g Protein 45.1 g

379. Chicken Meatballs

Prep Time: 10 Mins
Servings: 4

Cook Time: 25 mins

Ingredients:
- One lb ground chicken
- 1 teaspoon dried onion flakes
- One garlic clove, minced
- One egg, lightly beaten
- 2 tablespoons olive oil
- 1 tablespoon parsley, chopped
- 1/2 cup bread crumbs
- 1/2 cup parmesan, grated
- 1/4 teaspoon red pepper flakes
- 1/2 teaspoon dried oregano
- 1/2 teaspoon salt
- 1/4 teaspoon pepper

Directions: Line sheet with baking paper and set aside.
Select bake, set temperature 390 degrees F, timer for twenty-five mins. Press start to preheat the oven.
Add all ingredients to mixing bowl and mix until well combined.
Make balls from the meat mixture and arrange on a baking sheet.
Bake meatballs for twenty-five mins.

Nutrition: Cal 385 Fat 19.7 g Carbs 11.1 g Protein 39.8 g

380. Simple Chicken Thighs

Prep Time: 10 Mins
Servings: 6

Cook Time: 35 mins

Ingredients:
- *Six chicken thighs*
- *2 tsp. poultry seasoning*
- *2 tbsp olive oil*
- *Salt and Pepper*

Directions: Select bake, set temperature 390 degrees F, timer for forty mins.
Brush chicken with olive oil and rub with poultry seasoning, salt and pepper.
Place chicken on baking sheet and bake for 35-40 mins or until internal temperature reaches 165 degrees F.

Nutrition: Cal 319 Fat 15.5 g Carbs 0.3 g Protein 42.3 g

381. Simply Baked Chicken

Prep Time: 10 Mins
Servings: 4

Cook Time: 45 mins

Ingredients:
- *Four chicken breasts, skinless and boneless*
- *Five oz yogurt*
- *1/2 cup parmesan cheese, grated*
- *1 teaspoon garlic powder*
- *Salt and Pepper*

Directions: Select bake, set temperature 375 degrees F, timer for forty-five mins.
Spray the baking sheet with cook spray. Season chicken with salt and pepper and place in the baking dish.
Mix together garlic powder, yogurt, and parmesan cheese and pour over chicken.
Bake the chicken for forty-five mins.

Nutrition: Cal 341 Fat 13.7 g Carbs 3.4 g Protein 48 g

382. Spicy Chicken Meatballs

Prep Time: 10 Mins
Servings: 4

Cook Time: 25 mins

Ingredients:
- *One lb ground chicken*
- *1/2 cup cilantro, chopped*
- *Salt*
- *One jalapeno pepper, minced*
- *One habanero pepper, minced*
- *One poblano chili pepper, minced*

Directions: Select air fry, set temperature 400 degrees F, timer for twenty-five mins.
Add all ingredients into a bowl and mix until well combined.
Make small balls from meat mixture and place on the basket and air fry for twenty-five mins.

Nutrition: Cal 226 Fat 8.5 g Carbs 2.3 g Protein 33.4 g

383. Spicy Chicken Wings

Prep Time: 10 Mins
Servings: 4

Cook Time: 30 mins

Ingredients:
- *Two lbs fresh chicken wings*
- *Two tablespoon onion, chopped*
- *Four tablespoon cayenne pepper sauce*
- *One tablespoon Worcestershire sauce*
- *Four tablespoon butter*
- *One tablespoon brown sugar*
- *One teaspoon salt*

Directions: Line roasting pan with aluminum foil and set aside.

Select bake, set temperature 350 degrees F, timer for thirty mins. Place the chicken wings on roasting pan and bake for thirty mins.
In a bowl, mix together Worcestershire sauce, brown sugar, butter, cayenne pepper sauce, and salt.
Remove wings from oven and place in sauce bowl and mix until all wings are coated well with the sauce.
Garnish with onion.

Nutrition: Cal 563 Fat 29.3 g Carbs 6.2 g Protein 66.4 g

384. Tandoori Chicken

Prep Time: 10 Mins
Servings: 4

Cook Time: 15 mins

Ingredients:
- One lb chicken tenders, cut in half
- 1/4 cup parsley, chopped
- One teaspoon paprika
- One teaspoon garam masala
- One teaspoon turmeric
- One tablespoon garlic, minced
- One tablespoon ginger, minced
- 1/4 cup yogurt
- One teaspoon cayenne pepper
- One teaspoon salt

Directions: Select air fry, set temperature 350 degrees F, timer for fifteen mins.
Add all ingredients into a bowl and stir well. Place in refrigerator for thirty mins.
Add marinated chicken into the basket of the air fryer and cook for fifteen mins.

Nutrition: Cal 240 Fat 8.9 g Carbs 3.9 g Protein 34.2

385. Turkey Meatballs

Prep Time: 10 Mins
Servings: 6

Cook Time: 20 mins

Ingredients:
- One lb ground turkey
- Two eggs, lightly beaten
- One tablespoon basil, chopped
- 1/3 cup coconut flour
- 1 tablespoon dried onion flakes
- Two cups zucchini, grated
- 1 teaspoon dried oregano
- 1 tablespoon garlic, minced
- 1 teaspoon cumin
- 1 tablespoon nutritional yeast
- Salt and Pepper

Directions: Select bake, set temperature 390 degrees F, timer for twenty mins.
Add all ingredients into a bowl and mix until well combined.
Make small balls from meat mixture, place on a roasting pan and bake for twenty mins.

Nutrition: Cal 214 Fat 10.7 g Carbs 8.1 g Protein 24.9 g

386. Chicken Fajita Casserole

Prep Time: 10 Mins
Servings: 4

Cook Time: 15 mins

Ingredients:
- One lb cooked chicken, shredded
- One bell pepper, sliced
- 1/3 cup mayonnaise
- Seven oz cream cheese
- Seven oz cheddar cheese, shredded
- 2 tablespoon tex-mix seasoning
- One onion, sliced
- Salt and Pepper

Directions: Grease the baking sheet with butter. Set aside.
Select bake, set temperature 390 degrees F, timer for fifteen mins.
Mix all ingredients except 2 ounces cheddar in a baking dish.
Spread remaining cheese on top and bake for 15 mins.

Nutrition: Cal 641 Fat 44.1 g Carbs 13.3 g Protein 50.2 g

387. Chicken Tenders

Prep Time: 10 Mins
Servings: 4

Cook Time: 12 mins

Ingredients:
- *One lb chicken tenderloin*
- *Three eggs, lightly beaten*
- *1/2 cup all-purpose flour*
- *1/3 cup bread crumb*
- *Salt and Pepper*
- *Two tablespoon extra-virgin olive oil*

Directions: Select air fry, set temperature 330 degrees F, timer for twelve mins.
In a shallow dish, stir flour, salt, and pepper. Add bread crumbs in a separate dish. Add one egg in a small bowl.
Roll chicken in flour then dips in egg and coat with bread crumbs.
Place coated chicken on roasting pan and cook.

Nutrition: Cal 296 Fat 11.5 g Carbs 18.7 g Protein 29.9 g

RED MEAT

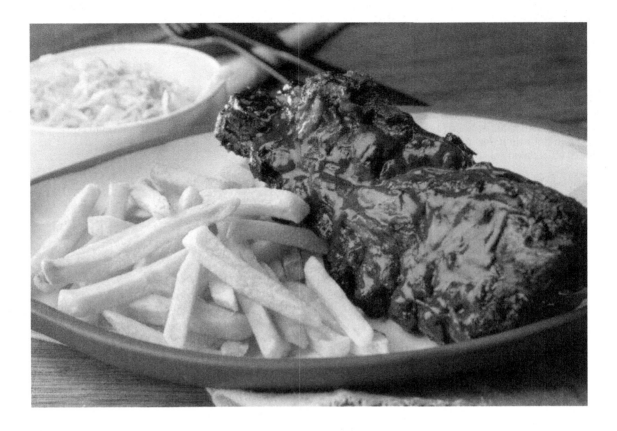

388. Lamb Kebabs

Prep Time: 10 Mins
Servings: 3

Cook Time: 60 Mins

Ingredients:

- *1 ½ pounds lamb shoulder, bones removed and cut into pieces*
- *Two tablespoons cumin seeds, toasted*
- *Two teaspoons caraway seeds, toasted*
- *One tablespoon Sichuan peppercorns*
- *One teaspoon sugar*
- *Two teaspoons crushed red pepper flakes*
- *Salt and pepper*

Directions: Place all ingredients in bowl and allow the meat marinate in the refrigerator for at least two hours.
Preheat the oven to 390 degrees F.
Grill the meat for fifteen mins per batch.
Flip the meat every eight mins for even grilling.

Nutrition: Cal: 465; Carbs: 7.7g; Protein: 22.8g; Fat: 46.9g

389. Air Fried Beef Schnitzel

Prep Time: 10 mins
Servings: 1

Cook Time:15 mins

Ingredients:

- *One lean beef schnitzel*
- *Olive oil: 2 tablespoon*
- *Breadcrumbs: ¼ cup*
- *One egg*
- *One lemon, to serve*

Directions: Let the air fryer heat to 370°F.

In a bowl, add oil and breadcrumbs, mix well until forms a crumbly mixture.

Dip beef steak in whisked egg and coat in breadcrumbs mixture.

Place the beef in the air fryer and cook for 15 mins or more until fully cooked through.

Nutrition: Cal 340, Protein 20 g, Carbs 14 g, Fat 10 g

390. Air Fryer Meatloaf

Prep Time: 10 mins
Servings: 8

Cook Time:40 mins

Ingredients

- Ground lean beef: 4 cups
- Bread crumbs: 1 cup (soft and fresh)
- Chopped mushrooms: ½ cup
- Cloves of minced garlic
- Shredded carrots: ½ cup
- Beef broth: ¼ cup
- Chopped onions: ½ cup
- Two eggs beaten
- Ketchup: 3 Tbsp.
- Worcestershire sauce: 1 Tbsp.
- Dijon mustard: 1 Tbsp.

For Glaze

- Honey: ¼ cup
- Ketchup: half cup
- Dijon mustard: 2 tsp

Directions: In a big bowl, add beef broth and breadcrumbs, stir well. And set it aside in a food processor, add garlic, onions, mushrooms, and carrots, and pulse on high until finely chopped.

In a separate bowl, add soaked breadcrumbs, Dijon mustard, Worcestershire sauce, eggs, lean ground beef, ketchup, and salt. With your hands, combine well and make it into a loaf.

Let the air fryer preheat to 390 °F.

Put Meatloaf in the Air Fryer and let it cook for 45 mins.

In the meantime, add Dijon mustard, ketchup, and brown sugar in a bowl and mix. Glaze this mix over Meatloaf when five mins are left.

Rest the Meatloaf for ten mins before serving.

Nutrition: Cal 330, Protein 19 g, Carbs 16 g, Fat 9.9 g

391. Air Fried Steak with Asparagus

Prep Time: 20 mins
Servings: 2

Cook Time:30 mins

Ingredients

- Olive oil spray
- Flank steak (2 pounds)- cut into 6 pieces
- Kosher salt and black pepper
- Two cloves of minced garlic
- Asparagus: 4 cups
  - Tamari sauce: half cup
  - Three bell peppers: sliced thinly
- Beef broth: 1/3 cup
- 1 Tbsp. of unsalted butter
- Balsamic vinegar: 1/4 cup

Directions: Sprinkle salt and pepper on steak and rub.

In a ziploc bag, add Tamari sauce and garlic, then add steak, toss well and seal the bag. Let it marinate for overnight.

Place bell peppers and asparagus in the center of the steak. Roll the steak around the vegetables and close with toothpicks.

Preheat the air fryer at 400°F.

Spray the steak with olive oil spray. And place steaks in the air fryer. Cook for 15 mins.

Take the steak out from the air fryer and let it rest for five minute.

Remove steak bundles and allow them to rest for 5 mins before serving/slicing.

In the meantime, add balsamic vinegar, butter, and broth over medium flame. Mix well and reduce it by half. Add salt and pepper to taste.

Pour over steaks right before serving.

Nutrition: Cal 471, Protein 29 g, Carbs 20 g, Fat 15 g

392. Air Fryer Hamburgers

Prep Time: 5 mins
Servings: 4

Cook Time:13 mins

Ingredients
- Buns:4
- Lean ground beef chuck: 4 cups
- Salt to taste
- Slices of any cheese: 4 slices
- Black Pepper, to taste

Directions: Let the air fryer preheat to 350 F.
In a bowl, add lean ground beef, pepper, and salt. Mix well and form patties.
Put them in the air fryer. Cook for 6 mins and flip them halfway through. One minute before you take out the patties, add cheese on top.
When cheese is melted, take out from the air fryer.
Add ketchup, any dressing to your buns, add tomatoes and lettuce and patties.

Nutrition: Cal: 520, Carbs: 22 g, Protein: 31 g, Fat: 34 g

393. Air Fryer Steak Kabobs with Vegetables

Prep Time: 30 mins
Servings: 4

Cook Time:10 mins

Ingredients
- Light Soy sauce: 2 tbsp.
- Lean beef chuck ribs: 4 cups, cut into one-inch pieces
- Low-fat sour cream: 1/3 cup
- Half onion
- 8 skewers: 6 inch
- One bell peppers

Directions: In a mixing bowl, add soy sauce and sour cream, and mix well. Add the lean beef chunks, coat well, and let it marinate for half an hour.
Cut onion, bell pepper into one-inch pieces. In water, soak skewers for ten mins.
Add bell peppers, onions, and beef on skewers; alternatively, sprinkle with Black Pepper
Let it cook for 10 mins in a preheated air fryer at 400F, flip halfway through.
Serve with yogurt dipping sauce.

Nutrition: Cal 268, Protein 20 g, Carbs 15 g, Fat 10 g

394. Air Fried Empanadas

Prep Time: 10 mins
Servings: 2

Cook Time:20 mins

Ingredients
- Square gyoza wrappers: eight pieces
- Olive oil: 1 tablespoon
- White onion: 1/4 cup, finely diced
- Mushrooms: 1/4 cup, finely diced
- Half cup lean ground beef
- Chopped garlic: 2 teaspoons
- Paprika: 1/4 teaspoon
- Ground cumin: 1/4 teaspoon
- Six green olives, diced
- Ground cinnamon: 1/8 teaspoon
- Diced tomatoes: half cup
- One egg, lightly beaten

Directions: In a skillet, over a medium heat, add oil, onions, and beef and cook for 3 mins, until beef turns brown.
Add mushrooms and cook for six mins until it starts to brown. Then add paprika, cinnamon, olives, cumin, and garlic and cook for 3 mins.
Add in the chopped tomatoes, and cook for 1 minute. Turn off the heat; let it cool for five mins.
Lay gyoza wrappers on a flat surface add one and a half tbsp. of beef filling in each wrapper. Brush edges with water or egg, fold wrappers, pinch edges.
Put four empanadas in an even layer in an air fryer basket, and cook for 7 mins at 400°F until nicely browned.
Serve with sauce and salad greens.

Nutrition: Cal 343, Fat 19 g, Protein 18 g Carbs 12.9 g

395. Air Fry Rib-Eye Steak

Prep Time: 5 mins
Servings: 2

Cook Time: 14 mins

Ingredients

- Lean rib eye steaks: 2 medium-sized
- Salt & freshly ground black pepper, to taste

Directions: Let the air fry preheat at 400 F. pat dry steaks with paper towels.
Season with any spice blend or just salt and pepper on both sides of the steak.
Put steaks in the air fryer basket. Cook according to the rareness you want. Or cook for 14 mins and flip after half time.
Take out from the air fryer and let it rest for about 5 mins.

Nutrition: Cal: 470, Protein: 45 g, Fat: 31 g, Carbs: 23 g

396. Beefsteak with Olives And Capers

Prep Time: 10 Mins
Servings: 4

Cook Time: 45 mins

Ingredients:

- One anchovy fillet, minced
- One clove of garlic, minced
- One cup pitted olives
- One tablespoon capers, minced
- 2 tablespoons fresh oregano
- 2 tablespoons garlic powder
- 2 tablespoons onion powder
- 2 tablespoons smoked paprika
- 1/3 cup extra-virgin olive oil
- Two pounds flank steak, pounded
- Salt and pepper

Directions: Preheat the air fryer to 390 F. Place the grill pan accessory in the air fryer.
Season the steak with pepper and salt. Sprinkle the onion powder, oregano, paprika, and garlic powder all over the steak.
Place on the grill and cook for forty-five mins. Be sure to turn the meat every ten mins for even cook.
Meanwhile, stir the olive oil, capers, garlic, olives, and anchovy fillets.

Nutrition: Cal: 553; Carbs: 11.6 g; Protein: 51.5 g; Fat: 33.4 g

397. Grilled Pork in Cajun Sauce

Prep Time: 10 Mins
Servings: 3

Cook Time: 12 mins

Ingredients:

- 1-lb pork loin, sliced into 1-inch cubes
- 2 tablespoons Cajun seasoning
- 3 tablespoons brown sugar + ¼ cup
- 1/4 cup cider vinegar

Directions: In a plate, mix pork loin, Cajun seasoning, and three tablespoons brown sugar. Stir well to coat. Marinate in the ref for three hours.
In a medium bowl mix well, brown sugar and vinegar to baste.
Thread pork pieces onto skewers. Baste with sauce and place on skewer rack in the oven.
Cook on 360 degrees F for twelve mins. Halfway through cook time, turn skewers over and baste with sauce. If necessary, bake in batches.

Nutrition: Cal: 428; Carbs: 30.3 g; Protein: 39 g; Fat: 16.7 g

398. Ribs with Cajun and Coriander

Prep Time: 10 Mins
Servings: 4

Cook Time: 60 Mins

Ingredients:

- Two slabs spareribs
- 2 teaspoon Cajun seasoning
- ¼ cup brown sugar

- *½ teaspoon lemon*
- *1 tablespoon paprika*
- *1 teaspoon coriander seed powder*
- *2 tablespoons onion powder*
- *1 tablespoon salt*

Directions: Preheat the air fryer to 390 degrees F.
Place the grill pan in the air fryer.
In a bowl, combine paprika, lemon, coriander, onion, and salt. Rub the spice mixture on to the spareribs.
Place the ribs on the grill pan and cook for twenty mins per batch.

Nutrition: Cal: 490; Carbs: 18.2 g; Protein: 24.4 g; Fat: 35.5 g

399. Roast Beef with Butter, Garlic and Thyme

Prep Time: 10 Mins   **Cook Time: 120 mins**
Servings: 12

Ingredients:
- *1 ½ tablespoon garlic*
- *One cup beef stock*
- *1 teaspoon thyme leaves, chopped*
- *3 tablespoons butter*
- *3-pound eye of round roast*
- *6 tablespoons extra-virgin olive oil*
- *1 teaspoon pepper*
- *1 teaspoon salt*

Directions: Place all ingredients in a Ziploc bag and let marinate in the refrigerator for 60 mins.
Preheat the oven for five mins.
Transfer all ingredients to a baking dish that fits in the air fryer.
Place in the air fryer and cook for 60 mins at 400 degrees F.
Baste the beef with sauce every thirty mins.

Nutrition: Cal: 273; Carbs: 0.8g; Protein: 34.2g; Fat: 14.7g

400. Marinated Beef BBQ

Prep Time: 10 Mins   **Cook Time: 1 hour**
Servings: 4

Ingredients:
- *2 pounds beef steak, pounded*
- *¼ cup bourbon*
- *1 tablespoon Worcestershire sauce*
- *¼ cup barbecue sauce*
- *Salt and pepper*

Directions: Place the ingredients in a Ziploc bag and let marinate in the ref for at least 60 mins.
Preheat the oven to 390 degrees F.
Place the beef steak on the grill pan and cook for twenty mins per batch.
Halfway through the cook time, give a stir to cook evenly.
Meanwhile, pour the marinade over saucepan and simmer until sauce stars to thicken.
Serve beef with the bourbon sauce.

Nutrition: Cal: 346; Carbs: 9.8 g; Protein: 48.2 g; Fat: 12.6 g

401. Steak with Chimichurri Sauce

Prep Time: 10 Mins   **Cook Time: 60 mins**
Servings: 6

Ingredients:
- *3 pounds steak*
- *One cup chimichurri*
- *Salt and pepper*

Directions: Place all ingredients in a Ziploc bag and let marinate in the refrigerator for 60 mins.
Preheat the oven to 390 degrees F.
Place the grill pan in the air fryer. Grill the steak for twenty mins per batch.

Turn the steak every ten mins for even grilling.

Nutrition: Cal: 507; Carbs: 2.8 g; Protein: 63 g; Fat: 27 g

402. Egg and Bell Pepper with Beef

Prep Time: 10 Mins
Servings: 4

Cook Time: 30 mins

Ingredients:
- 1-pound ground beef
- Six cups eggs, beaten
- One green bell pepper, seeded and chopped
- One onion, chopped
- Three cloves of garlic, minced
- 3 tablespoons olive oil
- Salt and pepper

Directions: Preheat the oven for five mins with baking pan insert.
In a baking dish stir the ground beef, olive oil, onion, garlic, and bell pepper. Dress with salt and pepper.
Pour in the beaten eggs and mix.
Place the dish with the beef and egg mixture in the air fryer.
Bake for thirty mins at 330 degrees F.

Nutrition: Cal: 579; Carbs: 14.5 g; Protein: 65.8 g; Fat: 28.6 g

403. Spanish Rice Casserole with Beef and Cheese

Prep Time: 10 Mins
Servings: 3

Cook Time: 50 mins

Ingredients:
- 1/2-pound lean ground beef
- 2 tablespoons chopped green bell pepper
- 1 tablespoon chopped fresh cilantro
- 1/4 cup shredded Cheddar cheese
- 1/2 teaspoon brown sugar
- 1/2 pinch ground pepper
- 1/3 cup uncooked long grain rice
- 1/4 cup finely chopped onion
- 1/4 cup chile sauce
- 1/4 teaspoon ground cumin
- 1/4 teaspoon Worcestershire sauce
- 1/2 (14.5 ounce) can canned tomatoes
- 1/2 cup water
- 1/2 teaspoon salt

Directions: Lightly grease air fryer pan with cook spray. Add the ground beef. For ten mins, cook on 360 degrees F. Halfway through cook, mix and crumble beef. Discard excess fat, stir in pepper, Worcestershire sauce, salt, chile sauce, rice, cumin, brown sugar, water, tomatoes, green bell pepper, and onion.
Cover pan with aluminum foil and cook for twenty-five mins. Stirring occasionally.
Give one last good stir, press down firmly and sprinkle with cheese.
Bake uncovered for fifteen mins at 390 degrees F until the tops are lightly browned.
Serve with cilantro.

Nutrition: Cal: 346; Carbs: 24.9 g; Protein: 18.5 g; Fat: 19.1 g

404. Beef Roast in Worcestershire-Rosemary

Prep Time: 10 Mins
Servings: 6

Cook Time: 60 mins

Ingredients:
- 1-pound beef chuck roast
- One onion, chopped
- Two cloves of garlic, minced
- 2 tablespoons olive oil
- Three cups water
- 1 tablespoon butter
- 1 tablespoon Worcestershire sauce
- 1 teaspoon rosemary
- 1 teaspoon thyme
- Three stalks of celery, sliced

Directions: Preheat the oven for five mins.
Place all ingredients in a deep pan that will fit in the air fryer.

Bake for 60 mins at 350 degrees F.
Braise the meat with its sauce every thirty mins until cooked.

Nutrition: Cal: 260; Carbs: 2.9 g; Protein: 17.5 g; Fat: 19.8 g

405. Beef with Honey and Mustard

Prep Time: 10 Mins   **Cook Time: 60 mins**
Servings: 6

Ingredients:
- 3 pounds beef steak sliced
- One clove of garlic, minced
- ½ cup honey
- ½ cup ketchup
- ½ teaspoon dry mustard
- 1 tablespoon chili powder
- Two onion, chopped
- Salt and pepper

Directions: Place all ingredients in a Ziploc bag and let to marinate in the ref for at least 60 mins.
Preheat the oven to 390 degrees F.
Place the grill pan in the air fryer.
Grill the beef for fifteen mins per batch being sure that you flip it every eight mins for even grilling.
Meanwhile, pour marinade over a saucepan and simmer over medium heat until sauce thickens.
Drizzle the beef with the sauce before serving.

Nutrition: Cal: 542; Carbs: 49 g; Protein: 37 g; Fat: 22 g

406. Texas Beef Brisket

Prep Time: 10 Mins   **Cook Time: 90 mins**
Servings: 8

Ingredients:
- 1 ½ cup beef stock
- 2 pounds beef brisket, trimmed
- One bay leaf
- 1 tablespoon garlic powder
- 1 tablespoon onion powder
- 2 teaspoons dry mustard
- Salt and pepper
- 4 tablespoons olive oil
- 2 tablespoons chili powder

Directions: Preheat the oven for five mins.
Place all ingredients in a baking pan that will fit in the air fryer.
Bake for 90 mins at 400 degrees F.
Mix the beef every after thirty mins to absorb in the sauce.

Nutrition: Cal: 306; Carbs: 3.8 g; Protein: 18.3 g; Fat: 24.1 g

407. Teriyaki BBQ Recipe

Prep Time: 10 Mins   **Cook Time: 15 mins**
Servings: 2

Ingredients:
- fourteen oz lean diced steak, with fat trimmed
- 1 thumb-sized piece of fresh ginger, grated
- 1 tablespoon honey
- 1 tablespoon mirin
- 1 tablespoon soy sauce

Directions: Stir all ingredients in a bowl and let marinate for at least 60 mins. Turn halfway through the marinating time.
Thread mead into skewers. Place on skewer rack.
Bake for 5 mins at 390 degrees F.

Nutrition: Cal: 460; Carbs: 10.6 g; Protein: 55.8 g; Fat: 21.6 g

408. Beef in Almond and Eggs Crust

Prep Time: 10 Mins
Servings: 1

Cook Time: 15 mins

Ingredients:
- 1/2-pound beef schnitzel
- One egg, beaten
- ½ cup almond flour
- One slice of lemon
- Two tablespoons vegetable oil

Directions: Preheat the air fryer for five mins.
Stir the oil and almond flour.
Dip the beef into the egg and dredge in the almond flour mixture. Press the almond flour so that it sticks on to the beef. Place in the oven and bake for fifteen mins at 350 degrees F.
Serve with a slice of lemon.

Nutrition: Cal: 732; Carbs: 1.1 g; Protein: 55.6 g; Fat: 56.1 g

409. Beef Casserole

Prep Time: 10 Mins
Servings: 4

Cook Time: 30 mins

Ingredients:
- 1-pound ground beef
- One green bell pepper, seeded and chopped
- One onion, chopped
- Three cloves of garlic, minced
- Six cups eggs, beaten
- Three tablespoons olive oil
- Salt and pepper

Directions: Preheat the air fryer for five mins.
In an ovenproof dish, mix the ground beef, garlic, olive oil, onion, and bell pepper. Season with salt and pepper.
Pour in the beaten eggs and toss well.
Place the dish with the beef and egg mixture in the air fryer.
Cook for 30 mins at 325 degrees F.

Nutrition: Cal: 1520; Carbs: 10.4 g; Protein: 87.9 g; Fat: 12.5 g

410. Beef and Pasta Casserole

Prep time: 10 mins
Servings: 4

Cook time: 20 mins

Ingredients:
- One pound ground beef
- Seventeen ounces pasta
- One yellow onion, peeled and chopped
- One carrot, peeled and chopped
- One celery stalk, chopped
- Thirteen ounces mozzarella cheese, shredded
- Sixteen ounces tomato puree
- 1 tablespoon red wine
- 2 tablespoons butter
- Salt and ground pepper

Directions: In a baking pan add the butter and melt. Add the onion carrot, and celery, stir and cook for five mins. Include the meat, salt and pepper and cook for ten mins. Add wine, stir and cook for one minute.
Add pasta, tomato puree and water to cover the pasta, stir, cover and cook for six mins.
Add cheese, stir, divide among plates.

Nutrition: Cal: 182, Fat: 1 g, Carbs: 31 g, Protein: 12 g

SEAFOOD

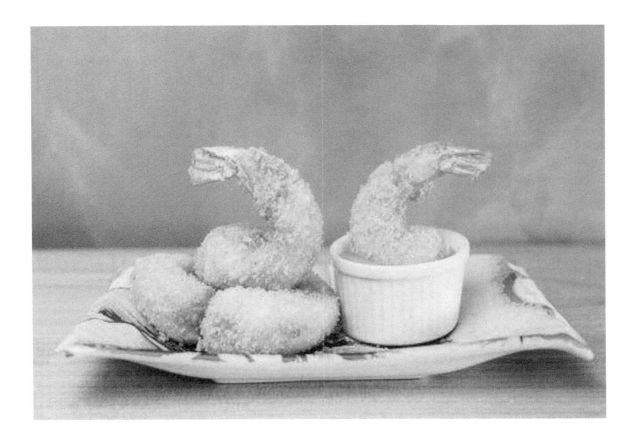

411. Air Fry Catfish

Prep Time: 5 mins
Serving: 4

Cook Time: 13 mins

Ingredients:
- *1 tbsp. chopped parsley*
- *1 tbsp. olive oil*
- *¼ C. seasoned fish fry*
- *4 catfish fillets*

Directions: Ensure your Air Fryer Oven is preheated to 400 degrees F.
Rinse off catfish fillets and pat dry.
Add fish fry seasoning to Ziploc baggie, then catfish. Shake the bag and ensure the fish gets well coated.
Spray each fillet with olive oil.
Add fillets to the air fryer basket.
Set temperature to 400°F, and the time to 10 mins. Cook 10 mins. Then flip and cook another 2-3 mins.

Nutrition: Cal: 208; Fat: 5 g; Protein: 17 g

412. Air Fried Fish Fillet

Prep Time: 10 mins
Servings: 2

Cook Time: 20 mins

Ingredients:
- *12 oz. white fish fillets*
- *1/2 tsp. lemon pepper seasoning*
- *1/2 tsp. garlic powder*

- *1/2 tsp. onion powder*
- *Salt and Pepper*

Directions: Place the air fryer Basket onto the Baking Pan and spray air fryer basket with cook spray.
Spray fish fillets with cook spray and season with onion powder, lemon pepper seasoning, garlic powder, pepper, and salt.
Place parchment paper in the bottom of the air fryer basket.
Place fish fillets into the air fryer basket. Place assembled baking pan. Set to air fry at 350° F for 10 mins.

Nutrition: Cal 298 Fat 13 g Carbs 1.4 g Protein 42 g

413. Salmon Cakes in Air Fryer

Prep Time: 10 mins   **Cook Time:10 mins**
Serving 2

Ingredients:
- *Fresh salmon fillet 8 oz.*
- *Egg 1*
- *Salt 1/8 tsp*
- *Garlic powder ¼ tsp*
- *Sliced lemon 1*

Directions: In the bowl, chop the salmon, add the egg & spices.
Form tiny cakes.
Let the Air fryer preheat to 390. On the bottom of the air fryer bowl lay sliced lemons and place cakes on top.
Cook them for seven mins.

Nutrition: Cal: 194, Fat: 9 g, Carbs: 1 g, Protein: 25 g

414. Coconut Shrimp

Prep Time: 10 mins   **Cook Time:30 mins**
Serving: 4

Ingredients:
- *Pork Rinds: ½ cup (Crushed)*
- *Jumbo Shrimp:4 cups. (deveined)*
- *Coconut Flakes preferably: ½ cup*
- *Eggs: two*
- *Flour of coconut: ½ cup*
- *Any oil of your choice for frying at least half-inch in pan*
- *Freshly ground black pepper & kosher salt to taste*

Dipping sauce (Pina colada flavor):
- *Powdered Sugar as Substitute: 2-3 tablespoon*
- *Mayonnaise: 3 tablespoons*
- *Sour Cream: ½ cup*
- *Coconut Extract or to taste: ¼ tsp*
- *Coconut Cream: 3 tablespoons*
- *Pineapple Flavoring as much to taste: ¼ tsp*
- *Coconut Flakes preferably unsweetened this is optional: 3 tablespoons*

Directions:

Pina Colada (Sauce): Mix all the ingredients into a tiny bowl for the Dipping sauce (Pina colada flavor). Combine well and put in the fridge.

Shrimps: Whip all eggs in a deep bowl, and a shallow bowl, add the coconut flour, crushed pork rinds, sea salt, coconut flakes, and freshly ground black pepper.
Put the shrimp in the mixed eggs for dipping, then in the coconut flour blend. Put them on your air fryer's basket.
Place the shrimp battered on your air fryer basket. Brush the shrimp with oil and cook for 8-10 mins at 360 ° F, flipping them through halfway.
Enjoy hot with dipping sauce.

Nutrition: Cal 340, Protein 25 g, Carbs 9 g, Fat 16 g

415. Fish Sticks in Air Fryer

Prep Time: 10 mins
Serving 4

Cook Time:15 mins

Ingredients
- *Whitefish such as cod 1 lb.*
- *Mayonnaise ¼ c*
- *Dijon mustard 2 tbsp.*
- *Water 2 tbsp.*
- *Pork rind 1&1/2 c*
- *Cajun seasoning ¾ tsp*
- *Kosher salt & pepper to taste*

Directions: Spray non-stick cook spray to the air fryer rack.
Pat the fish dry & cut into sticks about 1 inch by 2 inches' broad.
Stir together the mayo, mustard, and water in a tiny small dish. Mix the pork rinds & Cajun seasoning into another small container.
Adding kosher salt& pepper to taste.
Working on one slice of fish at a time, dip it into into the mayonnaise mix, then remove the excess. Dip in pork rind mixture, then turn to cover. Place on the rack of an air fryer.
Set at 400 °F to Air Fry & bake for 5 mins, then turn the fish with tongs and bake for another 5 mins.

Nutrition: Cal: 263, Fat: 16 g, Carbs: 1 g, Protein: 26.4 g

416. Honey-Glazed Salmon

Prep Time: 10 mins
Servings: 2

Cook Time:15 mins

Ingredients
- *Gluten-free Soy Sauce: 6 tsp*
- *Salmon Fillets: 2 pcs*
- *Sweet rice wine: 3 tsp*
- *Water: 1 tsp*
- *Honey: 6 tbsp.*

Directions: In a bowl, mix sweet rice wine, soy sauce, honey, and water.
Set half of it aside.
In the half of it, marinate the fish and let it rest for two hours.
Let the air fryer preheat to 370°F.
Cook the fish for 8 mins, flip halfway through and cook for another five mins.
Baste the salmon with marinade mixture after 4 mins.
The half of marinade, pour in a saucepan reduce to half.

Nutrition: Cal 254, Carbs 9.9 g, Fat 12 g, Protein 20 g

417. Basil-Parmesan Crusted Salmon

Prep Time: 5 mins
Servings: 4

Cook Time:15 mins

Ingredients
- *Grated Parmesan: 3 tablespoons*
- *Skinless four salmon fillets*
- *Salt: 1/4 teaspoon*
- *Freshly ground black pepper*
- *Low-fat mayonnaise: 3 tablespoons*
- *Basil leaves, chopped*
- *Half lemon*

Directions: Let the air fryer preheat to 400 °F. Spray the basket with olive oil.
With pepper, salt, and lemon juice, season the salmon.
In a bowl, mix two tablespoons of Parmesan cheese with mayonnaise and basil leaves.
Add this mix and parmesan on top of salmon and cook for seven mins or until fully cooked.

Nutrition: Cal: 289, Carbs: 1.5 g, Protein: 30 g, Fat: 18.5 g

418. Cajun Shrimp in Air Fryer

Prep Time: 10 mins
Servings: 4

Cook Time:20 mins

Ingredients

- Peeled, 24 extra-jumbo shrimp
- Olive oil: 2 tablespoons
- Cajun seasoning: 1 tablespoon
- one zucchini, thick slices (half-moons)
- Cooked Turkey: ¼ cup
- Yellow squash, sliced half-moons
- Kosher salt: 1/4 teaspoon

Directions: In a bowl, stir the shrimp with Cajun seasoning.
In another bowl, add turkey, salt, zucchini, squash, and coat with oil.
Let the air fryer preheat to 400 °F.
Move the shrimp and vegetable to the fryer basket and cook for three mins.

Nutrition: Cal: 284, Carbs: 8 g, Protein: 31 g, Fat: 14 g

419. Crispy Air Fryer Fish

Prep Time: 10 mins
Servings: 4

Cook Time:17 mins

Ingredients

- Old bay: 2 tsp
- 4-6, cut in half, Whiting Fish fillets
- Fine cornmeal: ¾ cup
- Flour: ¼ cup
- Paprika: 1 tsp
- Garlic powder: half tsp
- Salt: 1 and ½ tsp
- Freshly ground black pepper: half tsp

Directions: In a ziploc bag, add all ingredients and coat the fish fillets with it.
Spray oil on the basket of air fryer and put the fish in it.
Cook for ten mins at 400 F. flip fish if necessary and coat with oil spray and cook for another seven-minute.

Nutrition: Cal 254, Fat 12.7 g, Carbs 8.2 g, Protein 17.5 g

420. Air Fryer Lemon Cod

Prep Time: 5 mins
Servings: 1

Cook Time:10 mins

Ingredients

- One cod fillet
- Dried parsley
- Kosher salt and pepper to taste
- Garlic powder
- One lemon

Directions: In a bowl, mix all ingredients and coat the fish fillet with spices.
Slice the lemon and lay at the bottom of the air fryer basket.
Put spiced fish on top. Cover the fish with lemon slices.
Cook for ten mins at 375 °F, the internal temperature of fish should be 145 °F.
Serve with microgreen salad.

Nutrition: Cal: 101, Carbs: 10 g, Protein: 16 g, Fat: 1 g

421. Air Fryer Salmon Fillets

Prep Time: 5 mins
Servings: 2

Cook Time:15 mins

Ingredients

- Low-fat Greek yogurt: 1/4 cup
- Two salmon fillets
- Fresh dill: 1 tbsp. (chopped)
- One lemon and lemon juice
- Garlic powder: half tsp.
- Kosher salt and pepper

Directions: Cut the lemon in slices and lay at the bottom of the air fryer basket.
Season the salmon with salt and pepper. Put salmon on top of lemons.
Let it cook at 330 degrees for 15 mins.
In the meantime, mix lemon juice, garlic powder, salt, pepper with yogurt and dill.
Serve the fish with sauce.

Nutrition: Cal: 194, Carbs: 6 g, Protein: 25 g, Fat: 7 g

422. Air Fryer Fish & Chips

Prep Time: 10 mins
Servings: 4

Cook Time:35 mins

Ingredients
- 4 cups of any fish fillet
- flour: 1/4 cup
- Whole wheat breadcrumbs: one cup
- One egg
- Oil: 2 tbsp.
- 4 Potatoes
- Salt: 1 tsp.

Directions: Cut the potatoes in fries. Then coat with oil and salt.
Cook in the oven for 20 mins at 400 F, toss the fries halfway through.
In the meantime, coat fish in the flour, then in the whisked egg, and in breadcrumbs mix.
Place the fish in the air fryer and let it cook at 330 °F for 15 mins.
Flip it halfway through, if needed.

Nutrition: Cal: 409, Carbs: 44 g, Protein: 30 g, Fat: 11 g

423. Grilled Salmon with Lemon-Honey Marinade

Prep Time: 10 mins
Servings: 4

Cook Time:20 mins

Ingredients
- Olive oil: 2 tablespoons
- Two Salmon fillets
- Lemon juice
- Water: 1/3 cup
- Gluten-free light soy sauce: 1/3 cup
- Honey: 1/3 cup
- Scallion slices
- Cherry tomato
- Freshly ground black pepper, garlic powder, kosher salt to taste

Directions: Season salmon with pepper and salt.
In a bowl, mix honey, soy sauce, lemon juice, water, oil. Add salmon in this marinade and let it rest for least two hours.
Let the air fryer preheat at 370°F.
Place fish in the air fryer and cook for 8 mins.
Move to a dish and top with scallion slices.

Nutrition: Cal 211, Fat 9 g, Protein 15 g, Carbs 4.9 g

424. Air-Fried Fish Nuggets

Prep Time: 15 mins
Servings: 4

Cook Time:10 mins

Ingredients
- Fish fillets in cubes: 2 cups(skinless)
- 1 egg, beaten
- Flour: 5 tablespoons
- Water: 5 tablespoons
- Kosher salt and pepper to taste
- Breadcrumbs mix
- Smoked paprika: 1 tablespoon
- Whole wheat breadcrumbs: ¼ cup
- Garlic powder: 1 tablespoon

Directions: Season the fish cubes with kosher salt and pepper.
In a bowl, add flour and gradually add water, mixing as you add.
Then mix in the egg. And keep mixing but do not over mix.

Coat the cubes in batter, then in the breadcrumb mix. Coat well.
Place the cubes in a baking tray and spray with oil.
Let the air fryer preheat to 400 °F.
Place cubes in the air fryer and cook for 12 mins or until well cooked and golden brown.

Nutrition: Cal 184.2, Protein: 19 g, Fat: 3.3 g, Carbs: 10 g

425. Garlic Rosemary Prawns

Prep Time: 5 mins
Servings: 2

Cook Time:10 mins

Ingredients
- Melted butter: 1/2 tbsp.
- Green capsicum: slices
- Eight prawns
- Rosemary leaves
- Kosher salt& freshly ground black pepper
- 3-4 cloves of minced garlic

Directions: In a bowl, mix all the ingredients and marinate the prawns in it for at least 60 mins or more
Add two prawns and two slices of capsicum on each skewer.
Let the air fryer preheat to 370°F.
Cook for 5-6 mins. Then set the temperature to 400°F and cook for another minute.
Serve with lemon wedges.

Nutrition: Cal 194, Fat: 10 g, Carbs: 12 g, Protein: 26 g

426. Air-Fried Crumbed Fish

Prep Time: 10 mins
Servings: 2

Cook Time:12 mins

Ingredients
- Four fish fillets
- Olive oil: 4 tablespoons
- One egg beaten
- Whole wheat breadcrumbs: ¼ cup

Directions: Let the air fryer preheat to 370°F.
In a bowl, mix breadcrumbs with oil. Mix well.
First, coat the fish in the egg mix (egg mix with water) then in the breadcrumb mix. Coat well.
Place in the air fryer, let it cook for 10-12 mins.

Nutrition: per serving: 254 Cal| fat 12.7g|carbs10.2g |protein 15.5g.

427. Parmesan Garlic Crusted Salmon

Prep Time: 5 mins
Servings: 2

Cook Time:15 mins

Ingredients
- Whole wheat breadcrumbs: 1/4 cup
- 4 cups of salmon
- Butter melted: 2 tablespoons
- ¼ tsp of freshly ground black pepper
- Parmesan cheese: 1/4 cup(grated)
- Minced garlic: 2 teaspoons
- Half teaspoon of Italian seasoning

Directions: Let the air fryer preheat to 400 F, spray the oil over the air fryer basket.
Pat dry the salmon. In a bowl, mix Parmesan cheese, Italian seasoning, and breadcrumbs. In another pan, mix melted butter with garlic and add to the breadcrumbs mix. Mix well.
Add salt and ground black pepper to salmon. On top of every salmon piece, add the crust mix and press gently.
Let the air fryer preheat to 400 °F and add salmon to it. Cook until done to your liking.
Serve hot with vegetable side dishes.

Nutrition: Cal 330, Fat 19 g, Carbs 11 g, Protein 31 g

428. Air Fryer Salmon with Maple Soy Glaze

Prep Time: 5 mins
Servings: 4

Cook Time:8 mins

Ingredients

- *Pure maple syrup: 3 tbsp.*
- *Gluten-free soy sauce: 3 tbsp.*
- *Sriracha hot sauce: 1 tbsp.*
- *One clove of minced garlic*
- *Salmon: 4 fillets, skinless*

Directions: In a ziploc bag, mix sriracha, maple syrup, garlic, and soy sauce with salmon. Mix well and let it marinate for half an hour.
Let the air fryer preheat to 400 °F with oil spray the basket.
Take fish out from the marinade, pat dry.
Put the salmon in the air fryer, cook for 7 to 8 mins.
In the meantime, in a saucepan, add the marinade, let it simmer until reduced to half.
Add glaze over salmon and serve.

Nutrition: Cal 292, Carbs: 12 g, Protein: 35 g, Fat: 11 g

429. Air Fried Cajun Salmon

Prep Time: 10 mins
Servings: 1

Cook Time:20 mins

Ingredients

- *Fresh salmon: 1 piece*
- *Cajun seasoning: 2 tbsp.*
- *Lemon juice.*

Directions: Let the air fryer preheat to 370°F.
Pat dry the salmon fillet. Rub lemon juice and Cajun seasoning over the fish fillet.
Place in the air fryer, and cook for 7 mins.

Nutrition: 216 Cal, Fat 19 g, Carbs 5.6 g, Protein 19.2 g

430. Air Fryer Shrimp Scampi

Prep Time: 5 mins
Servings: 2

Cook Time:10 mins

Ingredients

- *Raw Shrimp: 4 cups*
- *Lemon Juice: 1 tablespoon*
- *Chopped fresh basil*
- *Red Pepper Flakes: 2 teaspoons*
- *Butter: 2.5 tablespoons*
- *Chopped chives*
- *Chicken Stock: 2 tablespoons*
- *Minced Garlic: 1 tablespoon*

Directions: Let the air fryer preheat with a metal pan to 330 °F.
In the hot pan, add garlic, red pepper flakes, and half of the butter. Let it cook for two mins.
Add the butter, shrimp, chicken stock, minced garlic, chives, lemon juice, basil to the pan. Let it cook for five mins. Bathe the shrimp in melted butter.
Take out from the air fryer and let it rest for one minute.
Add fresh basil leaves and chives and serve.

Nutrition: Cal 287, Fat 5.5 g, Carbs 7.5 g, Protein 18 g

431. Sesame Seeds Fish Fillet

Prep Time: 10 mins
Servings: 2

Cook Time:20 mins

Ingredients

- *Plain flour: 3 tablespoons*
- *One egg, beaten*
- *Five frozen fish fillets*

For Coating

- *Oil: 2 tablespoons*
- *Sesame seeds: 1/2 cup*
- *Rosemary herbs*
- *5-6 biscuit's crumbs*
- *Kosher salt & pepper, to taste*

Directions: For two-minute sauté the sesame seeds in a pan, without oil. Brown them and set it aside.
In a plate, mix all coating ingredients.
Place the aluminum foil on the air fryer basket and let it preheat at 400°F.
First, coat the fish in flour. Then in egg, then in the coating mix.
Place in the Air fryer. If fillets are frozen, cook for ten mins, then turn the fillet and cook for another four mins.

Nutrition: Cal 250, Fat: 8 g, Carbs: 12.4 g, Protein: 20 g

---

432. Lemon Pepper Shrimp in Air Fryer

Prep Time: 5 mins
Servings: 2

Cook Time:10 mins

Ingredients

- *Raw shrimp: 1 and 1/2 cup peeled, deveined*
- *Olive oil: 1/2 tablespoon*
- *Garlic powder: ¼ tsp*
- *Lemon pepper: 1 tsp*
- *Paprika: ¼ tsp*
- *Juice of one lemon*

Directions: Let the air fryer preheat to 400 F.
In a bowl, mix lemon pepper, olive oil, paprika, garlic powder, and lemon juice. Mix well. Add shrimps and coat well.
Add shrimps in the air fryer, cook for 6,8 mins and top with lemon slices.

Nutrition: per serving: Cal 237 |Fat 6g|Carbs 11g|Protein 36g

---

433. Lemon Garlic Shrimp in Air Fryer

Prep Time: 5 mins
Servings: 2

Cook Time:10 mins

Ingredients

- *Olive oil: 1 Tbsp.*
- *Small shrimp: 4 cups, peeled, tails removed*
- *One lemon juice and zest*
- *Parsley: 1/4 cup sliced*
- *Red pepper flakes (crushed): 1 pinch*
- *Four cloves of grated garlic*
- *Sea salt: 1/4 teaspoon*

Directions: Let air fryer heat to 400 °F.
Mix olive oil, lemon zest, red pepper flakes, shrimp, kosher salt, and garlic in a bowl and coat the shrimp well.
Place shrimps in the air fryer basket, coat with oil spray.
Cook at 400 F for 8 mins. Toss the shrimp halfway through.
Serve with lemon slices and parsley.

Nutrition: Cal 140, Fat: 18 g, Carbs: 8 g, Protein: 20 g

434. Parmesan Shrimp

Prep Time: 5 mins
Servings: 4

Cook Time:10 mins

Ingredients
- Olive oil: 2 tablespoons
- Jumbo cooked shrimp: 8 cups, peeled, deveined
- Parmesan cheese: 2/3 cup (grated)
- Onion powder: 1 teaspoon
- Pepper: 1 teaspoon
- Four cloves of minced garlic
- Oregano: 1/2 teaspoon
- Basil: 1 teaspoon
- Lemon wedges

Directions: Mix parmesan cheese, onion powder, oregano, olive oil, garlic, basil, and pepper in a bowl. Coat the shrimp in this mixture.
Spray oil on the air fryer basket put shrimp in it.
Cook for ten mins, at 350 F, or until browned.
Drizzle the lemon on shrimps before serving with a microgreen salad.

Nutrition: Cal 198, Fat: 13 g, Carbs: 5.6 g, Protein: 12.7 g

435. Juicy Air Fryer Salmon

Prep Time: 5 mins
Servings: 4

Cook Time:12 mins

Ingredients
- Lemon pepper seasoning: 2 teaspoons
- Salmon: 4 cups
- Olive oil: one tablespoon
- Seafood seasoning:2 teaspoons
- Half lemon's juice
- Garlic powder:1 teaspoon
- Kosher salt to taste

Directions: In a bowl, add one tbsp. of olive oil and half lemon's juice.
Pour this mixture over salmon and rub. Leave the skin on salmon. It will come off when cooked.
Rub the salmon with kosher salt and spices.
Put parchment paper in the air fryer basket. Put the salmon in the air fryer.
Cook at 360 F for ten mins. Cook until inner salmon temperature reaches 140 F.
Let the salmon rest five mins before serving.
Serve with lemon wedges.

Nutrition: 132 Cal, Fat 7.4 g, Carbs 12 g, Protein 22.1 g

436. Crispy Fish Sandwiches

Prep Time: 10 mins
Servings: 2

Cook Time:10 mins

Ingredients
- Cod:2 fillets.
- All-purpose flour: 2 tablespoons
- Pepper: 1/4 teaspoon
- Lemon juice: 1 tablespoon
- Salt: 1/4 teaspoon
- Garlic powder: half teaspoon
- One egg
- Mayo: half tablespoon
- Whole wheat bread crumbs: half cup

Directions: In a bowl, add salt, flour, pepper, and garlic powder.
In a separate bowl, add lemon juice, mayo, and egg.
In another bowl, add the breadcrumbs.
Coat the fish in flour, then in egg, and in breadcrumbs.
With cook oil, spray the basket and put the fish in the basket. Also, spray the fish with cook oil.
Cook at 400 F for ten mins. This fish is soft, be careful if you flip.

Nutrition: Cal 218, Carbs: 7 g, Fat: 12 g, Protein: 22 g

437. Air Fried Shrimp with Chili-Greek Yogurt Sauce

Prep Time: 10 mins
Servings: 4

Cook Time:20 mins

Ingredients
- Whole wheat bread crumbs: 3/4 cup
- Raw shrimp: 4 cups, deveined, peeled
- Flour: half cup
- Paprika: one tsp
- Chicken Seasoning, to taste
- 2 tbsp. of one egg white
- Kosher salt and pepper to taste

Sauce
- Sweet chili sauce: 1/4 cup
- Plain Greek yogurt: 1/3 cup
- Sriracha: 2 tbsp.

Directions: Let the Air Fryer preheat to 400 degrees F.
Add the seasonings to shrimp and coat well.
In three separate bowls, add flour, bread crumbs, and egg whites.
First coat the shrimp in flour, dab lightly in egg whites, then in the bread crumbs.
With cook oil, spray the shrimp.
Place the shrimps in an air fryer, cook for four mins, turn the shrimp over, and cook for another four mins. Serve with micro green and sauce.

Sauce
Mix all the ingredients.

Nutrition: 229 Cal, Fat 10 g, Carbs 13 g, Protein 22 g

438. Air Fryer Crab Cakes

Prep Time: 10 mins
Servings: 6

Cook Time:20 mins

Ingredients
- Crab meat: 4 cups
- Two eggs
- Whole wheat bread crumbs: ¼ cup
- Mayonnaise: 2 tablespoons
- Worcestershire sauce: 1 teaspoon
- Old Bay seasoning: 1 and ½ teaspoon
- Dijon mustard: 1 teaspoon
- Freshly ground black pepper to taste
- Green onion: ¼ cup, chopped

Directions: In a bowl, add Dijon mustard, Old Bay, eggs, Worcestershire, and mayonnaise mix it well. Then add in the chopped green onion and mix.
Fold in the crab meat to mayonnaise mix. Then add breadcrumbs, not to over mix.
Chill the mix in the refrigerator for at least 60 mins. Then shape into patties.
Let the air-fryer preheat to 350 °F. Cook for 10 mins. Flip the patties halfway through.
Serve with lemon wedges.

Nutrition: Cal 218, Fat: 13 g, Carbs: 5.6 g, Protein: 16.7 g

439. Air Fryer Tuna Patties

Prep Time: 15 mins
Servings: 10

Cook Time:10 mins

Ingredients
- Whole wheat breadcrumbs: half cup
- Fresh tuna: 4 cups, diced
- Lemon zest
- Lemon juice: 1 Tablespoon
- 1 egg
- Grated parmesan cheese: 3 Tablespoons
- One chopped stalk celery
- Garlic powder: half teaspoon
- Dried herbs: half teaspoon
- Minced onion: 3 Tablespoons
- Salt to taste
- Freshly ground black pepper

Directions: In a bowl, add lemon zest, bread crumbs, salt, pepper, celery, eggs, dried herbs, lemon juice, garlic powder, parmesan, cheese, and onion. Mix everything. Then add in tuna gently. Shape into patties.

Add air fryer baking paper in the air fryer basket. Spray the baking paper with cook spray. Spray the patties with oil.

Cook for ten mins at 360°F. turn the patties halfway over.

Serve with lemon slices.

Nutrition: Cal 214, Fat: 15 g, Carbs: 6 g, Protein: 22 g

440. Fish Finger Sandwich

Prep Time: 10 mins   **Cook Time:20 mins**
Servings: 3

Ingredients
- *Greek yogurt: 1 tbsp.*
- *Cod fillets: 4, without skin*
- *Flour: 2 tbsp.*
- *Whole-wheat breadcrumbs: 5 tbsp.*
- *Kosher salt and pepper to taste*
- *Capers: 10–12*
- *Frozen peas: 3/4 cup*
- *Lemon juice*

Directions: Let the air fryer preheat at 400°F.

Sprinkle kosher salt and pepper on the cod fillets, and coat in flour, then in breadcrumbs

Spray the fryer basket with oil. Put the cod fillets in the basket. Cook for 15 mins.

In the meantime, put the peas in boiling water for a few mins. Take out from the water and blend with Greek yogurt, lemon juice, and capers until well combined.

On a bun, add cooked fish with pea puree. Add lettuce and tomato.

Nutrition: Cal 240, Fat: 1 2g, Carbs: 7 g, Protein: 20 g

441. Lime-Garlic Shrimp Kebabs

Prep Time: 5 mins   **Cook Time:18 mins**
Servings: 2

Ingredients
- *One lime*
- *Raw shrimp: 1 cup*
- *Salt: 1/8 teaspoon*
- *1 clove of garlic*
- *Freshly ground black pepper*

Directions: In water, let wooden skewers soak for 20 mins.

Let the Air fryer preheat to 350 °F.

In a bowl, mix shrimp, minced garlic, lime juice, kosher salt, and pepper. Add shrimp on skewers.

Place skewers in the oven, and cook for 8 mins. Turn halfway over.

Top with cilantro and serve.

Nutrition: Cal: 76, Carbs: 4 g, Protein: 13 g, Fat 9 g

442. Air Fryer Sushi Roll

Prep Time: 1 hour 30 mins   **Cook Time:10 mins**
Servings: 3

Ingredients

For the Kale Salad
- *Rice vinegar: half teaspoon*
- *Chopped kale: one and a 1/2 cups*
- *Garlic powder:1/8 teaspoon*
- *Sesame seeds: 1 tablespoon*
- *Toasted sesame oil: 3/4 teaspoon*
- *Ground ginger: 1/4 teaspoon*
- *Soy sauce: 3/4 teaspoon*

Sushi Rolls
- *Half avocado - sliced*
- *Cooked Sushi Rice - cooled*
- *Whole wheat breadcrumbs: half cup*
- *Sushi: 3 sheets*

Directions:

Kale Salad: In a bowl, add vinegar, garlic powder, kale, soy sauce, sesame oil, and ground ginger. With your hands, mix with sesame seeds and set it aside.

Sushi Rolls: Lay a sheet of sushi on a flat surface. With damp fingertips, add a tablespoon of rice, and spread it on the sheet. Cover the sheet with rice, leaving a half-inch space at one end.
Add kale salad with avocado slices. Roll up the sushi, use water if needed.
Add the breadcrumbs in a bowl. Coat the sushi roll with Sriracha Mayo, then in breadcrumbs.
Add the rolls to the air fryer. Cook for ten mins at 390 F, shake the basket halfway through.
Take out from the fryer, and let them cool, then cut with a sharp knife.
Serve with light soy sauce.

Nutrition: Cal: 369, Fat: 13.9 g, Carbs: 15 g, Protein: 26.3 g

443. Roasted Salmon with Fennel Salad

Prep Time: 15 mins   **Cook Time:10 mins**
Servings: 4

Ingredients

- Skinless and center-cut: 4 salmon fillets
- Lemon juice: 1 teaspoon (fresh)
- Parsley: 2 teaspoons (chopped)
- Salt: 1 teaspoon, divided
- Olive oil: 2 tablespoons
- Chopped thyme: 1 teaspoon
- Fennel heads: 4 cups (thinly sliced)
- One clove of minced garlic
- Fresh dill: 2 tablespoons, chopped
- Orange juice: 2 tablespoons (fresh)
- Greek yogurt: 2/3 cup (reduced-fat)

Directions: In a bowl, add half teaspoon of salt, parsley, and thyme, mix well. Rub oil over salmon, and sprinkle with thyme mixture. Put salmon fillets in the air fryer basket, cook for ten mins at 350°F.
In the meantime, mix garlic, fennel, orange juice, yogurt, half tsp. of salt, dill, lemon juice in a bowl.
Serve with fennel salad.

Nutrition: Cal 364, Fat 30 g, Protein 38 g, Carbs 9 g

444. Catfish with Green Beans

Prep Time: 10 mins Cook Time:20 mins
Servings: 2

Ingredients

- Catfish fillets: 2 pieces
- Green beans: half cup, trimmed
- Honey: 2 teaspoon
- Ground black pepper and salt, to taste divided
- Crushed red pepper: half tsp.
- Flour: 1/4 cup
- One egg, lightly beaten
- Dill pickle relish: 3/4 teaspoon
- Apple cider vinegar: half tsp
- 1/3 cup whole-wheat breadcrumbs
- Mayonnaise: 2 tablespoons
- Dill
- Lemon wedges

Directions: In a bowl, add green beans, spray them with cook oil. Coat with crushed red pepper, 1/8 teaspoon of kosher salt, and half tsp. Of honey and cook in the air fryer at 400 F until soft and browned, for 12 mins. Take out from fryer and cover with aluminum foil
In the meantime, coat catfish in flour. Then in egg to coat, then in breadcrumbs. Place fish in an air fryer basket and spray with cook oil.
Cook for 8 mins, at 400°F, until cooked through and golden brown.
Sprinkle with pepper and salt. In the meantime, mix vinegar, dill, relish, mayonnaise, and honey in a bowl. Serve the sauce with fish and green beans.

Nutrition: Cal 243, Fat 18 g, Carbs 18 g, Protein 33 g

445. Honey & Sriracha Tossed Calamari

Prep Time: 10 mins
Servings: 2

Cook Time:20 mins

Ingredients

- Club soda: 1 cup
- Sriracha: 1-2 Tbsp.
- Calamari tubes: 2 cups
- Flour: 1 cup
- Pinches of salt, freshly ground black pepper, red pepper flakes, and red pepper
- Honey: 1/2 cup

Directions: Cut the calamari tubes into rings. Submerge them with club soda. Let it rest for ten mins.
In the meantime, in a bowl, add freshly ground black pepper, flour, red pepper, and kosher salt and mix well.
Drain the calamari and pat dry with a paper towel. Coat well the calamari in the flour mix and set aside.
Spray oil in the air fryer basket and put calamari in one single layer.
Cook at 375 for 11 mins. Toss the rings twice while cook. Meanwhile, to make sauce honey, red pepper flakes, and sriracha in a bowl, well.
Take calamari out from the basket, mix with sauce cook for another two mins more. Serve with salad green.

Nutrition: Cal 252, Fat: 38 g, Carbs: 3.1 g, Protein: 41 g

446. Scallops with Creamy Tomato Sauce

Prep Time: 5 mins
Servings: 2

Cook Time:10 mins

Ingredients

- Sea scallops eight jumbo
- Tomato Paste: 1 tbsp.
- Chopped fresh basil one tablespoon
- 3/4 cup of low-fat Whipping Cream
- Kosher salt half teaspoon
- Ground Freshly black pepper half teaspoon
- Minced garlic 1 teaspoon
- Frozen Spinach, thawed half cup
- Oil Spray

Directions

Take a seven-inch pan (heatproof) and add spinach in a single layer at the bottom
Rub olive oil on both sides of scallops, season with kosher salt and pepper.
On top of the spinach, place the seasoned scallops
Put the pan in the air fryer and cook for ten mins at 350F, until scallops are cooked completely, and internal temperature reaches 135F.
Serve immediately.

Nutrition: Cal: 259, Carbs: 6 g, Protein: 19 g, Fat: 13 g

447. Shrimp Spring Rolls in Air Fryer

Prep Time: 10 mins
Servings: 4

Cook Time:25 mins

Ingredients

- Deveined raw shrimp: half cup chopped (peeled)
- Olive oil: 2 and 1/2 tbsp.
- Matchstick carrots: 1 cup
- Slices of red bell pepper: 1 cup
- Red pepper: 1/4 teaspoon (crushed)
- Slices of snow peas: 3/4 cup
- Shredded cabbage: 2 cups
- Lime juice: 1 tablespoon
- Sweet chili sauce: half cup
- Fish sauce: 2 teaspoons
- Eight spring roll (wrappers)

Directions: In a skillet, add one and a half tbsp. of olive, until smoking lightly. Stir in bell pepper, cabbage, carrots, and cook for two mins. Turn off the heat, take out in a dish and cool for five mins.
In a bowl, add shrimp, lime juice, cabbage mixture, crushed red pepper, fish sauce, and snow peas. Mix well
Lay spring roll wrappers on a plate. Add 1/4 cup of filling in the middle of each wrapper. Fold tightly with water. Brush the olive oil over folded rolls. Put spring rolls in the basket of the Air Fryer and cook for 6 to 7 mins at 390°F until light brown and crispy.
You may serve with sweet chili sauce.

Nutrition: Cal 180, Fat 9 g, Protein 17 g, Carbs 9 g

448. Air Fryer Salmon

Prep Time: 10 mins
Serving: 2

Cook Time: 15 mins

Ingredients:
- ½ tsp. Salt
- ½ tsp. Garlic powder
- ½ tsp. smoked paprika
- Salmon

Directions:
Mix spices and sprinkle onto salmon.
Place seasoned salmon into the Air Fryer.
Pour into the basket. Set temperature to 400°F, and the time to 10 mins.

Nutrition: Cal: 185; Fat: 11 g; Protein: 21 g

449. Bacon-Wrapped Shrimp

Prep Time: 5 mins
Serving: 4

Cook Time: 10 mins

Ingredients:
- 1¼ pound tiger shrimp, peeled and deveined
- pound bacon

Directions: Wrap each shrimp with a slice of bacon.
Refrigerate for about 20 mins.
Preheat the Air Fryer to 390° F.
Arrange shrimp in the air fryer basket. Cook for about 5-7 mins.

450. Baked Salmon Rolls

Prep Time: 20mins
Servings: 4

Cook time: 8 mins

Ingredients:
- 1/2 pound (227 g) salmon fillet
- 1 teaspoon toasted sesame oil
- 1 onion, sliced
- 1 carrot, shredded
- 1 yellow bell pepper, thinly sliced
- 1/3 cup chopped fresh flat-leaf parsley
- ¼ cup chopped fresh basil
- 8 rice paper wrappers

Directions: Arrange the salmon in the air fry basket. Drizzle the sesame oil all over the salmon and scatter the onion on top.
Select Air Fry, set temperature to 370°F, and set time to 10 mins. Select Start to begin preheating.
Once preheated, place the basket on the air fry mode.
Meanwhile, fill a small shallow bowl with warm water. Dip the rice paper wrappers into the water for a few seconds or until moistened, then put them on a work surface.
When cook is complete, the fish should flake apart with a fork. Remove from the oven to a plate.
Make the spring rolls: Place 1/8 of the salmon and onion mixture, parsley, carrot, bell pepper, and basil into the rice wrapper's center and fold the sides over the filling. Roll up the wrapper carefully and tightly like you would a burrito. Repeat with the remaining wrappers and filling.
Transfer the rolls to the air fry basket.
Select Bake, set temperature to 380°F, and set time to 8 mins. Select Start to begin preheating.
Once preheated, place the basket on the bake position.
When cook is complete, the rolls should be crispy and lightly browned. Remove, and cut each roll in half, and serve warm.

451. Mahi Fillets

Prep Time: 10 mins
Servings: 4

Cook Time: 17 mins

Ingredients:

- *Four Mahi fillets*
- *1 tsp. paprika*
- *1 tsp. garlic powder*
- *3 tbsps. Olive oil*

- *1/2 cayenne*
- *1 tsp. oregano*
- *1 tsp. cumin*
- *1 tsp. onion powder*

- *1/2 tsp. pepper*
- *1/2 tsp. salt*

Directions: Line the Baking Pan with foil and set aside.
Place fish fillets on the baking pan and drizzle with oil.
In a small bowl, mix together cumin, onion powder, cayenne, paprika, oregano, garlic powder, pepper, and salt.
Rub fish fillets with a spice mixture.
Set to Bake at 450 degrees F for 12 mins.

Nutrition: Cal 189 Fat 12 g Carbs 2 g Protein 19 g

452. Cajun Catfish Fillets

Prep Time: 15 mins
Servings: 4

Cook Time: 20 mins

Ingredients:

- *lb. catfish fillets, cut ½-inch thick*
- *3/4 tsp. chili powder*

- *tsp. crushed red pepper*
- *tsp. onion powder*
- *1/2 tsp. ground cumin*

- *tbsps. dried oregano, crushed*
- *Salt and Pepper*

Directions: Line the Baking Pan with foil and set aside.
In a bowl, mix cumin, crushed red pepper, chili powder, onion powder, oregano, pepper, and salt.
Rub fish fillets with the spice mixture on both sides.
Place fish fillets in a baking pan.
Set to Bake at 350 degrees F for 15 mins.

Nutrition: Cal 165 Fat 9 g Carbs 2 g Protein 18 g

453. Cajun Salmon

Prep Time: 12 mins
Servings: 2

Cook Time: 8 mins

Ingredients:

- *2 (4-oz.) salmon fillets, skin removed*
- *2 tbsp. Unsalted butter; melted.*

- *1 tsp. Paprika*
- *1/8 tsp. Ground cayenne pepper*

- *¼ tsp. Ground black pepper*
- *½ tsp. Garlic powder*

Directions:
Brush the fillets with butter. Combine remaining ingredients and rub onto fish.
Place fillets into the air fryer basket.
Set the temperature to 390 Degrees F and the timer for 7 mins.

Nutrition: Cal: 253; Protein: 29 g; Fat: 16 g; Carbs: 4 g

454. Cheesy Tuna Patties

Prep Time: 5 mins
Servings: 4

Cook time: 17 mins

Ingredients:
Tuna Patties:
- 1 pound (454 g) canned tuna, drained
- 1 egg whisked

- 2 tablespoons shallots, minced
- 1 garlic clove, minced
- One cup grated Romano cheese

- 1 tablespoon sesame oil
- Sea salt and ground black pepper

Cheese Sauce:
- 1 tablespoon butter

- One cup beer

- 2 tablespoons grated Colby cheese

Directions: Mix the canned tuna, whisked egg, cheese, salt, shallots, garlic, and pepper in a bowl and toss to incorporate.
Divide the tuna mixture into four equal portions and form each piece into a patty with your hands. Refrigerate the patties for 2 hours.
When ready, brush both sides of each patty with sesame oil, and then place it in the air fry basket.
Select Bake, set temperature to 360°F and set time to 14 mins. Select Start to begin preheating.
Once preheated, place the basket on the bake position. Flip the patties halfway through the cook time.
Meanwhile, melt the butter in a saucepan.
Pour in the beer and whisk constantly, or until it begins to bubble. Add the grated Colby cheese and mix well. Continue cook for 3 to 4 mins or until the cheese melts. Remove from the heat.
When cook is complete, the patties should be lightly browned and cooked through. Remove the cakes from the oven to a plate. Drizzle them with the cheese sauce.

455. Chili Tuna Casserole

Prep Time: 10 mins
Servings: 4

Cook time: 16 mins

Ingredients:
- 1/2 tablespoon sesame oil
- 1/3 cup yellow onions, chopped
- 1/2 bell pepper, deveined and chopped
- Two cups canned tuna, chopped

- Cook spray
- 5 eggs, beaten
- 1/2 chili pepper, deveined and finely minced
- 11/2 tablespoons sour cream

- 1/3 teaspoon dried basil
- 1/3 teaspoon dried oregano
- Salt and ground black pepper

Directions: Heat the sesame oil in a nonstick skillet over medium heat until it shimmers.
Add the onions and bell pepper and sauté for 4 mins, stirring occasionally, or until tender.
Add the canned tuna and keep stirring until the tuna is heated through.
Meanwhile, coat a baking dish lightly with cook spray.
Transfer the tuna mixture to the baking dish, along with the beaten eggs, chili pepper, basil, sour cream, and oregano. Toss to combine and season with pepper and salt.
Select Bake, set temperature to 325 degrees F and set time to 12 mins. Select Start to begin preheating.
Once preheated, place the baking dish on the bake position.
When cook is complete, the eggs should be completely set and the top lightly browned.

456. Coconut Shrimp

Prep Time: 10 mins
Serving: 3

Cook Time: 15 mins

Ingredients:
- One cup almond flour
- One cup panko breadcrumbs

- 1 tbsp. coconut flour
- One cup unsweetened, dried coconut

- 1 egg white
- Twelve large raw shrimp

Directions: Put shrimp on paper towels to drain.
Stir coconut and panko breadcrumbs. Then mix in coconut flour and almond flour in a different bowl. Set to the side.
Dip shrimp into the flour mixture, then into egg white, and then into the coconut mixture.

Place into the air fryer basket. Repeat with remaining shrimp.
Set temperature to 350 degrees F, and the time to 10 mins. Turn halfway through the cook process.

Nutrition: Cal: 213; Fat: 8 g; Protein: 15 g

457. Cod and Endives

Prep Time: 25 mins   **Cook Time: 30 mins**
Servings: 4

Ingredients:
- *4 salmon fillets; boneless*
- *2 endives; shredded*
- *2 tbsp. extra-virgin olive oil*
- *½ tsp. sweet paprika*
- *Salt and pepper*

Directions: In a baking pan that fits the air fryer, combine the fish with the rest of the ingredients, stir, introduce in the fryer and bake at 350 degrees F for twenty mins, flipping the fish halfway

Nutrition: Cal: 243; Fat: 13 g; Carbs: 6 g; Protein: 14 g

458. Cod and Tomatoes

Prep Time: 20 mins   **Cook Time: 15 mins**
Servings: 4

Ingredients:
- *One cup cherry tomatoes; halved*
- *4 cod fillets, skinless and boneless*
- *2 tbsp. olive oil*
- *2 tbsp. Cilantro; chopped.*
- *Salt*
- *Pepper*

Directions: In a pan that fits your air fryer, mix all the ingredients, and mix gently.
Introduce in your oven and cook at 370 degrees F for fifteen mins
Divide everything between plates and serve right away.

Nutrition: Cal: 248; Fat: 11 g; Carbs: 5 g; Protein: 11 g

459. Crab Cakes

Prep Time: 20 mins   **Cook Time: 70 mins**
Servings: 2

Ingredients:
- *One large egg whites*
- *Two green onions, chopped*
- *1/2 celery rib, chopped*
- *3/4 cup crabmeat, drained*
- *1/4 cup breadcrumbs*
- *1 1/2 tbsp. mayonnaise*
- *1/2 sweet red pepper, chopped*
- *1/8 tsp. salt*

Directions: Place the air fryer Basket onto the Baking Pan and spray air fryer basket with cook spray.
Place breadcrumbs in a shallow dish.
In a bowl, add remaining ingredients except for crabmeat and stir well. Gently fold in crabmeat.
Drop a tablespoon of crabmeat mixture to the breadcrumbs and slowly coat and shape into patties.
Place crab cakes onto the air fryer basket.
Set to air fry at 375 degrees F for 12 mins.

Nutrition: Cal 151 Fat 4 g Carbs 21 g Protein 6 g

460. Crab Dip

Prep Time: 18 mins
Servings: 4

Cook Time: 8 mins

Ingredients:
- 8 oz. full-fat cream cheese; softened.
- 2 (6-oz.) can lump crabmeat
- ¼ cup chopped pickled jalapeños.
- ¼ cup full-fat sour cream.
- ½ cup shredded Cheddar cheese
- ¼ cup full-fat mayo
- 1 tbsp. Lemon juice
- ¼ cup sliced green onion
- ½ tsp. hot sauce

Directions: Place all ingredients into a 4-cup round baking dish and toss until thoroughly combined. Place dish into the air fryer basket.
Set the temperature to 400° F and set the timer for eight mins. The dip will be bubbling and hot when done.

Nutrition: Cal: 441; Protein: 18 g; Fat: 38 g; Carbs: 2 g

461. Crispy Paprika Fillets

Prep Time: 5 mins
Serving: 20

Cook Time: 15 mins

Ingredients:
- 2 fish fillets halved
- 1 egg, beaten
- 1/2 cup seasoned breadcrumbs
- 1 tablespoon balsamic vinegar
- 1/2 teaspoon seasoned salt
- 1 teaspoon paprika
- 1/2 teaspoon ground black pepper
- 1 teaspoon celery seed

Directions: In a bowl, dd the breadcrumbs, vinegar, pepper, salt, paprika, and celery seeds and mix well.
Coat the fish fillets with the beaten egg; then, coat them with the breadcrumbs mixture.
Pour into the basket. Set temperature to 350 degrees F, and time to fifteen mins.

462. Dijon Salmon

Prep Time: 20 mins
Servings: 4

Cook Time: 22mins

Ingredients:
- four salmon fillets
- 2 tbsp olive oil
- 1/4 cup Dijon mustard
- 1/4 cup maple syrup
- 2 garlic cloves, minced
- Salt and Pepper

Directions: Line the Baking Pan with foil and set aside.
Place salmon fillets into the baking pan.
Stir Dijon mustard, maple syrup, garlic, olive oil, pepper, salt, and pour over salmon. Coat well and let sit for ten mins.
Set to Bake at 400 degrees F for twelve mins.

Nutrition: Cal 360 Fat 18 g Carbs 14 g Protein 35 g

463. Baked Tilapia

Prep Time: 10 mins
Servings: 4

Cook Time: 20 mins

Ingredients:
- 1 lb. tilapia fillets
- 1 tbsp. garlic, minced
- 2 tbsp. dried parsley
- 1 tbsp. olive oil
- Salt and Pepper

Directions: Line the Baking Pan with foil and set aside.

Place fish fillets on a baking pan. Season with oil, salt and pepper.
Sprinkle parsley and garlic over fish fillets.
Set to Bake at 400 degrees F for fifteen mins.

Nutrition: Cal 160 Fat 8 g Carbs 1 g Protein 21 g

464. Garlic Lime Shrimp

Prep Time: 20 mins   **Cook Time: 20 mins**
Servings: 4

Ingredients:
- *1 lb. shrimp, peel and deveined*
- *Three garlic cloves, pressed*
- *2 tbsps. lime juice*
- *2 tbsps. butter, melted*
- *1/4 cup fresh cilantro, chopped*

Directions: Line the Baking Pan with foil and set aside.
Add shrimp into the baking dish. Stir together lime juice, garlic, and butter and pour over shrimp.
Toss shrimp well and let it sit for fifteen mins.
Set to Bake at 375 degrees F for fifteen mins.
Garnish with cilantro.

Nutrition: Cal 195 Fat 7.7 g Carbs 4.4 g Protein 26.1 g

465. Garlic Tilapia

Prep Time: 25 mins   **Cook Time: 20 mins**
Servings: 4

Ingredients:
- *4 tilapia fillets; boneless*
- *1 bunch kale; chopped.*
- *2 garlic cloves; minced*
- *1 tsp. Fennel seeds*
- *½ tsp. red pepper flakes, crushed*
- *3 tbsp. olive oil*
- *Salt and pepper*

Directions: In a bowl, stir all ingredients.
Put the pan in a fryer, set 360 degrees F, and cook for twenty mins

Nutrition: Cal: 240; Fat: 12 g; Carbs: 4 g; Protein: 12 g

466. Glazed Tuna and Fruits

Prep time: 15 mins   **Cook time: 10 mins**
Servings: 4

Ingredients:

Kebabs:
- *1-pound tuna steaks, cut into 1-inch cubes*
- *1/2 cup canned pineapple chunks, drained, juice reserved*
- *1/2 cup large red grapes*

Marinade:
- *1 tablespoon honey*
- *2 teaspoons grated fresh ginger*
- *1 teaspoon olive oil*
- *Pinch cayenne pepper*

Directions: Make the kebabs: Thread, pineapple chunks, alternating tuna cubes, and red grapes, onto the metal skewers.
Make the marinade: Whisk the honey, ginger, olive oil, and cayenne pepper in a small bowl. Brush the marinade generously over the kebabs and allow them to sit for ten mins.
When ready, transfer the kebabs to the air fry basket.
Select Air Fry, set the temperature to 370 degrees F, and set time to ten mins.

After five mins, remove and flip the kebabs and brush with the remaining marinade. Return the basket to the oven and continue cook for an additional five mins.

Remove, and discard any remaining marinade.

467. Golden Beer-Battered Cod

Prep Time: 5mins
Servings: 4

Cook time: 15 mins

Ingredients:
- 2 eggs
- 1 cup malty beer
- 1/2 cup cornstarch

- 1 teaspoon garlic powder
- 1 cup all-purpose flour
- Salt and pepper

- 4 (4-ounce / 113-g) cod fillets
- Cook spray

Directions: In a bowl, whisk together the eggs with the beer. In another bowl, thoroughly combine the flour and cornstarch. Season with garlic powder, pepper and salt.

Dredge each cod fillet in the flour mixture, then in the egg mixture. Dip each piece of fish in the flour mixture a second time.

Spritz the air fry basket with cook spray. Arrange the cod fillets in the basket in a single layer.

Select Air Fry, set temperature to 400 degrees F, and set time to fifteen mins. Select Start to begin preheating.

Once preheated, place the basket on the air fry position. Flip the fillets halfway through the cook time.

When cook is complete, the cod should reach an internal temperature of 145 degrees F on a meat thermometer, and the outside should be crispy. Let the fish cool for five mins.

468. Greek Pesto Salmon

Prep Time: 10 mins
Servings: 4

Cook Time: 30 mins

Ingredients:
- Four salmon fillets
- 1/2 cup pesto

- One onion, chopped
- 2 cups grape tomatoes, halved

- 1/2 cup feta cheese, crumbled

Directions: Line the Baking Pan with foil and set aside.

Place salmon fillet in baking pan and top with tomatoes, pesto, onion, and cheese.

Set to Bake at 350 degrees F for twenty mins.

Nutrition: Cal 447 Fat 28 g Carbs 8 g Protein 41 g

469. Grilled Salmon

Prep Time: 10 mins
Serving: 3

Cook Time: 15 mins

Ingredients:
- Two Salmon Fillets
- 1/2 Tsp. Lemon Pepper
- 1/2 Tsp. Garlic Powder

- 1/3 Cup Soy Sauce
- 1/3 Cup Sugar
- Salt and Pepper

- 1 Tbsp. Olive Oil

Directions: Season salmon fillets with garlic powder, lemon pepper, and salt. In a shallow bowl, add a third cup of water and combine the olive oil, soy sauce, and sugar. Place salmon in the bowl and immerse in the sauce. Cover with cling film and allow marinating in the refrigerator for at least 60 mins.

Preheat the oven at 350 degrees F.

Place salmon into the air fryer and cook for ten mins.

Serve with lemon wedges.

470. Fish And Chips

Prep Time: 5 mins
Serving: 3

Cook Time: 15 mins

Ingredients:
- 1 egg
- Old Bay seasoning
- ½ C. panko breadcrumbs
- 2 tbsp. almond flour
- 4-6 ounce tilapia fillets
- Frozen crinkle cut fries

Directions: Add almond flour to one bowl, beat egg in another bowl, and add panko breadcrumbs to the third bowl, mixed with Old Bay seasoning.
Dredge tilapia in flour, then egg, and then breadcrumbs.
Place coated fish in the oven along with fries.
Set temperature to 390 degrees F, and time to fifteen mins.

Nutrition: Cal: 219; Fat: 5 g; Protein: 25 g

471. Indian Fish Fingers

Prep Time: 35 mins
Serving: 4

Cook Time: 15 mins

Ingredients:
- 1/2 pound fish fillet
- 1 egg
- 1 tablespoon finely chopped fresh mint leaves or any fresh herbs
- 1/3 cup bread crumbs
- 1 teaspoon ginger garlic paste or ginger and garlic powders
- 1 hot green chili finely chopped
- 1/2 teaspoon paprika
- Generous pinch of black pepper
- 3/4 tablespoons lemon juice
- 3/4 teaspoons garam masala powder
- 1/3 teaspoon rosemary
- Salt

Directions: Start by removing any skin on the fish, washing, and patting dry. Cut the fish into fingers.
In a bowl, mix all ingredients except for fish, mint, and bread crumbs. Bury the fingers in the mixture and refrigerat for thirty mins.
Remove from the bowl from the fridge and mix in mint leaves.
In a separate bowl, beat the egg; pour bread crumbs into a third bowl. Dip the fingers in the egg bowl, and then stir them in the bread crumbs bowl.
Pour into the oven basket. Set the temperature to 360 degrees F, and set time to fifteen mins, toss the fingers halfway through.

Nutrition: Cal: 187; Fat: 7 g; Protein: 11 g

472. Mustard-Crusted Sole Fillets

Prep Time: 5 mins
Servings: 4

Cook time: 10 mins

Ingredients:
- 5 teaspoons low-sodium yellow mustard
- 1 tablespoon freshly squeezed lemon juice
- 4 (3.5-ounce / 99-g) sole fillets
- 1/8 teaspoon freshly ground pepper
- 1 slice low-sodium whole-wheat bread, crumbled
- 2 teaspoons olive oil
- ½ teaspoon dried marjoram
- ½ teaspoon dried thyme

Directions: Whisk together the lemon juice and mustard in a bowl until thoroughly mixed and smooth. Spread the mixture evenly over the sole fillets, and then transfer the fillets to the air fry basket.
In a separate bowl, combine the thyme, marjoram, olive oil, pepper, and bread crumbs and stir to mix well. Gently but firmly press the mixture over fillets, coating them completely.
Select Bake, set temperature to 320 degrees F, and set time to ten mins. Select Start to begin preheating.
Once preheated, place the basket on the bake position.
When cook is complete, the fish should reach an internal temperature of 145 degrees F on a meat thermometer. Remove the basket from the oven.

473. Parmesan Cod

Prep Time: 20 mins
Servings: 4

Cook Time: 14 mins

Ingredients:
- Four cod fillets; boneless
- A drizzle of olive oil
- Three spring onions; chopped.
- 1 cup parmesan
- 4 tbsp. balsamic vinegar
- Salt and pepper

Directions:
Season fish with pepper, salt, grease with the oil, and coat it in parmesan.
Put the fillets in your air fryer's basket and cook at 370 degrees F for forty mins. Meanwhile, in a bowl, toss the spring onions with salt, pepper, the vinegar and whisk.
Divide the cod between plates, drizzle the spring onions mix all over and serve with a side salad.

Nutrition: Cal: 220; Fat: 12 g; Carbs: 5 g; Protein: 13 g

474. Parmesan Walnut Salmon

Prep Time: 10 mins
Servings: 4

Cook Time: 25 mins

Ingredients:
- Four salmon fillets
- 1/4 cup walnuts
- 1/4 cup parmesan cheese, grated
- 1 tbsp. lemon rind
- 1 tsps. olive oil

Directions: Line the Baking Pan with foil and set aside.
Place salmon fillets in the baking pan.
Add walnuts into the blender and blend until ground.
Mix together walnuts, cheese, oil, and lemon rind and spread on top of salmon fillets.
Place the baking pan into rack position 2.
Set to Convection Bake at 400°F for 15 mins.

Nutrition: Cal 312 Fat 18 g Carbs 1 g Protein 38 g

475. Parmesan-Crusted Halibut Fillets

Prep Time: 5 mins
Servings: 4

Cook time: 10 mins

Ingredients:
- 2 medium-sized halibut fillets
- Dash of Tabasco sauce
- 1/2 teaspoon hot paprika
- 1 teaspoon curry powder
- 1/2 teaspoon ground coriander
- Kosher salt and freshly cracked mixed peppercorns
- One eggs
- 11/2 tablespoons olive oil
- 1/2 cup grated Parmesan cheese

Directions:
Drizzle the halibut fillets with the Tabasco sauce. Sprinkle with the curry powder, coriander, hot paprika, salt, and cracked mixed peppercorns. Set aside.
In a bowl, beat the eggs. In another bowl, combine the oil and Parmesan cheese.
One at a time, dredge the fillets in the eggs, remove any excess, then roll them over the Parmesan cheese until evenly coated.
Arrange the halibut fillets in the air fry basket in a single layer.
Select Roast, set temperature to 365 degrees F, and set time to ten mins. Select Start to begin preheating.
Once preheated, place the basket on the roast position.
When cook is complete, the fish should be golden brown and crisp. Cool for five mins before serving.

476. Parmesan-Crusted Salmon Patties

Prep Time: 10 mins
Servings: 4

Cook time: 13 mins

Ingredients:

- 1 pound (454 g) salmon, chopped into ½-inch pieces
- Two tablespoons coconut flour
- Two tablespoons grated Parmesan cheese
- 1 ½ tablespoons milk
- 1/2 onion, peeled and finely chopped
- 1/2 teaspoon butter, at room temperature
- 1/2 teaspoon chipotle powder
- 1/2 teaspoon dried parsley flakes
- One teaspoon acceptable salt
- 1/3 teaspoon ground black pepper
- 1/3 teaspoon smoked cayenne pepper

Directions: Put all the ingredients for the salmon patties in a bowl and stir to combine well.
Scoop out two tablespoons of the salmon mixture and shape into a patty with your palm, about 1/2 inches thick
Repeat until all the combination is used. Transfer to the refrigerator for about 120 mins until firm.
When ready, arrange the salmon patties in the air fry basket.
Select Bake, set temperature to 395°F, and set time to thirteen mins. Select Start to begin preheating.
Once preheated, place the basket on the bake position. Flip the patties halfway through the cook time.
When cook is complete, the patties should be golden brown.

477. Paella

Prep Time: 7 mins
Serving: 22

Cook Time: 15 mins

Ingredients:

- (10-ounce) package frozen cooked rice, thawed
- (6-ounce) jar artichoke hearts, drained and chopped
- ½ teaspoon turmeric
- ½ teaspoon dried thyme
- ¼ cup vegetable broth
- cup frozen cooked small shrimp
- ½ cup frozen baby peas
- 1 tomato, diced

Directions: In a 6-by-6-by-2-inch pan, combine the rice, artichoke hearts, vegetable broth, turmeric, and thyme, and stir gently.
Place in the Cuisinart Air Fryer Oven and bake for 8 to 9 mins or until the rice is hot. Remove from the air fryer and gently stir in the shrimp, peas, and tomato. Cook for 5 to 8 mins or until the shrimp and peas are hot, and the paella is bubbling.

Nutrition: Cal: 345; Fat: 1 g; Protein: 18 g

478. Salmon and Cauliflower Rice

Prep Time: 30 mins
Servings: 4

Cook Time: 40 mins

Ingredients:

- Four salmon fillets; boneless
- ½ cup chicken stock
- 1 cup cauliflower, riced
- 1 tsp. turmeric powder
- Salt and pepper
- 1 tbsp. butter; melted

Directions: In a pan that fits your air fryer, mixes the cauliflower rice with the other ingredients except the salmon, and toss.
Arrange the salmon fillets over the cauliflower rice, put the pan in the fryer, and bake at 360 degrees F for twenty-five mins, flipping the fish after fifteen mins.

Nutrition: Cal: 241; Fat: 12 g; Carbs: 6 g; Protein: 12 g

479. Salmon with Coconut Sauce

Prep Time: 25 mins
Servings: 4

Cook Time: 20 mins

Ingredients:

- 4 salmon fillets; boneless
- ½ cup coconut; shredded
- ¼ cup coconut cream

- 1/3 cup heavy cream
- ¼ cup lime juice
- 1 tsp. lime zest; grated
- A pinch of salt and pepper

Directions: Take a bowl and mix all the ingredients except the salmon and whisk.
Arrange the fish in a pan that fits your air fryer, drizzle the coconut sauce all over, put the pan in the machine, and cook at 360 degrees F for twenty mins.

Nutrition: Cal: 227; Fat: 12 g; Carbs: 4 g; Protein: 9 g

480. Salmon and Dill Sauce

Prep Time: 25 mins
Servings: 4

Cook Time: 20 mins

Ingredients:
- 4 salmon fillets; boneless
- 2 garlic cloves; minced
- 1 tbsp. Chives; chopped.
- 1 tsp. lemon juice
- ¼ cup ghee; melted
- ½ cup heavy cream
- 1 tsp. Dill; chopped.
- A pinch of salt and black pepper

Directions: Take a bowl and stir all the ingredients except the salmon, and whisk well.
Arrange the salmon in a pan that fits the air fryer, drizzle the sauce all over, introduce the pan in the machine, and cook at 360 degrees F for twenty mins.

Nutrition: Cal: 220; Fat: 14 g; Carbs: 5 g; Protein: 12 g

481. Salmon Dill Patties

Prep Time: 10 mins
Servings: 2

Cook Time: 15 mins

Ingredients:
- One egg
- tsp. dill weeds
- 1/2 cup almond flour
- 14 oz. salmon
- 1/4 cup onion, diced

Directions: Place the air fryer Basket onto the Baking Pan and spray air fryer basket with cook spray.
Add all ingredients into a bowl and stir well.
Make patties from bowl mixture and place onto the air fryer basket.
Set to air fry at 375 degrees F for ten mins.

Nutrition: Cal 350 Fat 18 g Carbs 3 g Protein 44 g

482. Salmon Patties

Prep Time: 20 mins
Servings: 2

Cook Time: 7 mins

Ingredients:
- One egg, lightly beaten
- 8 oz. salmon fillet, minced
- Salt and Pepper
- 1/4 tsp. garlic powder
- 1/4 tsp. onion powder

Directions: Place the air fryer Basket onto the Baking Pan and spray air fryer basket with cook spray.
Add all ingredients into the bowl and mix until just combined.
Make small patties from salmon mixture and place onto the air fryer basket.
Set to air fry at 400 degrees F for seven mins.

Nutrition: Cal 184 Fat 9 g Carbs 1 g Protein 25 g

483. Sesame Shrimp

Prep Time: 15 mins
Servings: 4

Cook Time: 12 mins

Ingredients:
- 1 lb. shrimp; peeled and deveined
- 1 tbsp. olive oil
- 1 tbsp. Sesame seeds, toasted
- ½ tsp. Italian seasoning
- A pinch of salt and pepper

Directions: Take a bowl and mix the shrimp with the rest of the ingredients and stir well
Put the shrimp in the air fryer's basket, cook at 370 degrees F for twelve mins, divide into bowls

Nutrition: Cal: 199; Fat: 11 g; Carbs: 4 g; Protein: 11 g

484. Air Fry Salmon

Prep Time: 22 mins
Servings: 2

Cook Time: 15 mins

Ingredients:
- 2 (4-oz.salmon fillets, skin removed
- 2 tbsp. unsalted butter; melted
- ½ tsp. Dried dill
- One medium lemon
- ½ tsp. Garlic powder

Directions: Place each fillet on a 5" × 5" square of foil. Drizzle with butter and garlic powder.
Zest half of the lemon and sprinkle zest over salmon. Slice the other half of the lemon and lay two slices on each piec of salmon. Sprinkle dill on top of the salmon.
Gather and fold foil at the top and sides to fully close packets. Place foil packets into the air fryer basket. Adjust the temperature to 400° F and set the timer for twelve mins.

Nutrition: Cal: 252; Protein: 29 g; Fat: 15 g; Carbs: 2 g

485. Sole and Cauliflower Fritters

Prep Time: 5 mins
Servings: 2

Cook time: 24 mins

Ingredients:
- ½ pound (227 g) sole fillets
- ½ pound (227 g) mashed cauliflower
- ½ cup red onion, chopped
- 1 egg, beaten
- 2 garlic cloves, minced
- Cook spray
- 2 tablespoons fresh parsley, chopped
- 1 tablespoon olive oil
- 1 tablespoon coconut amino
- ½ teaspoon scotch bonnet pepper, minced
- ½ teaspoon paprika
- 1 bell pepper, finely chopped
- Salt and white pepper

Directions: Spray the air fry basket with cook spray. Place the sole fillets in the basket.
Select Air Fry, set temperature to 395 degrees F, and set time to ten mins. Select Start to begin preheating.
Once preheated, place the basket on the air fry position. Flip the fillets halfway through.
When cook is complete, transfer the fish fillets to a bowl. Mash the fillets into flakes. Add remaining ingredients and toss to combine.
Make the patties: Scoop out two tablespoons of the fish mixture and shape into a patty about ½ inches thick with your hands.
Repeat with the remaining fish mixture. Place the cakes in the air fry basket.
Select Bake, set temperature to 380 degrees F, and set time to fourteen mins. Select Start to begin preheating.
Once preheated, place the basket on the bake position. Flip the patties halfway through.
When cook is complete, they should be golden brown and cooked through. Remove the basket from the oven and cool for five mins before serving.

486. Spicy Shrimp

Prep Time: 10 mins
Servings: 2

Cook Time: 16 mins

Ingredients:
- 1/2 lb. shrimp, peeled and deveined
- 1/2 tsp. old bay seasoning
- 1/2 tsp. cayenne pepper
- 1/4 tsp. paprika
- 1 tbsp. extra-virgin olive oil
- Pinch of salt

Directions: Place the air fryer Basket onto the Baking Pan and spray air fryer basket with cook spray.
Add shrimp and remaining ingredients into the bowl and mix well to coat.
Add shrimp into the air fryer basket.
Set to air fry at 400 degrees F for six mins.

Nutrition: Cal 197 Fat 9 g Carbs 2 g Protein 26 g

487. Spicy Tilapia

Prep Time: 20 mins
Servings: 4

Cook Time: 25 mins

Ingredients:
- Four tilapia fillets
- 1/2 tsp. red chili powder
- 1 tbsp. fresh lemon juice
- 2 tsps. fresh parsley, chopped
- 1 tsp. garlic, minced
- 3 tbsp. butter, melted
- One lemon, sliced
- Salt and Pepper

Directions: Line the Baking Pan with foil and set aside.
Place fish fillets in the baking pan and season with pepper and salt.
Mix together butter, garlic, red chili powder, and lemon juice and pour over fish fillets.
Arrange lemon slices over the fish fillets.
Set to Bake at 350 degrees F for fifteen mins.
Garnish with parsley.

Nutrition: Cal 149 Fat 12 g Carbs 4 g Protein 6 g

488. Sticky Hoisin Tuna

Prep Time: 15mins
Servings: 4

Cook time: 5 mins

Ingredients:
- 1/2 cup hoisin sauce
- 2 tablespoons rice wine vinegar
- 1 teaspoon garlic powder
- 3 cups cooked jasmine rice
- ¼ teaspoon red pepper flakes
- 1/2 onion, quartered and thinly sliced
- ounces (227 g) fresh tuna, cut into 1-inch cubes
- Cook spray
- 2 teaspoons sesame oil
- 2 teaspoons dried lemongrass

Directions: In a bowl, mix together the hoisin sauce, sesame oil, vinegar, lemongrass, garlic powder, and red pepper flakes. Add the sliced onion and tuna cubes and gently toss until the fish is evenly coated.
Arrange the coated tuna cubes in the air fry basket in a single layer.
Select Air Fry, set temperature to 390 degrees F, and set time to five mins. Select Start to begin preheating.
Once preheated, place the basket on the air fry position. Flip the fish halfway through the cook time.
When cook is complete, the fish should begin to flake. Remove from the oven and serve over hot jasmine rice.

489. Sweet and Savory Breaded Shrimp

Prep Time: 5 mins
Serving: 2

Cook Time: 20 mins

Ingredients:
- ½ pound of fresh shrimp, peeled from their shells and rinsed
- Two raw eggs
- ½ teaspoon of turmeric powder
- ½ teaspoon of red chili powder
- ½ teaspoon of cumin powder
- ½ cup of breadcrumbs
- ½ white onion, peeled and rinsed and finely chopped
- One teaspoon of ginger-garlic paste
- ½ teaspoon of black pepper powder
- ½ teaspoon of dry mango powder
- Pinch of salt

Directions: Cover the air fryer's basket with a lining of tin foil, leaving the edges.
Preheat the oven to 350 degrees F.
In a mixing bowl, beat the eggs until fluffy until the yolks and whites are thoroughly combined.
Dunk all the shrimp in the egg mixture, fully submerging.
In a separate mixing bowl, combine the bread crumbs with all the dry ingredients until evenly blended.
One by one, coat the egg-covered shrimp in the mixed dry ingredients fully covered, and place on the foil-lined air fryer basket. Set the timer to twenty mins.
Halfway through the cook time, shake the air fryer's handle so that the breaded shrimp jostles inside and fry-coverage is even.
After twenty mins the shrimp will be perfectly cooked. Using tongs, remove from the air fryer and set on a serving dish to cool.

490. Shrimp Fajitas

Prep Time: 10 mins
Servings: 4

Cook Time: 25 mins

Ingredients:
- lb. shrimp, peeled and deveined
- One medium onion, sliced
- 1/2 lime juice
- 1 1/2 tbsp. taco seasoning
- One bell pepper, sliced
- 1 1/2 tbsp. extra-virgin olive oil

Directions: Line the Baking Pan with foil and set aside.
In a bowl, mix shrimp with remaining ingredients.
Spread shrimp mixture on a baking pan.
Set to Bake at 400 degrees F for fifteen mins.

Nutrition: Cal 229 Fat 8 g Carbs 12 g Protein 27 g

491. Tilapia and Salsa

Prep Time: 20 mins
4

Cook Time: 15 mins Servings:

Ingredients:
- 4 tilapia fillets; boneless
- 2 tbsp. Sweet red pepper; chopped.
- 1 tbsp. balsamic vinegar
- 12 oz. Canned tomatoes; chopped.
- 2 tbsp. Green onions; chopped.
- 1 tbsp. olive oil
- A pinch of salt and black pepper

Directions: Arrange the tilapia in a pan that fits the air fryer and season with salt and pepper.
In a bowl, combine all the other ingredients, stir and spread over the fish.
Introduce the baking pan in the oven and cook at 350 degrees F for fifteen mins.

Nutrition: Cal: 221; Fat: 12 g; Carbs: 5 g; Protein: 14 g

492. Tilapia with Vegetables

Prep time: 10 mins
Servings: 4

Cook time: 20 mins

Ingredients:

- 10 ounces Yukon Gold potatoes, sliced ¼-inch thick
- Five tablespoons unsalted butter, melted, divided
- One teaspoon kosher salt, divided
- 4 (8-ounce) tilapia fillets
- 1/2 pound green beans, trimmed
- Two tablespoons chopped fresh parsley, for garnish
- Juice of one lemon

Directions: Drizzle the potatoes with 2 tablespoons of melted butter and ¼ teaspoon of kosher salt in a bowl. Transfer the potatoes to the sheet pan.
Select Roast, set temperature to 375 degrees F, and set time to twenty mins.
Meanwhile, season both sides of the fillets with 1/2 teaspoon of kosher salt. Put the green beans in a bowl and sprinkle with the remaining ¼ teaspoon of kosher salt and one tablespoon of butter, tossing to coat.
After ten mins, remove the pan and push the potatoes to one side. Put the fillets in the middle of the pan and add the green beans on the other side.
Drizzle the rest of the 2 tablespoons of butter over the fillets. Return it and cook until the fish flakes easily with a fork, and the green beans are crisp-tender.
Once cooked, remove and drizzle the lemon juice over the fillets and sprinkle the parsley on top for garnish.

Nutrition: Cal: 172 Carbs: 24 g Fat: 2 g Protein: 24 g

493. Trout with Mint

Prep Time: 21 mins
Servings: 4

Cook Time: 8 mins

Ingredients:

- 1 avocado, peeled, pitted, and roughly chopped.
- 4 rainbow trout
- 1/3 pine nuts
- 3 garlic cloves; minced
- ½ cup mint; chopped.
- 1 cup olive oil+ 3 tbsp.
- 1 cup parsley; chopped
- Zest of 1 lemon
- Juice of 1 lemon
- A pinch of salt and pepper

Directions: Pat dry the trout, season with salt and pepper, and rub with 3 tbsp. oil
Put the fish in the basket and cook for eight mins on each side. Divide the fish between plates and drizzle half of the lemon juice all over
In a blender, combine the rest of the oil with the remaining lemon juice, parsley, garlic, mint, pine nuts, lemon zest, and the avocado and pulse well. Spread this over the trout.

Nutrition: Cal: 240; Fat: 12 g; Carbs: 6 g; Protein: 9 g

494. Tuna Veggie

Prep Time: 5 mins
Serving: 4

Cook Time: 12 mins

Ingredients:

- 1 tablespoon olive oil
- 1 red bell pepper, chopped
- 1 cup green beans, cut into 2-inch pieces
- 2 tablespoons low-sodium soy sauce
- 1 onion, sliced
- 2 cloves garlic, sliced
- 1 tablespoon honey
- ½ pound fresh tuna, cubed

Directions: In a 6-inch metal bowl, combine the olive oil, onion, pepper, green beans, and garlic.
Pour into the basket. Set temperature to 350 degrees F, and set time to 4 to 6 mins, stirring once, until crisp and tender. Add honey, soy sauce, and tuna, and mix. Cook for another 3 to 6 mins, stirring once until the tuna is cooked as desired.

Nutrition: Cal: 187; Fat: 8 g; Protein: 17 g

495. Bacon Shrimps

Prep Time: 5-10 min.
Servings: 5-6

Cook Time: 10 min.

Ingredients:
- *1 package bacon*
- *1 pound shrimp*
- *1/2 teaspoon cayenne pepper*
- *1/2 teaspoon ground cumin*
- *1/2 teaspoon onion powder*
- *1 teaspoon garlic powder*
- *1/2 teaspoon lemon zest*
- *1 tablespoon lemon juice*
- *1 tablespoon Worcestershire sauce*

Directions: In a mixing bowl, whisk the Worcestershire sauce, cumin, lemon zest, cayenne pepper, onion powder, and garlic powder. Add and combine the shrimp. Refrigerate for 1-2 hours to marinate.
Take the bacon, slice into 2 parts, and wrap each shrimp with them.
Press Air Fry, set the temperature to 400 degrees F and set the timer to five mins to preheat.
In the inner pot, place the Air Fryer basket. In the basket, add the wrapped shrimps.
Press the "Air Fry" setting. Set temperature to 380 degrees F and set the timer to ten mins.
Halfway down, shake the basket and close to continue cook for the remaining time.

Nutrition: Cal: 138 Fat: 3 g Carbs: 6 g Protein: 17 g

496. Cajuned Salmon

Prep Time: 5-10 mins
Servings: 2

Cook Time: 8 mins

Ingredients:
- *Two salmon fillets (6 ounce each and with skin)*
- *1 tablespoon Cajun seasoning*
- *1 teaspoon brown sugar*

Directions: In a mixing bowl, combine Cajun seasoning and brown sugar. Add the fillets and coat well.
Press Air Fry, set the temperature to 400 degrees F and set the timer to five mins to preheat.
Spray the Air Fryer basket with some cook oil, and add the fillets.
Press the "Air Fry" setting. Set temperature to 390 degrees F and set the timer to eight mins.
Halfway down, flip the fillets, and continue cook for the remaining time.

Nutrition: Cal: 145 Fat: 5 g Carbs: 2 g Protein: 19 g

497. Coconut Chili Shrimp

Prep Time: 5-10 mins
Servings: 5-6

Cook Time: 6 mins

Ingredients:
- *Three cups panko breadcrumbs*
- *½ cup all-purpose flour*
- *Two large eggs*
- *¼ cup honey*
- *2 teaspoon fresh cilantro, chopped*
- *3 cups flaked coconut, unsweetened*
- *12 ounce medium-size raw shrimps, peeled, and deveined*
- *One serrano chili, thinly sliced*
- *¼ cup lime juice*
- *½ teaspoon kosher salt*
- *½ teaspoon ground black pepper*

Directions: In a mixing bowl, combine honey, Serrano chili with lime juice.
In another bowl, combine the pepper and flour. In a mixing bowl, beat the eggs.
In another bowl, combine the breadcrumbs and coconut. Coat the shrimps with the eggs, then with the flour, and then with the crumbs. Coat with some cook spray.
Press Air Fry, set the temperature to 400 degrees F and set the timer to five mins to preheat.
Line with a parchment paper, add the shrimps.
Press the "Air Fry" setting. Set temperature to 200 degrees F and set the timer to six mins.
Halfway down, shake the basket and continue cook for the remaining time.
Serve the shrimps warm with the chili sauce.

Nutrition: Cal: 233 Fat: 8.5 g Carbs: 28 g Protein: 13 g

498. Creamed Cod

Prep Time: 5-10 mins   **Cook Time:** 10 mins
Servings: 2

Ingredients:
- 1 tablespoon lemon juice
- 1 pound cod fillets
- 2 tablespoons olive oil
- ½ teaspoon ground black pepper
- ½ teaspoon salt

Sauce:
- 3 tablespoons ground mustard
- ½ cup heavy cream
- 1 tablespoon butter
- ½ teaspoon salt

Directions: Spread some olive oil on the fillets. Season with the pepper, salt, and lemon juice.
Grease Air Fryer Basket with some cook spray. Place the fillets over.
Press Air Fry, set the temperature to 400 degrees F and set the timer to five mins to preheat.
Press the "Air Fry" setting. Set temperature to 350 degrees F and the timer to ten mins.
Halfway down, flip the fillets, and continue cook for the remaining time.
In a bowl, add the heavy cream, mustard sauce, heavy cream, and salt. Cook for 3-4 mins.
Pour it over the fish and serve warm.

Nutrition: Cal: 523 Fat: 31.5 g Carbs: 17.5 g Protein: 29.5 g

499. Garlic Lemon Shrimp

Prep Time: 5-10 mins   **Cook Time:** 5 mins
Servings: 4

Ingredients:
- ¼ teaspoon, crushed red pepper flakes
- Four cloves garlic, finely grated
- 1 tablespoon olive oil
- 1 pound small shrimps, peeled and deveined
- 1 lemon juice, zested
- ¼ cup, parsley, chopped
- ¼ teaspoon salt

Directions: Remove the tails of the shrimps. In a mixing bowl, add shrimps, the garlic, lemon zest, red pepper flakes, salt, and oil.
Combine the ingredients to stir well with each other.
Press Air Fry, set the temperature to 400 degrees F and set the timer to five mins to preheat.
In the Air Fryer basket, add the shrimps. Press the "Air Fry" setting and et temperature to 400 degrees F. Set the timer to six mins.
Halfway down, shake the basket and continue cook for the remaining time.
Serve warm with the lemon juice and parsley on top.

Nutrition: Cal: 134 Fat: 5 g Carbs: 3.5 g Protein: 17 g

500. Mustard Salmon

Prep Time: 5-10 mins   **Cook Time:** 10 mins
Servings: 2

Ingredients:
- Two salmon fillets
- One garlic clove, grated
- Two tablespoons mustard, whole grain
- Two teaspoon olive oil
- ½ teaspoon ground black pepper
- One tablespoon brown sugar
- ½ teaspoon thyme leaves

Directions: Rub the salmon with salt and pepper. In a mixing bowl, combine the mustard grain, thyme, brown sugar, garlic, and oil. Coat the salmon with the mixture.
Press Air Fry, set the temperature to 400 degrees F and set the timer to five mins to preheat.
In the basket of the oven, add the salmon. Press the "Air Fry" setting. Set temperature to 400 degrees F and set the timer to ten mins. Halfway down, flip the salmon, and continue cook for the remaining time.

Nutrition: Cal: 247 Fat: 10 g Carbs: 51.5 g Protein: 17 g

501. Fennel Cod

Prep Time: 5-10 mins
Servings: 2

Cook Time: 15 mins

Ingredients:
- ½ cup red pepper, thinly sliced
- ½ cup carrots, julienned
- 2 ½ ounces cod fillets, frozen and thawed
- ½ cup fennel bulbs, julienned
- Two tablespoons butter, melted
- Two sprigs tarragon
- 1 tablespoon vegetable oil
- One tablespoon lemon juice
- ½ teaspoon black pepper powder
- 1 tablespoon salt

Directions: In a mixing bowl, combine the tarragon, lemon juice, melted butter, and ½ teaspoon salt. Mix the fennel bulbs, carrots and toss well.
Coat the codfish fillets with the oil. Rub pepper and salt evenly.
Place the fillets over a baking pan. Add the veggies on top.
Press Air Fry, set the temperature to 400 degrees F and set the timer to five mins to preheat.
In the Air Fryer basket, add the baking pan with the fish. Press the "Air Fry" setting. Set temperature to 350 degrees F and set the timer to fifteen mins. Halfway down, flip the fillets, and continue cook for the remaining time.

Nutrition: Cal: 288 Fat: 19 g Carbs: 24 g Protein: 6.5 g

502. Air Fryer Salmon (2nd Version)

Prep time: 10 mins
Servings: 2

Cook time: 10 mins

Ingredients:
- Salmon
- ½ teaspoon. salt
- ½ teaspoon. garlic powder
- ½ teaspoon. smoked paprika

Directions: Stir spices together and sprinkle onto salmon.
Place seasoned salmon into the Air Fryer Oven.
Pour into the basket. Set temperature to 400 degrees F, and set time to ten mins.

Nutrition: Cal 296 Fat 11.5 g Carbs 18.7 g Protein 29.9 g

503. Air Fryer Salmon Patties

Prep time: 10 mins
Servings: 4

Cook time: 7 mins

Ingredients:
- 1 C. almond flour
- 1 tablespoon. ghee
- ¼ teaspoon. salt
- 1/8 teaspoon. pepper
- One egg
- 1 tablespoon. olive oil
- 1 can wild Alaskan pink salmon

Directions: Drain can of salmon into a bowl and keep liquid. Discard skin and bones.
Add pepper, salt, and egg to salmon, stirring well with hands to incorporate. Make patties.
Dredge in flour and remaining egg. If it seems dry, spoon reserved salmon liquid from the can onto patties.
Pour the patties into the basket. Set temperature to 378 degrees F, and set time to seven mins. Cook till golden, making sure to flip once during cook process.

Nutrition: Cal 296 Fat 11.5 g Carbs 18.7 g Protein 29.9 g

504. Bang Panko Breaded Fried Shrimp

Prep time: 10 mins
Servings: 4

Cook time: 8 mins

Ingredients:
- Montreal chicken seasoning
- 1 pound raw shrimp (peeled and deveined)
- 1 teaspoon paprika
- ¾ C. panko bread crumbs
- ½ C. almond flour
- One egg white

Bang Bang Sauce:
- 1/3 C. plain Greek yogurt
- ¼ C. sweet chili sauce
- 2 tablespoons sriracha sauce

Directions: Preheated your Air Fryer Oven to 400° F.
Season all shrimp with seasonings.
Add flour to a bowl, egg white in another, and breadcrumbs to a third.
Dip seasoned shrimp in flour, then egg whites, and then breadcrumbs. Spray coated shrimp with oil and add to air fryer basket.
Set temperature to 400 degrees F, and set time to four mins. Flip, and cook an additional four mins.
To make the sauce, stir together all sauce ingredients until smooth.

Nutrition: Cal 296 Fat 11.5 g Carbs 18.7 g Protein 29.9 g

505. Flying Fish

Prep time: 10 mins
Servings: 6

Cook time: 12 mins

Ingredients:
- Four Fish Fillets
- A Lemon
- 4 Tablespoon Oil
- 3–4 oz Bread crumbs
- 1 Whisked Whole Egg in a Saucer/Soup Plate

Directions: Preheat the air fryer to 350 degrees F.
Mix the crumbs and oil until it looks nice and loose.
Dip the fish in the egg and coat lightly, then move on to the crumbs. Make sure the fillet is covered evenly.
Cook in the Air Fryer Oven basket for roughly twelve mins.
Serve with lemon.

Nutrition: Cal 296 Fat 11.5 g Carbs 18.7 g Protein 29.9 g

506. Grilled Salmon

Prep time: 10 mins
Servings: 3

Cook time: 10 mins

Ingredients:
- Two Salmon Fillets
- 1/2 Teaspoon Garlic Powder
- 1/3 Cup Soy Sauce
- 1/2 Teaspoon Lemon Pepper
- 1/3 Cup Sugar
- 1 Tablespoon Olive Oil
- Salt and Pepper

Directions: Season salmon fillets with garlic powder, lemon, pepper, and salt. In a bowl, add a third cup of water and combine the soy sauce, oil, and sugar. Place salmon the bowl and immerse in the sauce. Cover with cling film and allow to marinate in the refrigerator for at least 60 mins.
Preheat the Air Fryer Oven at 350° F.
Place salmon into the air fryer and bake for ten mins.

Nutrition: Cal 296 Fat 11.5 g Carbs 18.7 g Protein 29.9 g

507. Soy Salmon Fillets

Prep time: 10 mins
Servings: 4

Cook time: 8 mins

Ingredients:
- Four salmon fillets
- 1 teaspoon onion powder
- 1/4 teaspoon ground black pepper
- 1/2 teaspoon cayenne pepper
- 1 tablespoon lemon juice
- 1/2 cup soy sauce
- 1/2 cup water
- 1 tablespoon honey
- 1 tablespoons olive oil
- 1/2 teaspoon salt

Directions: Firstly, pat the salmon fillets dry using kitchen towels. Season the salmon with pepper, salt, cayenne pepper, and onion powder.
To make the marinade, combine together the soy sauce, lemon juice, water, honey, and oil. Marinate the salmon for at least 120 mins in your refrigerator.
Arrange the fish fillets on the basket of your Air Fryer. Bake at 330° F for 8 to 9 mins, or until salmon fillets are easily flaked with a fork.
Work with batches and serve warm.

Nutrition: Cal 296 Fat 11.5 g Carbs 18.7 g Protein 29.9 g

508. Lemony Tuna

Prep time: 10 mins
Servings: 4

Cook time: 10 mins

Ingredients:
- 2 (6-ounce) cans water packed plain tuna
- One egg
- Two teaspoons Dijon mustard
- Hot sauce
- 1/2 cup bread crumbs
- One tablespoon fresh lime juice
- Two tablespoons fresh parsley, chopped
- Three tablespoons canola oil
- Salt and freshly ground black pepper

Directions: Drain the liquid from the canned tuna.
In a bowl, add the fish, crumbs, mustard, citrus juice, parsley and hot sauce and stir till well combined. Add a little
canola oil if it seems too dry. Add egg, salt and toss to combine. Make the patties from tuna mixture. Refrigerate the tuna patties for about 120 mins.
Pour into the Air Fryer basket. Set temperature to 355 degrees F, and set time to twelve mins.

Nutrition: Cal 296 Fat 11.5 g Carbs 18.7 g Protein 29.9 g

509. Shrimp Po Boy

Prep time: 10 mins
Servings: 6

Cook time: 10 mins

Ingredients:
- 1 pound deveined shrimp
- Lettuce leaves
- One teaspoon creole seasoning
- Eight slices of tomato
- ¼ C. buttermilk
- ½ C. Louisiana Fish Fry

Remoulade sauce:
- ½ teaspoon creole seasoning
- One chopped green onion
- One teaspoon hot sauce
- One teaspoon Worcestershire sauce
- One teaspoon Dijon mustard
- Juice of ½ a lemon
- ½ C. mayo

Directions: Combine all sauce ingredients until well incorporated. Chill while you cook shrimp.
Stir seasonings together and liberally season shrimp.
Add buttermilk to a bowl. Dip each shrimp into milk and place in a Ziploc bag. Chill half an hour to marinate.
Add Louisiana fish fry to a bowl. Take shrimp from marinating bag and dip into fish fry, then add to air fryer.
Ensure your air fryer is preheated to 400° F.

Spray shrimp with oil. Pour into the basket. Set temperature to 400 degrees F, and set time to five mins. Flip and then cook another five mins. Assemble Po Boy by adding sauce to lettuce leaves, along with shrimp and tomato.

Nutrition: Cal 296 Fat 11.5 g Carbs 18.7 g Protein 29.9 g

510. Old Bay Crab Cakes

Prep time: 10 mins
Servings: 4

Cook time: 20 mins

Ingredients:
- One pound lump crabmeat
- Slices dried bread, crusts removed
- Small amount of milk
- One egg
- One tablespoon mayo
- One tablespoon Worcestershire sauce
- One tablespoon baking powder
- One tablespoon parsley flakes
- One teaspoon Old Bay® Seasoning
- 1/4 teaspoon salt

Directions: Crush your bread into a bowl until it is broken down into small pieces. Add milk and mix until bread crumbs are moistened. Mix mayo and Worcestershire sauce. Add remaining ingredients and stir well. Shape into four patties.
Pour into the basket. Set temperature to 360 degrees F, and set time to twenty mins, flip half way through.

Nutrition: Cal 296 Fat 11.5 g Carbs 18.7 g Protein 29.9 g

511. Pistachio-Crusted Lemon-Garlic Salmon

Prep time: 10 mins
Servings: 6

Cook time: 20 mins

Ingredients:
- Four medium-sized salmon filets
- Three ounces of melted butter
- One clove of garlic, peeled and finely minced
- One large-sized lemon
- Two raw eggs
- One tablespoon of parsley, rinsed, patted dry and chopped
- One teaspoon of dill, rinsed, patted dry and chopped
- ½ cup of pistachio nuts, shelled and coarsely crushed
- One teaspoon of salt

Directions: Cover the basket of the air fryer with a lining of tin foil, leaving the edges.
Preheat the Air Fryer Oven to 350 degrees.
In a mixing bowl, beat the eggs until the yolks and whites are fully combined. Add the melted butter, the juice of the lemon, the minced garlic, the parsley and the dill to the beaten eggs, and stir thoroughly.
One by one, dunk the salmon filets into the wet mixture, then roll them in the crushed pistachios, coating completely.
Place the coated salmon fillets in the Smart Air Fryer Oven basket. Set the Smart Air Fryer Oven timer for 10 mins.
When the air fryer shuts off, after 10 mins, the salmon will be partly cooked and the crust beginning to crisp. Using tongs, turn each of the fish filets over.
Reset the Air Fryer Oven to 350 degrees for another 10 mins.
After 10 mins, when the air fryer shuts off, the salmon will be perfectly cooked and the pistachio crust will be toasted and crispy.
Using tongs, remove from the air fryer and serve.

Nutrition: Cal 296 Fat 11.5 g Carbs 18.7 g Protein 29.9 g

512. Salmon Noodles

Prep time: 10 mins
Servings: 4

Cook time: 16 mins

Ingredients:
- One Salmon Fillet
- One Cup Broccoli
- One Tablespoon Teriyaki Marinade
- Seven Ozs Mixed Salad
- 3 ½ Ozs Soba Noodles, cooked and drained
- Ten Ozs Firm Tofu
- Olive Oil
- Salt and Pepper

Directions: Season the salmon with salt and pepper, then coat with the teriyaki marinate. Set aside for fifteen mins.
Preheat the Air Fryer Oven at 350° F, then cook the salmon for eight mins.
Whilst the air fryer is cook the salmon, start slicing the tofu into small cubes.
Next, slice the broccoli into smaller chunks. Drizzle with oil.
Once the salmon is cooked, put the broccoli and tofu into the Air Fryer Oven tray for eight mins.
Plate the salmon and broccoli tofu mixture over the soba noodles. Add the mixed salad to the side.

513. Salmon Quiche

Prep time: 10 mins
Servings: 4

Cook time: 12 mins

Ingredients:
- *Five Ozs Salmon Fillet*
- *Quiche Pan*
- *1/2 Cup Flour*
- *1/2 Tablespoon Lemon Juice*
- *1/4 Cup Butter, melted*
- *One Eggs and 1 Egg Yolk*
- *Three Tablespoons Whipped Cream*
- *Two Teaspoons Mustard*
- *Pepper*
- *Salt*

Directions: Clean and cut the salmon into small cubes.
Heat the Air Fryer Oven to 375° F.
Pour the lemon juice over the salmon cubes and allow to marinate for 60 mins.
Combine a tablespoon of water with the flour, butter, and yolk in a bowl. Knead the mixture until smooth.
Use a rolling pin to form a circle of dough. Place this into the quiche pan, using your fingers to adhere the pastry to the edges.
Whisk the cream, mustard and eggs together. Season with salt and pepper. Add the marinated salmon into the bowl and combine.
Pour the content of the bowl into the dough lined quiche pan.
Put the pan in the oven tray and cook for twenty-five mins until browned and crispy.

514. Scallops and Vegetables

Prep time: 10 mins
Servings: 4

Cook time: 8 mins

Ingredients:
- *One pound sea scallops*
- *½ pound asparagus, ends trimmed, cut into 2-inch pieces*
- *One cup sugar snap peas*
- *One tablespoon lemon juice*
- *½ teaspoon dried thyme*
- *Two teaspoons olive oil*
- *Pinch of salt*
- *Ground black pepper*

Directions: Place the asparagus and sugar snap peas in the air fryer basket. Cook for 2 to 3 mins.
Meanwhile, check the scallops for a small muscle attached to the side, and pull it off and discard.
In a bowl, mix the scallops with the lemon juice, thyme, olive oil, salt, and pepper. Place into the Air Fryer basket over the vegetables.
Steam for 5 to 7 mins, tossing the basket once during cook time, until the scallops are opaque in the center, and the vegetables are tender.

Nutrition: Cal 296 Fat 11.5 g Carbs 18.7 g Protein 29.9 g

515. Tuna Stuffed Potatoes

Prep time: 10 mins
Servings: 4

Cook time: 30 mins

Ingredients:
- *One scallion, chopped and divided*
- *Four starchy potatoes*
- *½ tablespoon olive oil*
- *1 (6-ounce) can tuna, drained*
- *Two tablespoons plain Greek yogurt*
- *One tablespoon capers*
- *One teaspoon red chili powder*
- *Salt and ground black pepper*

Directions: In a bowl with water, soak the potatoes for about thirty mins. Drain well and pat dry with paper towel.
Preheat the air fryer to 355° F. Place the potatoes in the air fryer basket.
Cook for about thirty mins.
Meanwhile in a bowl, add tuna, red chili powder, yogurt, salt, pepper and half of scallion and with a potato masher, mash the mixture completely.
Remove the potatoes from the Air Fryer and place onto a smooth surface.
Carefully, cut each potato from top side lengthwise.
With your fingers, press the open side of potato halves slightly. Stuff the potato open portion with tuna mixture evenly.
Sprinkle with the capers and remaining scallion.

Nutrition: Cal 296 Fat 11.5 g Carbs 18.7 g Protein 29.9 g

VEGETABLES

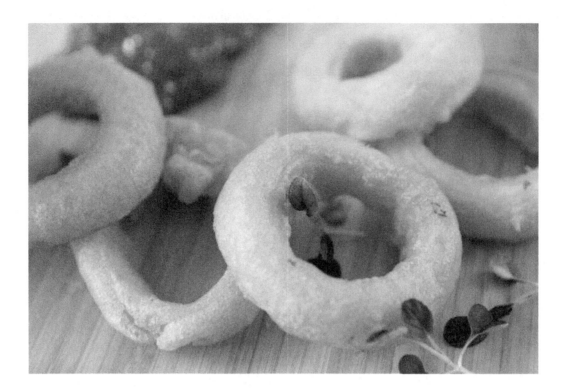

516. Air Fried Asparagus

Prep Time: 5 mins
Serving: 4

Cook Time: 5 mins

Ingredients:
- *1 pound (454 g) fresh asparagus spears, trimmed*
- *Salt and pepper*
- *1 tablespoon olive oil*

Directions: Press Start. Preheat the Air Fryer Oven to 375 degrees F.
Combine all the ingredients and transfer them to the fry basket. Insert the fry basket at mid position.
Select Air Fry, and set time to five mins, or until soft.

517. Air Fried Brussels Sprouts

Prep Time: 5 mins
Servings: 1

Cook time: 10 mins

Ingredients:
- *1 pound (454 g) Brussels sprouts*
- *1 tablespoon unsalted butter, melted*
- *1 tablespoon coconut oil, melted*

Directions: Preheat the Air Fryer to 400 degrees F.
Prepare the Brussels sprouts by halving them, discarding any loose leaves.
Combine with the melted coconut oil and transfer to the air fryer basket.
Place the air basket onto the baking pan, select Air Fry, and set time to ten mins, shaking the basket once cook. The sprouts are ready when they are partially caramelized.
Remove from the oven and serve with a topping of melted butter.

518. Air Fried Carrots, Squash & Zucchini

Prep Time: 10 Mins   **Cook Time: 35 mins**
Servings: 4

Ingredients:
- ½ pound carrots
- 1 tablespoon chopped tarragon leaves
- 1 pound yellow squash
- 1 pound zucchini
- 6 teaspoons olive oil
- ½ teaspoon white pepper
- 1 teaspoon salt

Directions: Stem and root the end of squash and zucchini and cut in ¾-inch half-moons. Peel and cut carrots into 1-inch cubes.
Combine carrot cubes with 2 teaspoons of oil, stirring to combine.
Pour into the Air Fryer basket, set temperature to 400 degrees F, and set time to five mins.
As carrots cook, drizzle remaining oil over squash and zucchini pieces, then season with salt and pepper. Stir well to coat. Add squash and zucchini when the timer for carrots goes off. Cook thirty mins, making sure to toss 2-3 times during the cook process. Once done, take out vegetables and stir with tarragon. Serve up warm.

Nutrition: Cal: 122 Fat: 9 g Carbs: 0 g Protein: 6 g

519. Cauliflower in an Almond Crust with Avocado Ranch Dip

Prep time: 10 mins   **Cook time: 15 mins**
Servings: 4

Ingredients:
- Almond-crusted Cauliflower Bites
- Avocado Ranch Dip
- One cup heaping mashed avocado
- Two tbsp. unsweetened non-dairy milk
- One tsp. onion powder
- One tsp. garlic powder
- One tbsp. white vinegar
- ¾ cup almond meal
- One tbsp. lemon juice
- ½ tsp. onion powder
- ½ tsp. dried parsley
- ½ tsp. nutritional yeast
- ¼-½ tsp. sea salt to taste
- ¼ tsp. garlic powder
- ¼ tsp. agave nectar
- Pinch of dried dill
- One piece large head cauliflower florets chopped into bite-sized
- ½ cup unsweetened non-dairy milk
- Six tbsp. vegan mayo soy-free
- ¼ cup chickpea flour
- ¼ cup cornmeal
- ½ tsp. paprika
- One tsp. of salt
- Pinch of black pepper

Directions for Avocado Ranch Dip: Place all ingredients in a prepared mixing bowl and mix together until combined and mostly smooth. Refrigerate until ready to serve.

Directions for Almond-crusted Cauliflower Bites: Preheat oven at temperature of 400 degrees F and line a baking sheet with parchment paper.
Stir together the non-dairy milk, vegan mayo and chickpea flour in a mixing bowl until smooth and thick enough to cover a spoon.
Mix the cornmeal, onion powder, almond meal, garlic powder, paprika salt, and pepper in another mixing bowl until mixed.
Take each piece of cauliflower and first dunk it into the wet mixture, then press into crumb mixture, covering evenly and shaking off loose bits; place onto a baking pan. Repeat until all pieces are coated and then on the baking pan.
Coat cauliflower bites lightly with cook oil spray and place in the oven. Bake for fifteen mins, flip pieces over and lightly spray with oil again, bake for an additional fifteen mins. The cool baking pan on a rack for five mins before serving with avocado ranch dip.

Nutrition: Cal: 485 Protein: 7.6 g Fat: 41.1 g Carbs: 25.6 g

520. Air Fried Kale Chips

Prep Time: 10 Mins   **Cook Time: 10 mins**
Servings: 6

Ingredients:
- One bunch of kale
- Three tablespoon yeast
- ¼ teaspoon Himalayan salt
- Avocado oil

Directions: Tear kale leaves into large pieces.
Place them in a bowl and drizzle with avocado oil. Sprinkle with yeast and salt.
With your hands, mix kale leaves well to combine.

Pour half of the kale mixture into the Air Fryer basket, set temperature to 350 degrees F, and set time to five mins. Remove and repeat with another half of kale.

Nutrition: Cal: 55 Fat: 10 g Carbs: 0 g Protein: 1 g

521. Cauliflower Rice

Prep Time: 10 Mins
Servings: 4

Cook Time: 20 mins

Ingredients:
Round 1:
- One C. diced carrot
- ½ C. diced onion

- One Teaspoon turmeric
- Two tablespoons soy sauce

- ½ block of extra firm tofu

Round 2:
- Three C. riced cauliflower
- Two minced garlic cloves
- ½ C. chopped broccoli

- ½ C. frozen peas
- One tablespoon minced ginger
- One tablespoon rice vinegar

- One ½ teaspoon toasted sesame oil
- Two tablespoons soy sauce

Directions: Crumble tofu in a bowl and stir with the entire Round one ingredient.
Preheat the Air Fryer to 370° F, place the baking pan in the oven basket, set temperature to 370 degrees F, and set time and cook to ten mins, making sure to shake once.
In another bowl, mix ingredients from Round 2 together.
Add Round 2 mixture to air fryer and cook another ten mins.

Nutrition: Cal: 67 Fat: 8 g Carbs: 0 g Protein: 3 g

522. Steamed Broccoli

Prep Time: 10 Mins
Servings: 2

Cook Time: 3 mins

Ingredients:
- 1 pound broccoli florets
- 1 teaspoon olive oil

- 1 ½ cups water
- Salt and pepper

Directions: Add water to the bottom of the air fryer and set the basket on top.
Stir the broccoli florets with pepper, salt, and oil until evenly combined. Then transfer to the basket.
Cook at 350° F for five mins.

Nutrition: Cal: 160 Carbs: 6.1 g Fat: 12 g Protein: 13 g

523. Pasta with Artichoke Pesto and Chickpeas (Vegan)

Prep time: 10 mins
Servings: 4

Cook time: 15 mins

Ingredients:
- Eight ounces vegan pappardelle or other pasta
- One batch roasted chickpeas
- One clove garlic

- One packed cup (1 ounce) fresh basil leaves
- Six jarred artichoke hearts drained and squeezed slightly to remove excess liquid

- 2 Tbsp. shelled pumpkin seeds
- 1 Tbsp. juice of half a lemon
- ½ tsp. white miso paste
- One tsp. olive oil

Directions: Cook the pasta according to package directions.
While pasta is cook, you can combine garlic, basil leaves, lemon juice, artichoke hearts, shelled pumpkin seeds, and white miso paste in a food processor until it is thoroughly combined. Scrape down the sides, and then continue processing until the pesto is mostly smooth.

If the pasta is already cooked, drain in a colander. Then transfer the noodles to a bowl and add olive oil to keep them from sticking together. Spoon over the pasta with the artichoke pesto, and toss until evenly mixed.
Serve pasta topped with chickpeas which are roasted.

Nutrition: Cal: 196 Protein: 7.9 g Fat: 3.8 g Carbs: 38.4 g

524. Almond Asparagus

Prep Time: 10 Mins   **Cook Time: 6 mins**
Servings: 3

Ingredients:
- 1 lb. asparagus
- 1/3 cup almonds, sliced
- 2 tablespoons balsamic vinegar
- 2 tablespoons olive oil
- Salt and ground black pepper

Directions: In a bowl, toss the asparagus, vinegar, oil, salt, and pepper.
Select the "Air Fry" mode. Press the Time button and set the cook time to six mins. Set the temperature at 400° F.
Press the Start button to start. Arrange the vegetable mixture in a greased "Air Fry Basket" and insert it in the oven.

Nutrition: Cal 173 Fat 14.8 g Carbs 8.2 g Protein 5.6 g

525. Onion Rings with Almond Four Battered

Prep Time: 10 Mins   **Cook Time: 15 mins**
Servings: 3

Ingredients:
- ½ cup almond flour
- One egg, beaten
- ¾ cup coconut milk
- One tablespoon baking powder
- One tablespoon smoked paprika
- One big white onion, sliced into rings
- Salt and pepper

Directions: Preheat the Air Fryer Oven for five mins.
In a mixing bowl, stir the smoked paprika, almond flour, baking powder, salt, and pepper.
In another bowl, combine the eggs and coconut milk.
Soak the onion slices into the egg mixture. Dredge the onion slices in the almond flour mixture.
Pour into the Air Fryer basket. Set temperature to 325 degrees F, and set time to fifteen mins. Select START to begin. Shake the oven basket for even cook.

Nutrition: Cal: 217 Fat: 17.9 g Carbs: 0 g Protein: 5.3 g

526. Coconut Artichokes

Prep time: 5 mins   **Cook time: 15 mins**
Servings: 2

Ingredients:
- Two artichokes, washed, trimmed and halved
- ¼ cup coconut, shredded
- Two garlic cloves, minced
- One tbsp. coconut oil, melted
- Juice of 1 lemon

Directions: In a bowl, toss the artichokes with the oil, garlic, and lemon juice.
Put the artichokes into your air fryer and cook at 360° F for fifteen mins.
Divide the artichokes between plates and sprinkle the coconut on top.

Nutrition: Cal 213 Fat 8 g Carbs 13 g Protein 6 g

527. Baby Potatoes

Prep Time: 10 mins
Serve: 2

Cook Time: 20 mins

Ingredients:
- 12 oz. baby potatoes
- 1/2 tbsp. olive oil
- 1/4 tsp. paprika
- 1/4 tsp. chili powder
- 1/4 tsp. cumin
- 1/4 tsp. garlic salt
- 1/4 tsp. pepper
- 1/2 tsp. kosher salt

Directions: Add all ingredients into a zip-lock bag and shake well.
Transfer baby potatoes into the air fryer basket.
Place air fryer basket into the oven and select air fry mode with 370 degrees F for twenty mins. Toss twice.

Nutrition: Cal 133 Fat 3.8 g Carbs 22 g Protein 4.6 g

528. Baked Eggplant with Marinara and Cheese

Prep Time: 10 Mins
Servings: 3

Cook Time: 45 mins

Ingredients:
- One clove garlic, sliced
- One large eggplant
- 3 1/2 tablespoon olive oil
- 1/2 pinch salt, or as needed
- 1/4 cup and two tablespoons ricotta cheese
- Two tablespoons shredded pepper jack cheese
- 1/4 cup and two tablespoons dry bread crumbs
- 1/4 cup grated Parmesan cheese
- 1/4 teaspoon red pepper flakes
- 1-1/2 cups prepared marinara sauce
- Salt and ground black pepper
- 1/4 cup water, plus more as needed

Directions: Cut eggplant crosswise into five pieces. Peel and chop two pieces into ½-inch cubes.
Lightly grease the air fryer's baking pan with one tablespoon of olive oil for 5 mins, heat oil at 390 degrees F. Add half eggplant strips and cook for two mins per side. Transfer to a plate.
Add 1 ½ teaspoon olive oil and add garlic. Cook for a minute. Add chopped eggplants. Season with salt and pepper flakes. Cook for four mins to 330 degrees F and continue cook eggplants until soft, around eight mins more.
Mix in water and marinara sauce. Cook for seven mins until heated through. Stirring every now and then.
Transfer to a bowl.
In a bowl, whisk well pepper, pepper jack cheese, salt, Parmesan cheese, and ricotta. Evenly spread cheeses over eggplant strips and then fold in half.
Lay folded eggplant in a baking pan. Pour the marinara sauce on top.
In a small bowl whisk well olive oil and bread crumbs. Sprinkle all over the sauce.
Place the baking pan in the Air Fryer Oven basket. Cook for fifteen mins at 390 degrees F until tops are lightly browned.

Nutrition: Cal: 405 Fat: 21.4 g Carbs: 0 g Protein: 12.7 g

529. Polenta Roll with Cheese Sauce

Prep Time: 5 mins
Servings: 1

Cook Time: 10 mins

Ingredients:
- One polenta roll, sliced
- One tablespoon chili powder
- One cup cheddar cheese sauce

Directions: Arrange the polenta slices in the baking pan.
Add the chili powder and cheddar cheese sauce.
Cook for ten mins at 390 degrees F.

Nutrition: Cal: 206; Carbs: 25.3 g; Protein: 3.2 g; Fat: 4.2 g

530. Baked Vegan Eggplant

Prep time: 10 mins
Servings: 4

Cook time: 30 mins

Ingredients:
- 4 eggplants
- 2 yellow onions
- 0.4 cup soy milk
- 1 carrot
- 0.44 lbs. tofu
- 0.22 lbs. soy cheese
- One tsp. basil
- One tsp. oregano
- 1.76 oz. parsley
- 0.2 cup water
- 1 tsp. olive oil
- One tsp. black pepper
- One tsp. salt

Directions: Wash the eggplants and cut into 2 parts. Then rub it with salt and leave it. Meanwhile, peel the onions and chop them. Peel the carrot and grate it. Combine chopped the onion and grated carrot together. Sprinkle it with basil, pepper, oregano and mix it carefully.
Take the eggplants and remove the meat from them. Chop the meat and combine it with carrot and onion. Toss it.
Chop the parsley and then put it into the mixture too. Stir it again. Grate the tofu. Preheat the air fryer to 380 degrees F. Pour the soy milk and water into the air fryer and stir it with a wooden spoon's help.
Fill the eggplants with the vegetable mass and sprinkle each half with grated tofu cheese. Transfer all eggplant to the air fryer. Cook it for twenty mins. Then remove the pan from the air fryer and chill it a little.

Nutrition: Cal 248 Protein 12.0 g Fat 6.2 g Carbs 43.2 g

531. Baked Potato with Cream Cheese (Vegan)

Prep Time: 10 mins
Servings: 1
Ingredients:

Cook Time: 40 mins

- 1 medium russet potato, scrubbed and peeled
- ¼ teaspoon onion powder
- 1 tablespoon chives, chopped
- 1 tablespoon Kalamata olives
- A dollop of vegan butter
- A dollop of vegan cream cheese
- 1 teaspoon olive oil
- 1/8 teaspoon salt

Directions: Preheat the oven to 400 degrees F.
Put the potatoes together in a baking pan and pour in onion powder, olive oil, salt, and vegan butter. Place the pan in the Air Fryer. Cook for forty mins. Be sure to turn the potatoes once halfway.
Serve the potatoes with vegan cream cheese, chives, and Kalamata olives.

Nutrition: Cal: 504; Carbs: 68.3 g; Protein: 9.1 g; Fat: 21.3 g

532. Baked Egg Tomato

Prep Time: 5 mins
Serving: 2

Cook Time: 30 mins

Ingredients:
- Two large fresh tomatoes
- Two eggs
- 1 tsp. fresh parsley
- Salt and Pepper

Directions: Cut the top of the tomato and spoon out the tomato innards.
Break the egg in each tomato. Place tomatoes on a baking pan.
Select bake mode and set the oven to 350 degrees F for thirty mins, then place the pan into the Air Fryer.
Season with salt and pepper.
Garnish with parsley.

Nutrition: Cal 96 Fat 4.7 g Carbs 7.5 g Protein 7.2 g

533. Baked Macaroni with Cheese

Prep Time: 10 Mins   **Cook Time: 25 mins**
Servings: 4

Ingredients:

- 1 pound elbow macaroni
- ½ pound Cheddar cheese, shredded
- Two eggs
- Four tablespoons butter
- One teaspoon Dijon mustard
- 12 oz. evaporated milk
- ½ c. breadcrumbs
- Salt and pepper

Directions: Cook macaroni according to package directions.
A spray baking dish with cook spray.
Add all ingredients except for bread crumbs to the dish and stir well to combine. Sprinkle with bread crumbs.
Cover with foil and place the pan on the rack. Bake at 350° F for 15-20 mins. Remove the foil, and cook for another 5-10 mins.

Nutrition: Cal: 480 Fat: 19 g Carbs: 31 g Protein: 24 g

534. Baked Zucchini with Cheese

Prep Time: 10 mins   **Cook Time: 30 mins**
Servings: 4

Ingredients:

- 1 1/2 pounds zucchini, cubed
- 3/4 cup shredded Cheddar cheese
- 1/2 cup chopped onion
- 1/2 teaspoon garlic salt
- 1/2 teaspoon paprika
- 1/2 teaspoon dried oregano
- 1/2 teaspoon cayenne pepper
- 1/2 cup cooked long-grain rice
- 1/2 cup cooked pinto beans
- 1/4 cups salsa
- 1 tablespoon olive oil

Directions: Drizzle a baking pan with olive oil. Add onions and zucchini and place the pan in a bowl.
Cook in the oven for ten mins at 360 degrees F. Halfway through cook time, stir.
Season with cayenne pepper, paprika, oregano, and garlic salt. Stir well. Toss in salsa, beans, and rice and cook for five mins. Stir in cheddar cheese and mix well.
Cover pan with foil. Cook for fifteen mins at 390 degrees F until bubbly.

Nutrition: Cal: 263; Carbs: 24.6 g; Protein: 12.5 g; Fat: 12.7 g

535. Baked Sweet Potatoes

Prep Time: 10 Mins   **Cook Time: 40 mins**
Servings: 4

Ingredients:

- Four sweet potatoes, scrubbed and washed
- ½ teaspoon salt
- ½ tablespoon. butter, melted

Directions: Prick potatoes using a fork and rub them with melted butter. Then, season with salt.
Arrange sweet potatoes on instant vortex air fryer drip pan and bake at 400 degrees F for forty mins.

Nutrition: Cal: 125 Fat: 1.5 g Carbs: 26.2 g Protein: 2.1 g

536. Baked Salad (Vegan)

Prep time: 10 mins   **Cook time: 20 mins**
Servings: 4

Ingredients:

- 1 red onion
- 1 red apple
- 0.44 lbs. tomatoes

- 1.76 oz. chopped chives
- 0.35 oz. garlic
- 1.76 oz. quinoa
- 0.22 lbs. tofu
- 2 tsp. lemon juice
- 0.2 cup soy sauce
- 0.4 cup water
- 0.2 cup soy milk
- 1 tsp. rice flour
- 2 red sweet peppers
- 1 sweet green pepper

Directions: Get the seeds from the sweet peppers and chop the pepper. Put it in a large bowl and sprinkle the vegetables with chopped chives and soy sauce. Stir it.

Chop the tomatoes and apples. Peel the onion and chop it too. All the vegetables should be chopped at the same size. Add them to the bowl with pepper mixture and stir it. Add quinoa, rice flour, and garlic. Stir the mass.

Chop the tofu roughly and add it to the bowl too. Preheat the air fryer to 390 degrees F. Then pour soy milk into it and transfer the vegetable mixture to the air fryer.

Cover with the lid and cook it for ten mins, not more. Open the lid and remove the salad from it. Sprinkle the salad with lemon juice.

Nutrition: Cal 159 Protein 7.4 g Fat 2.6 g Carbs 28.4 g

537. Balsamic Mushrooms

Prep Time: 5 mins
Serve: 6

Cook Time: 20 mins

Ingredients:
- One lb. button mushrooms, scrubbed and stems trimmed
- 3 garlic cloves, crushed
- 4 tbsp. balsamic vinegar
- 1/2 tsp. dried basil
- 1/2 tsp. dried oregano
- Two tbsp. extra-virgin olive oil
- 1/4 tsp. black pepper
- One tsp. salt

Directions: Spray a baking pan with cook spray and set aside.

In a bowl, mix together basil, oregano, garlic, vinegar, oil, pepper, and salt.

Stir in mushrooms and let sit for fifteen mins.

Spread mushrooms onto the prepared pan.

Select bake mode and set the Air fryer to 425 degrees F for twenty mins and place the cook pan into the oven.

Nutrition: Cal 61 Fat 4.9 g Carbs 3.2 g Protein 2.5 g

538. Asparagus and Prosciutto

Prep time: 5 mins
Servings: 4

Cook time: 5 mins

Ingredients:
- Eight ounces prosciutto slices
- Eight asparagus spears, trimmed
- A pinch of salt and black pepper

Directions: Wrap the asparagus in prosciutto slices and then season with salt and pepper.

Put all in your air fryer's basket and cook at 400° F for five mins.

Nutrition: Cal 100 Fat 2 g Carbs 8 g Protein 4 g

539. Balsamic Cabbage

Prep time: 5 mins
Servings: 4

Cook time: 8 mins

Ingredients:
- 1 red cabbage head, shredded
- 1 carrot, grated
- 1 tbsp. extra-virgin olive oil
- Salt and pepper
- ¼ cup balsamic vinegar

Directions: Place all ingredients in a pan that fits your air fryer, and stir well.
Put the pan in the fryer and cook at 380° F for eight mins.

Nutrition: Cal 100 Fat 4 g Carbs 7 g Protein 2 g

540. Basil Tomatoes

Prep Time: 10 Mins   **Cook Time: 10 mins**
Servings: 2

Ingredients:
- *Three tomatoes, halved*
- *One tablespoon fresh basil, chopped*
- *Olive oil cook spray*
- *Salt and ground black pepper*

Directions: Drizzle cut sides of the tomato halves with cook spray evenly.
Sprinkle with pepper, salt, and basil.
Select the "Air Fry" mode and set the cook time to ten mins.
Set the temperature at 320° F.
Arrange the tomatoes in "Air Fry Basket" and insert them in the oven.

Nutrition: Cal 34 Fat 0.4 g Carbs 7.2 g Protein 1.7 g

541. Beet Salad

Prep time: 10 mins   **Cook time: 14 mins**
Servings: 4

Ingredients:
- *4 beets, trimmed*
- *2 tbsp. balsamic vinegar*
- *A bunch of parsley, chopped*
- *1 garlic clove, chopped*
- *2 tbsp. capers*
- *1 tbsp. olive oil*
- *Salt and black pepper*

Directions: Put beets in your air fryer's basket and cook them at 360° F for fourteen mins.
In a bowl, mix parsley with salt, pepper, garlic, oil and capers. Leave beets to cool down. Now peel them, slice and put them in a bowl. Next, add vinegar and the parsley mix.

Nutrition: Cal: 33 Protein: 0.87 g Fat: 1.68 g Carbs: 3.8 g

542. Beet Salad and Parsley

Prep time: 10 mins   **Cook time: 14 mins**
Servings: 4

Ingredients
- *4 beets*
- *Two tbsp. balsamic vinegar*
- *A bunch of parsley*
- *One garlic clove*
- *2 tbsp. capers*
- *Salt and pepper*
- *1 tbsp. olive oil*

Directions: Insert beets in the air fryer and cook them at 360 degrees F for fifteen mins.
Combine parsley with pepper, salt, garlic, oil and capers in a bowl and mix well.
Move beets to a cutting board peel them after cooling and slice. Transfer them to a salad bowl.
Sprinkle the parsley all over after putting in vinegar.

Nutrition: Cal: 27 Protein: 0.3 g Fat: 1.8 g Carbs: 2.9 g

543. Beets and Arugula Salad

Prep time: 5 mins
Servings: 4

Cook time: 15 mins

Ingredients:

- One and ½ pounds beets
- Two tbsp. orange zest
- Two tbsp. cider vinegar
- ½ cup of orange juice
- Two scallions
- A sprinkle of olive oil
- Two tbsp. mustard
- Two cups arugula
- Two tbsp. brown sugar

Directions: Chafe beets with the orange juice and oil put in the air fryer and cook at 350 degrees F for ten mins.
Move beet quarters to a bowl, put in arugula, orange Zest and scallions. Mix well.
Blend sugar with mustard and vinegar in another bowl, beat, and add to salad. Toss.

Nutrition: Cal: 95 Protein: 2.8 g Fat: 0.8 g Carbs: 20.6 g

544. Tortilla with Bell Pepper-Corn Wrapped

Prep Time: 10 Mins
Servings: 4

Cook Time: 15 mins

Ingredients:

- Four large tortillas
- Two cobs grilled corn kernels
- Four pieces nuggets, chopped
- One small red bell pepper, chopped
- One small yellow onion, diced
- Mixed greens
- One tablespoon water

Directions: Preheat the Air Fryer Oven to 400 degrees F.
In a skillet heated over medium heat, water sauté the nuggets with the bell peppers, onions, and corn kernels. Set aside.
Place filling inside the corn tortillas.
Pour the tortillas into the Air Fryer basket. Set temperature to 400 degrees F, and set time to fifteen mins until the tortilla wraps are crispy.
Serve with mix greens on top.

Nutrition: Cal: 548 Cal Fat: 20.7 g Carbs: 0 g Protein: 46 g

545. Bell Peppers and Kale Leaves

Prep time: 5 mins
Servings: 4

Cook time: 15 mins

Ingredients:

- 2 red bell peppers, cut into strips
- 2 green bell peppers, cut into strips
- ½ pound kale leaves
- 2 yellow onions, roughly chopped
- ¼ cup vegetable stock
- 2 tbsp. tomato sauce
- Salt and pepper

Directions: Add all ingredients to a pan that fits your air fryer; mix well.
Place the pan in the fryer and cook at 360° F for fifteen mins.

Nutrition: Cal 161 Fat 7 g Carbs 12 g Protein 7 g

546. Jalapeño Poppers

Prep Time: 10 Mins
Servings: 4

Cook Time: 10 mins

Ingredients:
- 12-18 whole fresh jalapeño
- Two large eggs
- One cup nonfat refried beans
- One cup shredded Monterey Jack
- One scallion, sliced
- 1/4 cup all-purpose flour
- 1/2 cup fine cornmeal
- Olive oil cook spray
- One teaspoon salt, divided

Directions: Start by slicing each jalapeño lengthwise on one side. Place the jalapeños side by side in a microwave safe bowl and microwave them around five mins.
While your jalapeños cook; mix refried scallions, beans, 1/2 teaspoon salt, and cheese in a bowl.
Once your jalapeños are softened you can scoop out the seeds and add 1 tablespoon of your refried bean mixture.
Press the jalapeño closed around the filling.
Beat your eggs in a bowl and place the flour in a separate bowl. In a third bowl mix cornmeal and the remaining salt.
Roll each pepper in the flour, dip it in the egg, and finally roll it in the cornmeal.
Place the peppers on a flat surface and coat them with a cook spray; olive oil cook spray is suggested.
Pour into the Air Fryer basket and set temperature to 400 degrees F
Set time to five mins. Turn each pepper and cook for another five mins.

Nutrition: Cal: 244 Fat: 12 g Carbs: 0 g Protein: 12 g

547. Tomato Chili and Black Beans

Prep time: 15 mins
Servings: 6

Cook time: 23 mins

Ingredients:
- 1 medium onion, diced
- 3 garlic cloves, minced
- 2 tsp. chilli powder
- One cup vegetable broth
- 3 cans of black beans must drained and rinsed
- 2 cans of diced tomatoes
- 1 tsp. dried oregano
- 1 tbsp. olive oil
- 2 chipotle peppers, chopped
- ½ tsp. salt

Directions: Over medium heat, fry the garlic add onion in the oil for three mins.
Add the remaining ingredients, tossing and scraping the bottom to prevent sticking.
Preheat and set the temperature at 400 degrees F.
Take a dish and place the mixture inside. On top put a pan of aluminum foil.
Select bake and set time to twenty mins.

Nutrition: Cal: 362 Protein: 1.2 g Fat: 38.5 g Carbs: 6.5 g

548. Brown Rice, Spinach and Frittata

Prep Time: 10 Mins
Servings: 4

Cook Time: 55 mins

Ingredients:
- 1 ¾ cups brown rice, cooked
- ½ cup baby spinach, chopped
- ½ cup kale, chopped
- ½ onion, chopped
- Three big mushrooms, chopped
- Three tablespoons nutritional yeast
- Four cloves garlic, crushed
- Four spring onions, chopped
- ½ teaspoon turmeric
- One flax egg
- One tablespoon olive oil
- One yellow pepper, chopped
- Two tablespoons soy sauce
- Two teaspoons arrowroot powder
- Two teaspoons Dijon mustard
- 2/3 cup almond milk
- A handful of basil leaves, chopped

Directions: Preheat the Air Fryer to 375 degrees F. Grease a pan that will fit inside the oven.
Prepare the frittata crust by mixing the brown rice and flax egg. Press the rice onto the baking pan until you form a crust. Brush with a little oil and cook for ten mins.
Meanwhile, heat olive oil in a skillet over medium flame and sauté the garlic and onions for two mins. Add the pepper and mushroom and continue tossing for three mins. Stir in the kale, onions, spinach, and basil. Remove from the pan and set aside.

In a food processor, pulse together mustard, soy sauce, turmeric, nutritional yeast, almond milk and arrowroot powder. Pour in a mixing bowl and mixing in the sautéed vegetables.
Pour the frittata mixture over the rice crust and cook in the Air Fryer for forty mins.

Nutrition: Cal: 226 Fat: 8 g Carbs: 0 g Protein: 10.6 g

549. Broccoli Salad

Prep time: 5 mins   **Cook time: 12 mins**
Servings: 4

Ingredients:
- 1 broccoli head, florets separated
- 6 garlic cloves
- One tbsp. Chinese rice wine vinegar
- One tbsp. peanut oil
- Salt
- Pepper

Directions: Combine broccoli with pepper, salt, and half of the oil in a bowl. Toss, put in the air fryer and cook at 350 degrees F for eight mins while shaking fryer halfway.
Get broccoli to a salad bowl, put the garlic, rice vinegar, and the rest of the peanut oil. Toss thoroughly.

Nutrition: Cal: 42 Fat: 3.3 g Carbs: 2.6 g

550. Brussels Sprouts with Pine Nuts

Prep Time: 10 Mins   **Cook Time: 15 mins**
Servings: 6

Ingredients:
- fifteen oz brussels sprouts, stems cut off and cut in half
- 1 ¾ oz toasted pine nuts
- 1 ¾ oz raisins, drained
- Juice of one orange
- One tablespoon olive oil
- Salt

Directions: Take raisins and soak in orange juice for twenty mins.
Meanwhile, in a bowl, pop the sprouts with oil and salt and mix to combine.
Preheat your Air Fryer to 390° F.
Add the sprouts to the oven and roast for fifteen mins. Check often and remove Brussel sprouts from the oven. Mix with toasted pine nuts and soaked raisins. Drizzle with remaining orange juice.

551. Brussels Sprouts And Tomatoes

Prep time: 5 mins   **Cook time: 10 mins**
Servings: 4

Ingredients:
- One pound Brussels sprouts
- 6 cherry tomatoes halved
- ¼ cup green onions
- One tbsp. olive oil
- Salt
- Pepper

Directions: Spice Brussels sprouts with salt and pepper, get them in the oven. Cook at 350 degrees F for ten mins.
Move them to a bowl; add green onions, cherry tomatoes, pepper, salt and oil. Stir properly.

Nutrition: Cal: 85 Protein: 4.4 g Fat: 3.7 g Carbs: 11.5 g

552. Burritos

Prep Time: 10 mins
Serving: 4

Cook Time: 35 mins

Ingredients:

Refried beans:
- 4-5 flour tortillas
- 1/2 cup red kidney beans
- 1/2 small onion
- 2 tbsp. Tomato puree
- ¼ tsp. red chili powder
- 1 tbsp. olive oil
- 1 tsp. of salt

Vegetable Filling:
- 1 medium onion
- 3 flakes garlic crushed
- 1/2 cup French beans
- One cup cottage cheese
- 1/2 cup shredded cabbage
- 2 carrots
- One tbsp. coriander
- One tbsp. vinegar
- One tsp. white wine
- 1/2 tsp. red chili flakes
- One tsp. freshly ground peppercorns
- 1/2 cup pickled Jalapeños
- 1 tbsp. Olive oil
- A pinch of salt

Salad:
- 1-2 lettuce leaves shredded
- 1 cup of cheddar
- One or two spring onions
- 1 green chili

Directions: Cook the beans with the garlic and onion and mash them.
For the filling, sauté the ingredients in a pan.
Mix the salad ingredients together.
Lay the tortilla on a flat surface and put a layer of sauce and filling inside.
Wrap the tortilla to create a burrito.
Preheat the oven to 200 degrees F. Place the burritos inside.
Cook for fifteen mins. Flip the burritos halfway through.

553. Cajun Asparagus

Prep time: 5 mins
Servings: 4

Cook time: 5 mins

Ingredients:
- 1 bunch asparagus, trimmed
- ½ tbsp. Cajun seasoning
- 1 tsp. olive oil

Directions: In a bowl, stir the asparagus with the oil and Cajun seasoning; coat the asparagus.
Put the asparagus in your Air Fryer and cook at 400° F for five mins.

Nutrition: Cal 151 Fat 3 g Carbs 9 g Protein 4 g

554. Buttery Potatoes

Prep Time: 10 Mins
Servings: 4

Cook Time: 20 mins

Ingredients:
- 1½ pounds of small potatoes, halved
- ½ teaspoon garlic powder
- ¼ teaspoon dried thyme
- ¼ teaspoon dried rosemary
- Three tablespoons butter, melted
- Salt and pepper

Directions: In a bowl, add all the ingredients and stir to coat well.
Preheat the Air Fryer.
Arrange the potatoes in the basket. Set the temperature to 380° F for 20 mins.
Shake the potatoes once halfway through.

Nutrition: Cal: 195 Fat: 8.8 g Carbs: 27.1 g Protein: 3 g

555. Cajun Mushrooms and Beans

Prep time: 10 mins
Servings: 4

Cook time: 15 mins

Ingredients:

- Eight ounces white mushrooms, sliced
- Fifteen ounces canned kidney beans, drained
- One zucchini, chopped
- One tbsp. Cajun seasoning
- One green bell pepper, chopped
- One yellow onion, chopped
- Two celery stalks, chopped
- Three garlic cloves, minced
- Fifteen ounces canned tomatoes, chopped
- Two tbsp. olive oil
- Salt
- Pepper

Directions: In the air fryer's pan, toss oil with bell pepper, celery, garlic, tomatoes, onion, mushrooms, beans, zucchini, Cajun seasoning, salt and pepper.
Stir, cover and cook on at 370° F for fifteen mins.

Nutrition: Cal: 192 Protein: 5.01 g Fat: 13.2 g Carbs: 15.8 g

556. Carrot Mix

Prep time: 5 mins
Servings: 4

Cook time: 30 mins

Ingredients:

- One cup Shredded carrots
- Two cups Coconut milk
- Five cups Steel-cut oats
- Five tsp. Agave nectar
- One pinch Saffron
- One tsp. Ground cardamom

Directions: Lightly spritz the Air Fryer sheet using a cook oil spray.
Warm the oven to reach 365 degrees F.
When it's hot, whisk and add the fixings.
Set the timer for fifteen mins.
Portion into the serving dishes with a sprinkle of saffron.

Nutrition: Cal: 202 Protein: 3 g Carbs: 4 g Fat: 7 g

557. Cheddar Muffins

Prep Time: 10 Mins
Servings: 3

Cook Time: 8 mins

Ingredients:

- Three split English muffins, toasted
- One cup cheddar cheese smoked and shredded
- One mashed avocado
- One tomato, chopped
- One sweet onion, chopped
- ¼ cup ranch-style salad dressing
- One cup alfalfa sprouts
- ¼ cup sesame seeds, toasted

Directions: Arrange the muffins open-faced in the cook tray. Spread the mashed avocado on each half of the muffin.
Place the halves close to each other. Cover the muffins with tomatoes, sprouts, onion, sesame seeds, dressing, and the cheese. Cook for 7-8 mins at 350 degrees F.

Nutrition: Cal 340 Fat 15 g Carbs 38 g Protein 14 g

558. Cauliflower, Chickpea, and Avocado Mash

Prep time: 10 mins
Servings: 4

Cook time: 25 mins

Ingredients:

- 1 medium head cauliflower, cut into florets
- 1 can chickpeas, drained and rinsed
- 2 tbsp. lemon juice
- 4 flatbreads, toasted
- 2 ripe avocados, mashed
- 1 tbsp. olive oil
- Salt
- Pepper

Directions: Preheat the Vortex and set the temperature at 425 degrees F
In a bowl, mix the cauliflower, lemon juice chickpeas, and oil. Sprinkle salt and pepper as desired. Transfer to the air fryer basket.
Place the air fryer basket onto the baking pan and select air fry mode.
Set time to twenty-five mins.
Spread on top of the flatbread with the mashed avocado. Sprinkle with more pepper and salt

Nutrition: Cal: 285 Protein: 7.9 g Fat: 18.4 g Carbs: 28.3 g

559. Cheese and Bean Enchiladas

Prep Time: 10 mins
Serving: 4

Cook Time: 25 mins

Ingredients:
- Flour tortillas

Red sauce:
- 3 medium tomatoes
- 1 1/2 tsp. of garlic
- 1 1/2 cups of readymade tomato puree
- A few red chili flakes to sprinkle
- One tsp. of oregano
- Four tbsp. of olive oil
- A pinch of salt
- One tsp. of sugar

Filling:
- Two tbsp. oil
- Two tsp. chopped garlic
- 2 onions
- 2 capsicums
- Two cups of readymade baked beans
- A few drops of Tabasco sauce
- 1 cup cottage cheese
- 1 cup grated cheddar
- 1 1/2 tsp. red chili flakes
- 1 tbsp. of finely chopped Jalapeños
- 1 tsp. oregano
- A pinch of salt
- 1/2 tsp. pepper

Directions: In a skillet, heat 2 tbsp. Of oil. Add garlic and the rest of the sauce ingredients.
Cook until the sauce reduces and ends up being thick.
For the filling, warm one tbsp. of oil in another skillet.
Add garlic and onions and cook till the onions are caramelized.
Add the filling ingredients. Remove from heat and sprinkle cheddar over the sauce.
Take a tortilla and spread a portion of the sauce on it. Roll up the tortilla cautiously and then repeat for each.
Line a baking pan with a foil. Preheat the oven to 320 degrees F and cook for fifteen mins.
Turn the tortillas over in the middle to cook uniformly.

560. Cauliflower Chickpea Tacos

Prep time: 10 mins
Servings: 4

Cook time: 20 mins

Ingredients:
- Four cups of cauliflower florets, cut into bite-sized pieces
- 19-oz. can of chickpeas drained and rinsed
- 2 tbsp. taco seasoning
- 2 tbsp. olive oil

To Serve:
- *Eight small flour tortillas*
- *Four cups cabbage, finely shredded*
- *Two Haas avocados, sliced*
- *Coconut yogurt, for drizzling*

Directions: Preheat the Vortex at temperature of 390° F.
In a bowl, toss the chickpeas and cauliflower with taco seasoning and oil.
Put them into the basket and cook for twenty mins. Make sure to check often to ensure the cauliflower and chickpeas are evenly cooked through.
Serve in tacos with avocado slices, cabbage, and coconut yogurt drizzled on top.

Nutrition: Cal: 760 Protein: 22.4 g Fat: 30.8 g Carbs: 103.5 g

561. Cheesy Broccoli Casserole

Prep Time: 5 mins
Serve: 6

Cook Time: 30 mins

Ingredients:
- *16 oz. frozen broccoli florets, defrosted and drained*
- *10.5 oz. can cream of mushroom soup*
- *1/2 tsp. onion powder*
- *One cup cheddar cheese, shredded*
- *1/3 cup unsweetened almond milk*

For topping:
- *1 tbsp. butter, melted*
- *1/2 cup cracker crumbs*

Directions: Add all ingredients except topping ingredients into the casserole pan.
In a bowl, mix cracker crumbs and melted butter and sprinkle over the casserole mixture.
Select bake mode and set the oven to 350 degrees F for thirty mins. Then, put the casserole inside.

Nutrition: Cal 193 Fat 12.9 g Carbs 10.5 g Protein 6.9 g

562. Cherry Tomatoes Skewers

Prep time: 10 mins
Servings: 4

Cook time: 26 mins

Ingredients:
- *Three tbsp. balsamic vinegar*
- *Twenty-four cherry tomatoes*
- *3 garlic cloves*
- *1 tbsp. thyme*
- *2 tbsp. olive oil*
- *Salt and pepper*

For dressing:
- *2 tbsp. balsamic vinegar*
- *Four tbsp. olive oil*
- *Salt*
- *Pepper*

Directions: Mix in 2 tbsp. vinegar with three tbsp. oil, 3 garlic cloves, thyme, pepper, salt in a bowl and beat properly. Put tomatoes. Stir to coat and allow for thirty mins.
Assemble 6 tomatoes on one skewer. Do the same with the remaining tomatoes.
Put into oven and cook at 360 degrees F for six mins.
Mix in 2 tbsp. vinegar with four tbsp. oil, salt, and pepper. Beat properly.
Serve with dressing sprinkled over.

Nutrition: Cal: 210 Protein: 0.61 g Fat: 20.34 g Carbs: 6.53 g

563. Cheesy Macaroni Balls

Prep Time: 10mins
Serving: 2

Cook Time: 10 mins

Ingredients:
- two cups leftover macaroni
- One cup shredded Cheddar cheese
- One cup bread crumbs
- 3 large eggs
- One cup milk
- 1/2 cup flour
- 1/2 teaspoon salt
- ¼ teaspoon pepper

Directions: Preheat the air fryer oven to 365 degrees F.
In a bowl, combine the leftover macaroni and shredded cheese.
Pour the flour into a separate bowl. Put the breadcrumbs in a third bowl. Finally, in a fourth bowl, mix the eggs and milk with a whisk.
With an ice-cream scoop, create balls from the macaroni mixture. Coat them the flour, then in the egg mixture, and lastly in the breadcrumbs.
Arrange the balls in the Air Fryer basket. Select Air Fry and set time to ten mins, giving them an occasional stir. Ensure they crisp up nicely.

564. Cherry Tomato Salad

Prep time: 5 mins
Servings: 6

Cook time: 25 mins

Ingredients:
- 1 pint mixed cherry tomatoes, halved
- 8 small beets, trimmed, peeled and cut into wedges
- 1 red onion, sliced
- 1 tbsp. balsamic vinegar
- 2 ounces pecans, chopped
- Two tbsp. olive oil
- Salt
- Pepper

Directions: Put the beets in your air fryer's basket, and add the pepper, salt, and one tbsp. of the oil.
Cook at 400° F for fifteen mins.
Transfer the beets to a pan that fits your air fryer, and add the tomatoes, onions, pecans, and remaining one tbsp. of the oil; mix well.
Cook at 400° F for 10 more mins.

Nutrition: Cal 144 Fat 7 g Carbs 8 g Protein 6 g

565. Cheesy Asparagus and Potatoes

Prep Time: 5 mins
Servings: 4

Cook time: 23 mins

Ingredients:
- 1 bunch asparagus
- 4 medium potatoes
- 1/3 cup cottage cheese
- 1/3 cup low-fat crème Fraiche
- 1 tablespoon wholegrain mustard
- Salt and pepper
- Cook spray

Directions: Preheat the air fryer oven to 390 degrees F. Spritz the air fryer basket with cook spray.
Place the potatoes in the basket. Place the air fryer basket onto the baking pan, select Air Fry, and set time to twenty mins.
Meanwhile, boil the asparagus in water for three mins.
Remove the potatoes and mash them with the rest of the ingredients. Sprinkle with pepper and salt.

566. Cheesy Spinach

Prep Time: 10 Mins
Servings: 3

Cook Time: 15 mins

Ingredients:

- 1 (10-ounce) package frozen spinach, thawed
- ½ cup onion, chopped
- Four ounces cream cheese, chopped
- ¼ cup Parmesan cheese, shredded
- Two teaspoons garlic, minced
- ½ teaspoon ground nutmeg
- Salt and pepper

Directions: In a bowl, mix well spinach, garlic, cream cheese, onion, nutmeg, salt, and pepper.
Place spinach mixture into a baking pan.
Preheat the Air Fryer Oven and arrange the baking pan in the basket. Select "Air Fry" mode and set the temperature to 350° F for ten mins.

Nutrition: Cal: 194 Fat: 15.5 g Carbs: 7.3 g Protein: 8.4 g

567. Chinese Beans

Prep time: 10 mins
Servings: 6

Cook time: 30 mins

Ingredients:

- One pound green beans, halved
- One cup tomato sauce
- ¼ cup tomato paste
- ¼ cup mustard
- One cup maple syrup
- ¼ cup olive oil
- ¼ cup apple cider vinegar
- 2 tbsp. coconut aminos
- 4 tbsp. stevia

Directions: Stir beans with maple syrup, stevia, tomato paste, mustard, tomato paste, oil, vinegar and amino.
Cover and cook at 365° F for thirty-five mins.

Nutrition: Cal: 301 Protein: 2.92 g Fat: 9.94 g Carbs: 51.5 g

568. Chili Potatoes

Prep Time: 10 mins
Servings: 4

Cook time: 16 mins

Ingredients:

- 1 pound potatoes, rinsed and cut into wedges
- One teaspoon cayenne pepper
- One teaspoon nutritional yeast
- 1/2 teaspoon garlic powder
- One teaspoon olive oil
- One teaspoon salt
- One teaspoon black pepper

Directions: Preheat the oven to 400 degrees F. Coat the potatoes with the rest of the ingredients. Transfer to the air fryer basket. Select Air Fry, and set time to sixteen mins, shaking the basket halfway through the cook time.

569. Coconut Mix

Prep time: 5 mins
Servings: 8

Cook time: 8 mins

Ingredients:

- One pound mushrooms, halved
- One small onion, chopped
- Two tbsp. olive oil
- Fourteen ounces of coconut milk
- Salt and pepper

Directions: Add all ingredients to a pan that fits your air fryer and mix well. Place the pan in the fryer and cook at 400 degrees F for 8 mins.

Nutrition: Cal 202 Fat 4 g Carbs 13 g Protein 4 g

570. Indian Cilantro Potatoes with Pepper

Prep Time: 10 Mins
Servings: 2

Cook Time: 15 mins

Ingredients:

- 4 potatoes, cubed
- 3 tablespoon lemon juice
- 1 bell pepper, sliced
- 2 onions, chopped
- ½ cup mint leaves, chopped
- 2 cups cilantro, chopped
- 4 tablespoon fennel
- 5 tablespoon flour
- 2 tablespoon ginger-garlic paste
- Salt and black pepper

Directions: Preheat the oven to 360 degrees F, and in a bowl, mix coriander, ginger garlic paste, mint, fennel, flour, salt, and lemon juice.
Stir to form a paste and add potato cubes. In another bowl, mix the onions, capsicum, and fennel mixture. Blend the mixture.
Divide the mixture evenly into 5-6 cakes.
Add the prepared potato cakes to the Air Fryer and bake for fifteen mins.

Nutrition: 328 Cal; 12.4 g Fat; 50.7 g Carbs; 8.1 g Protein

571. Collard Green Mix

Prep time: 5 mins
Servings: 4

Cook time: 15 mins

Ingredients:

- One bunch collard greens
- 2 tbsp. tomato puree
- One onion
- Three garlic cloves
- 2 tbsp. olive oil
- 1 tbsp. balsamic vinegar
- 1 tbsp. sugar
- Salt and pepper

Directions: Mix oil, garlic, vinegar, tomato puree and onion in a bowl and whisk.
Add pepper, salt, collard greens and sugar. Stir and place in the air fryer. Bake at 320 degrees F for ten mins.
Spread the collard greens mixture on the plates.

Nutrition: Cal: 82 Protein: 0.46 g Fat: 6.81 g Carbs: 5.24 g

572. Corn and Cabbage Salad

Prep time: 10 mins
Servings: 4

Cook time: 15 mins

Ingredients:

- One small onion, chopped
- Two garlic cloves, minced
- One and ½ cups mushrooms, sliced
- Three tsp. ginger, grated
- 2 cups corn
- 4 cups red cabbage, chopped
- One tbsp. nutritional yeast
- Two tsp. tomato paste
- One tsp. coconut aminos
- One tsp. sriracha sauce
- One tbsp. olive oil
- A pinch of salt and pepper

Directions: In fryer pan, mix oil with garlic, mushrooms, onion, ginger, salt, pepper, corn, cabbage, yeast and tomato paste. Stir, cover and cook at 365 degrees F for 15 mins.
Add sriracha sauce and amino, stir, divide between plates.

Nutrition: Cal: 387 Protein: 10.9 g Fat: 7.57 g Carbs: 73.8 g

573. Broccoli with Cream Cheese

Prep Time: 10 mins
Servings: 2

Cook Time: 30 mins

Ingredients:

- 1-pound fresh broccoli, coarsely chopped
- Two tablespoons all-purpose flour
- Salt
- One tablespoon dry bread crumbs
- 1/2 large onion, coarsely chopped
- 1/2 (14 ounces) can evaporate milk, divided
- 1/2 cup Cheddar cheese
- One teaspoon butter
- 1/4 cup water

Directions: Grease the baking pan with cook spray.
Mix half the milk and flour in the pan and place in the oven.
Cook for 5 mins at 360 degrees F. Halfway through cook, stir well. Add the broccoli and the remaining milk. Stir well and cook for 5 mins.
Stir in the cheese and mix well until melted.
In a small bowl mix well, butter and breadcrumbs. Sprinkle over the broccoli.
Bake for 20 mins at 360 degrees F until the tops are lightly browned.

574. Creamy Spinach Quiche

Prep Time: 10 Mins
Servings: 4

Cook Time: 20 mins

Ingredients:

- Premade quiche crust, chilled and rolled flat to a 7-inch round
- ½ cup of cooked spinach, drained and coarsely chopped
- 2 Eggs
- ¼ cup of milk
- 1 garlic clove, peeled and finely minced
- ¼ cup of shredded mozzarella cheese
- ¼ cup of shredded cheddar cheese
- Pinch of salt and pepper

Directions: Preheat the Vortex Oven to 360° F.
Press the premade crust into a 7-inch pie tin. Press down and trim edges if necessary. Using a fork, poke some holes in the dough to allow air to circulate and prevent the crust from breaking during baking.
In a bowl, beat the eggs until fluffy and until the yolks and white are evenly combined.
Add spinach, milk, garlic, salt and pepper, and half the cheddar and mozzarella to the eggs. Set the rest of the cheese aside for now, and stir the mixture until completely blended. Make sure the spinach is not clumped together, but rather spread among the other ingredients.
Pour the mixture into the pie crust, slowly and carefully to avoid splashing. The mixture should almost fill the crust, but not completely – leaving a ¼ inch of crust at the edges.
Place the baking dish in oven basket. Set the time at 15 mins. After 15 mins, the quiche will already be firm and the crust beginning to brown. Sprinkle the rest of the cheddar and mozzarella over the quiche filling. Reset the Air Fryer at 360 degrees F for 5 mins.

Nutrition: Cal: 371 Fat: 33 g Carbs: 6 g Protein: 14 g

575. Creamy Brussels sprouts

Prep time: 3 mins
Servings: 4

Cook time: 11 mins

Ingredients

- 1 pound Brussels sprouts, cut up
- One tablespoon mustard
- Two tablespoons of coconut cream
- Two tablespoons chopped dill
- Salt and black pepper

Directions: Place the Brussels sprouts in the basket of your air fryer.
Cook at 350 degrees F for 10 mins.
In a bowl, mix the mustard with cream, dill, salt and pepper and whisk.
Add the Brussels sprouts and stir.

Nutrition: Protein: 4.48 g Fat: 3.09 g Carbs: 11.94 g

576. Crispy Cheese Baked In Chilli

Prep time: 10 mins
Portions: 3

Cook time: 30 mins

Ingredients:
- 1 (7 ounce) can whole green chile peppers, drained
- One beaten egg
- One tablespoon all-purpose flour
- 1/2 (5 ounces) can evaporated milk
- 1/2 (8 ounces) can tomato sauce
- 1/4 pound Monterey Jack cheese, shredded
- 1/4 pound Longhorn or Cheddar cheese, shredded
- 1/4 cup milk

Directions: Grease the baking pan with cook spray. Evenly distribute chiles and sprinkle with cheddar cheese and Monterey Jack. Place the baking tray in the oven.
In a bowl, whisk well the flour, milk and eggs. Pour over the chillies.
The air fryer should close the lid and cook for 20 mins at 360 degrees F.
Add the tomato sauce on top.
Cook for 10 mins at 390 degrees F until the tops are lightly browned.

Nutrition: Cal: 392; Carbs: 12 g; Protein: 23.9 g; Fat: 27.6 g

577. Crispy Potatoes with Parsley

Prep time: 5 mins
Portions: 4

Cook time: 15 mins

Ingredients:
- 1 lb. golden potatoes, cut into wedges
- 2 tbsp olive oil
- Juice of ½ lemon
- ¼ cup of parsley leaves
- Salt and black pepper

Directions: Dab potatoes with salt, pepper, lemon juice and olive oil, place in air fryer, then bake at 350 degrees F for 10 mins. Distribute on plates and sprinkle parsley on top.

Nutrition: Cal: 100 Protein: 2.63 g Fat: 0.63 g Carbs: 21.84 g

578. Crispy Chickpeas

Prep time: 5 mins
Servings: 4

Cook time: 15 mins

Ingredients:
- 1 (15-ounces) canned chickpeas, drained but not rinsed
- Two tablespoons olive oil
- Two tablespoons lemon juice
- One teaspoon salt

Directions: Preheat the fryer oven to 400 degrees F.
Combine all ingredients in a bowl. Then transfer them to the basket of the fryer. Place the frying basket in the center position. Select Air Fry and set the time to 15 mins, making sure the chickpeas get nice and crispy.

579. Jicama Chips

Prep time: 5 mins
Servings: 1

Cook time: 20 mins

Ingredients:
- One small jicama, peeled
- ¼ teaspoon of onion powder
- ¾ teaspoon chilli powder

214

- ¼ teaspoon of garlic powder
- ¼ teaspoon ground black pepper

Directions: Preheat the fryer oven to 350 degrees F.
To make the chips, cut the jicama into matchsticks of desired thickness.
In a bowl, stir in the chili powder, onion powder, garlic powder and black pepper. Transfer the chips to the basket of the air fryer. Place the air fryer basket on the baking tray, select Air Fry and set the time to 20 mins, giving the basket an occasional shake during the cook process. The chips are ready when they are hot and golden brown.

580. Vegan Broccoli

Prep time: 10 mins
Servings: 4

Cook time: 20 mins

Ingredients:
- 0.88 lbs. broccoli
- ½ cup soya milk
- ½ cup mushrooms
- One yellow onion
- 1 tablespoon almond flakes
- One teaspoon white pepper
- ½ cup grated tofu
- 3 tablespoons of chopped dill

Directions: Cut the florets from the broccoli and sprinkle them with white pepper. Then take the large bowl and combine the almond flakes and chopped dill in it.
Add the soy milk and mix the mass very gently. Then chop the tofu cheese and slice the mushrooms. Peel the onion and cut it into small pieces. Combine the chopped ingredients and mix.
Preheat the fryer to 190 C / 380 degrees F and put the broccoli florets in. Then pour in the liquid mass and add the chopped vegetable mass.
Stir with the aid of a wooden or plastic spoon and close the lid. Cook for 15 mins.

Nutrition: Cal 116 Protein 8.8 g Fat 3.5 g Carbs 17,1 g

581. Curried Cauliflower

Prep time: 10 mins
Servings: 4

Cook time: 15 mins

Ingredients:
- 2 lbs. cauliflower, cut into florets
- 1 1/2 teaspoons curry powder
- 1 tablespoon coriander, chopped
- 2 tablespoons fresh lemon juice
- 1 teaspoon kosher salt
- 1 tablespoon olive oil

Directions:
Brush cauliflower florets in a bowl with olive oil.
Sprinkle the cauliflower florets with curry powder and salt.
Spread the cauliflower florets over a cook pan.
Select the cook mode and set the oven to 425 degrees F for 15 mins, once the oven sounds, place the cook pan in the oven.
Return the roasted cauliflower florets to the bowl and stir in the cilantro and lemon juice.

Nutrition: Cal 90 Fat 3.9 g Carbs 12,5 g Protein 4,6 g

582. Curried Courgette Chips

Prep time: 10 mins
Servings: 2

Cook time: 24 mins

Ingredients:
- 1 medium-sized courgette, sliced
- 1 tbsp. virgin olive oil
- 1/8 teaspoon. garlic powder
- ¼ teaspoon. curry powder
- 1/8 teaspoon salt

Directions: Lightly grease a paper-lined baking sheet. Arrange the courgette slices in a layer on the baking tray. Drizzle with olive oil and sprinkle with curry powder, salt and garlic powder.
Place the baking sheet on a 1-inch rack and bake on 350 degrees F for 12 mins. Flip courgette and bake for an additional 10 mins or until very crispy. Cool and store in an airtight container.

Nutrition: Cal: 152 Carbs: 17 g Fat: 3 g Protein: 2 g

583. Portobello Mushrooms

Prep time: 5 mins   **Cook time: 17 mins**
Servings: 4

Ingredients:
- Ten basil leaves
- 1 cup spinach
- Three cloves of garlic
- 1 cup almonds
- 1 tablespoon of parsley
- ¼ cup olive oil
- Eight cherry tomatoes
- Salt and pepper
- 4 Portobello mushrooms

Directions: Blend basil with spinach, garlic, parsley, almonds, fat, pepper, salt and mushrooms. Mix thoroughly.
Infuse each mushroom with mixture, place in the air fryer and cook at 350 degrees F for 12 mins.

Nutrition: Cal: 135 kcal Protein: 1.21 g Fat: 13.8 g Carbs: 2.88 g

584. Roasted Garlic Mushrooms

Prep time: 5 mins   **Cook time: 25 mins**
Servings: 2

Ingredients:
- 8 oz. package of crimini or button mushrooms
- 2 cloves. garlic, minced
- 1 tablespoon. chopped thyme
- 2 tbsp. olive oil
- Salt and pepper

Directions: In a bowl, combine the olive oil, garlic, and fresh thyme. Whisk until well combined. Add pepper and salt to taste. Pour marinade over mushrooms and mix well until mushrooms are well coated. Place marinated mushrooms directly on lined baking sheet.
Roast for about 20-25 mins.

Nutrition: Cal: 260 Fat: 18 g Carbs: 44 g Protein: 6 g

585. Grilled Zucchini with Feta

Prep time: 10 mins   **Cook time: 25 mins**
Servings: 4

Ingredients:
- 1 medium zucchini, sliced
- 12 ounces of thawed puff pastry
- 4 large eggs, beaten
- 4 ounces feta cheese, drained and crumbled
- 2 tablespoons fresh dill, chopped
- Salt and pepper

Directions: Preheat the Air Fryer to 360 degrees F, and in a bowl, add the beaten eggs and season with salt and pepper.
Stir in zucchini, dill and feta cheese. Grease 8 muffin pans with cook spray. Roll up dough and arrange to cover sides of muffin pans. Divide the egg mixture evenly between the holes. Place the prepared pans in your air fryer and bake for 15 mins.

Nutrition: Cal 95 Fat 1 g Carbs 18 g Protein 6 g

586. Vegan Falafel

Prep time: 10 mins   **Cook time: 15 mins**
Servings: 4

Ingredients:
- One 16-ounce can of chickpeas, rinsed
- 1/3 cup fresh chopped parsley
- Four garlic cloves, minced
- Two shallots, minced (3/4cup)
- 2 tablespoons raw sesame seeds or can use

- 1 ½ teaspoons cumin, plus more to taste
- ¼ teaspoon sea salt
- black pepper
- 3-4 tablespoons all-purpose flour
- 3-4 tablespoons (45-60 ml) of grapeseed oil for cook
- Garlic and dill sauce for serving

Directions: In a blender, add the chickpeas, sesame seeds, parsley, shallots, garlic, cumin, salt, pepper, scraping down the sides if necessary, until fully combined.

Add a tablespoon of flour at a time and mix until the dough is no longer wet and you can form a ball without it sticking to your hands. Taste the seasonings and change them if needed. Add a little more salt, pepper, and a sprinkle of cilantro and cardamom.

To firm up, move to a bowl, cover and refrigerate for 1-2 hours.

Once chilled gently shape into 11-12 small discs.

Heat a skillet over medium heat and add enough oil to coat the pan - about 2 tbsp. generously. Turn to coat.

If the oil is hot, add only as many falafels as will comfortably fit in the pan at a time.

Cook for 4-5 mins in all, flipping when golden brown is deep on the underside. Repeat until all falafels are golden brown. When they cool slightly, they will firm up further.

Serve hot with garlic dill sauce or hummus, inside a pita with desired toppings or over a bed of vegetables.

Nutrition: Cal: 347 Protein: 10.54 g Fat: 18 g Carbs: 37.48 g

587. Potato Croquettes

Prep time: 15 mins
Portion size: 10

Cook time: 15 mins

Ingredients:
- 2 cups boiled potatoes, mashed
- ¼ cup nutritional yeast
- One flax egg
- One tablespoon flour
- Two tablespoons chopped chives
- Two tablespoons vegetable oil
- ¼ cup breadcrumbs
- Salt and ground black pepper

Directions: Preheat the fryer oven to 400 degrees F.

In a bowl, combine the potatoes, nutritional yeast, flax egg, flour and chives. Sprinkle with salt and pepper.

In a separate bowl, mix vegetable oil and bread crumbs to a crumbly consistency.

Form the potato mixture into small balls and dip them into the breadcrumb mixture. Place the croquettes in the basket of the air fryer.

Place the air fryer basket on the baking sheet and select Air Fry. Set the time to 15 mins, making sure the croquettes turn golden brown.

588. Polenta Roll with Cheese

Prep Time: 5 mins
Servings: 1

Cook Time: 10 mins

Ingredients:
- One commercial polenta roll, sliced
- 1 cup cheddar cheese sauce
- One tablespoon chilli powder

Directions: Arrange the polenta slices in the baking pan.

Add the chilli powder and cheddar cheese sauce.

Cook for 10 mins at 390 degrees F.

Nutrition: Cal: 206; Carbs: 25.3 g; Protein: 3.2 g; Fat: 4.2 g

589. Potato with Cheese

Prep Time: 10 mins
Servings: 1

Cook Time: 40 mins

Ingredients:
- ¼ teaspoon onion powder
- One medium russet potato, scrubbed and peeled
- One tablespoon chives, chopped
- One tablespoon Kalamata olives
- A dollop of butter
- A dollop of cream cheese
- One teaspoon olive oil
- 1/8 teaspoon salt

Directions: Preheat the oven at 400 degrees F.

Put the potatoes all together in a baking pan and pour in onion powder, olive oil, salt, and butter. Place the baking dish in the oven. Cook for 40 mins. Be sure to turn the potatoes once halfway.

Serve the potatoes with cream cheese, chives, and Kalamata olives.

Nutrition: Cal: 504; Carbs: 68.4 g; Protein: 9.3 g; Fat: 21.5 g

590. Banana with Tofu 'n Spices

Prep Time: 5 mins
Servings: 8

Cook Time: 10 mins

Ingredients:
- ½ teaspoon red chilli powder
- ½ teaspoon turmeric powder
- One onion, finely chopped
- One package firm tofu, crumbled
- One teaspoon coriander powder
- Three tablespoons coconut oil
- Eight banana peppers, top-end sliced and seeded
- Salt

Directions: Preheat the oven at 325 degrees F for 5 mins.

In a mixing bowl, combine the tofu, coconut oil, turmeric powder, onion, red chilli powder, coriander powder, and salt. Mix until well combined.

Scoop the tofu mixture into the hollows of the banana peppers.

Place the stuffed peppers in an air fryer basket. Cook for 10 mins.

Nutrition: Cal: 72; Carbs: 4.1 g; Protein: 1.2 g; Fat: 5.6 g

591. Vegetables with Tandoori Spice

Prep Time: 10 mins
Servings: 6

Cook Time: 20 mins

Ingredients:
- ½ head cauliflower, cut into florets
- ½ cup yoghurt
- One carrot, peeled and shaved to 1/8-inch thick
- 1 cup young ears of corn
- One handful of sugar snap peas
- One small zucchini, cut into thick slices
- One sweet yellow pepper, seeded and chopped
- Two small onions, cut into wedges
- 2-inch fresh ginger, minced
- Three tablespoons Tandoori spice blend
- Six cloves of garlic, minced
- Two tablespoons canola oil

Directions: Preheat the oven at 330 degrees F.

In a Ziploc bag, put all ingredients and give a shake to season all vegetables.

Dump all ingredients on the baking pan, and cook for 20 mins.

Make sure to give the vegetables a shake halfway through the cook time.

Nutrition: Cal: 126; Carbs: 17.9 g; Protein: 2.9 g; Fat: 6.1 g

592. Honey Seasoned Vegetables

Prep Time: 5 mins
Servings: 5

Cook Time: 15 mins

Ingredients:
- ¼ cup honey
- ¼ cup yellow mustard
- One large red bell pepper, sliced
- Two large yellow squashes, cut into ½ inch thick slices
- Two medium zucchinis, cut into ½ inch thick slices
- Two teaspoons creole seasoning
- Two teaspoons smoked paprika
- Three tablespoons olive oil
- One teaspoon black pepper
- One teaspoon salt

Directions: Preheat the Air Fryer at 330 degrees F.

In a Ziploc bag, put the zucchini, olive oil, squash, red bell pepper, salt and pepper. Give a shake to season all vegetables. Place on the baking pan and cook for 15 mins.

Meanwhile, prepare the sauce by combining the mustard, honey, and paprika, and creole seasoning season with salt to taste. Serve the vegetables with the sauce.

Nutrition: Cal: 164; Carbs: 21.5 g; Protein: 2.6 g; Fat: 8.9 g

593. Carrots and Zucchinis with Mayo Butter

Prep Time: 10 mins
Servings: 4

Cook Time: 25 mins

Ingredients:
- 1/2 pound carrots, sliced
- 1/2 zucchinis, sliced
- One tablespoon grated onion
- Two tablespoons butter, melted
- 1/4 cup water
- 1/4 cup mayo
- 1/4 teaspoon prepared horseradish
- 1/4 cup bread crumbs
- 1/4 teaspoon salt
- 1/4 teaspoon ground black pepper

Directions: Grease baking pan of the Air Fryer with cook spray.
Add carrots and place the baking pan in the oven.
Cook for 8 mins at 360 degrees F. Add zucchinis and continue cook for another 5 mins.
Meanwhile, in a bowl stir horseradish, pepper, salt, onion, mayo, and water. Pour into the pan of veggies. Toss well to coat. Sprinkle over vegetables. Cook for 10 mins at 390 degrees F until tops are lightly browned.

Nutrition: Cal: 223; Carbs: 13.8 g; Protein: 2.7 g; Fat: 17.4 g

594. Easy Brussels Sprouts

Prep Time: 5 mins
Servings: 4

Cook Time: 15 mins

Ingredients:
- 2 cups Brussels sprouts, halved
- ¼ teaspoon salt
- One tablespoon balsamic vinegar
- Two tablespoons olive oil

Directions: Preheat the oven at 350 degrees F for 5 mins.
Put and mix ingredients all together in a bowl until well coated.
Put some mixture in the air fryer basket and place it in the oven.
Cook for 15 mins.

Nutrition: Cal: 82; Carbs: 4.6 g; Protein: 1.5 g; Fat: 6.8 g

595. Yellow Squash 'n Zucchini

Prep Time: 10 mins
Servings: 4

Cook Time: 30 mins

Ingredients:
- 1/2 pound yellow squash, sliced
- 1/2 pound zucchini, sliced
- One egg
- Five saltine crackers, or as needed, crushed
- Two tablespoons bread crumbs
- 1/2 cup shredded Cheddar cheese
- 1/2 teaspoons white sugar
- 1/4 onion, diced
- 1/4 cup biscuit baking mix
- 1/4 cup butter
- 1/2 teaspoon salt

Directions: Grease baking pan of the oven with cook spray. Add zucchini, onion, and yellow squash, stir well.
Cover the pan with foil and place the baking pan in the oven.
Cook for 15 mins at 360oF or until tender.
Stir in butter, baking mix, salt, sugar, egg, and cheddar cheese. Mix well. Fold in crushed crackers. Top with bread crumbs. Cook for 15 mins at 390 degrees F until tops are lightly browned.

Nutrition: Cal: 285; Carbs: 16.4 g; Protein: 8.6 g; Fat: 20.5 g

596. Veggie Burger with Spices

Prep Time: 5 mins
Servings: 1

Cook Time: 15 mins

Ingredients:

- ¼ cup desiccated coconut
- ½ cup oats
- ½ pound cauliflower, steamed and diced
- 1 cup bread crumbs
- 1 flax egg (1 flaxseed egg + 3 tablespoon water)
- One teaspoon mustard powder
- Two teaspoons chives
- Two teaspoons coconut oil, melted
- Two teaspoons garlic, minced
- Two teaspoons parsley
- Two teaspoons thyme
- Three tablespoon plain flour
- Salt and pepper

Directions: Preheat the Air Fryer to 390 degrees F.
Place some of the cauliflower in a dish towel and discard excess water. Place in a bowl and add all ingredients except breadcrumbs. Mix well until well combined.
Form 8 hamburger patties with the mixture using your hands.
Roll the patties in the breadcrumbs and place them in the basket of the fryer. Make sure they don't overlap.
Cook for 10-15 mins or until the meatballs are crispy.

Nutrition: Cal: 70; Carbs: 10.8 g; Protein: 2.5 g; Fat: 1.5 g

597. Buffalo Sauce Cauliflower

Prep Time: 5 mins
Servings: 1

Cook time: 5 mins

Ingredients:

- 1/2 packet dry ranch seasoning
- Two tablespoons salted butter, melted
- 1 cup cauliflower florets
- ¼ cup buffalo sauce

Directions: Preheat the oven to 400ºF.
In a bowl, combine the dry ranch seasoning and butter. Stir with the cauliflower florets to coat and transfer them to the air fryer basket.
Select Air Fry, and set time to 5 mins, shaking the basket occasionally to ensure the florets cook evenly.
Remove the cauliflower and place it on a platter. Pour the buffalo sauce over it.

598. Zucchini Balls

Prep Time: 5 mins
Servings: 4

Cook time: 10 mins

Ingredients:

- Four zucchinis
- One egg
- 1/2 cup grated Parmesan cheese
- One tablespoon Italian herbs
- 1 cup grated coconut

Directions: Thinly grate the zucchinis and pat dry with cheesecloth. Making sure to remove all the moisture.
In a bowl, combine the zucchinis with egg, Parmesan, Italian herbs, and grated coconut, mixing well to incorporate everything.
Shape the mixture into balls.
Preheat the air fryer oven to 400ºF. Lay zucchini balls in the air fryer basket.
Select Air Fry, and set time to 10 mins.

599. Potatoes with Tofu

Prep Time: 15mins
Serving: 8

Cook Time: 35 mins

Ingredients:

- Eight sweet potatoes, scrubbed
- Two tablespoons olive oil
- One large onion, chopped
- Two green chilies, deseeded and chopped

- 8 ounces tofu, crumbled
- Two tablespoons Cajun seasoning
- 1 cup chopped tomatoes
- One can of kidney beans, drained and rinsed
- Salt and ground pepper

Directions: Preheat the fryer oven to 400°F.
Pierce the skin of the potatoes and transfer them to the fryer basket. Place the fry basket in the center position. Select Air Fry and set the time to 30 mins.
Remove from air fryer oven, halve each potato and set to one side.
Fry the onions and chiles in the olive oil in a skillet for 2 mins until fragrant.
Add the tofu and Cajun seasoning and sauté for another 3 mins before incorporating the beans and tomatoes. Sprinkle with salt and pepper as desired.
Top each sweet potato half with a spoonful of the tofu mixture and serve.

600. Gold Ravioli

Prep Time: 10mins
Serving: 4

Cook Time: 6 mins

Ingredients:
- 1/2 cup panko bread crumbs
- Two teaspoons nutritional yeast
- One teaspoon dried basil
- One teaspoon dried oregano
- One teaspoon garlic powder
- Salt and ground black pepper
- ¼ cup aquafaba
- 8 ounces ravioli
- Cook spray

Directions: Cover the fry basket with aluminum foil and coat with a light coat of oil.
Preheat the fryer oven to 400°F. Combine panko bread crumbs, nutritional yeast, basil, oregano and garlic powder. Sprinkle with salt and pepper.
Place the aquafaba in a separate bowl. Dip the ravioli in the aquafaba before tossing in the panko mixture. Spray with cook spray and transfer to frying basket. Insert the frying basket in the center position.
Select Air Fry and set the time to 6 mins. Shake the fry basket halfway through.

601. Mediterranean Vegetables

Prep Time: 10mins
Serving: 4

Cook Time: 6 mins

Ingredients:
- One large zucchini, sliced
- 1 cup cherry tomatoes, halved
- One parsnip, sliced
- One green pepper, sliced
- One carrot, sliced
- One teaspoon mixed herbs
- One teaspoon mustard
- One teaspoon garlic purée
- Six tablespoons olive oil
- Salt and ground black pepper

Directions: Preheat the air fryer oven to 400°F.
Combine all the ingredients in a bowl, and coat the vegetables well.
Transfer to the fry basket. Select Air Fry, and set time to 6 mins.

602. Veg Rolls

Prep Time: 20mins
Serving: 6

Cook Time: 10 mins

Ingredients:
- Two potatoes, mashed
- ¼ cup peas
- ¼ cup mashed carrots
- One small cabbage, sliced
- ¼ cups beans
- Two tablespoons sweet corn
- One small onion, chopped
- 1/2 cup bread crumbs
- One packet spring roll sheets
- 1/2 cup cornstarch slurry

Directions: Preheat the air fryer oven to 390°F.
Boil all the vegetables in water over low heat. Rinse and allow drying.
Unroll the spring roll sheets and pour an equal amounts of vegetables in the center of each. Fold into spring rolls and

coat each one with the slurry and bread crumbs. Transfer to the fry basket.
Insert the fry basket at mid position. Select Air Fry, and set time to 10 mins.

603. Rice and Eggplant

Prep Time: 15mins
Serving: 4

Cook Time: 10 mins

Ingredients:
- ¼ cup sliced cucumber
- Seven tablespoons Japanese rice vinegar
- Three medium eggplants, sliced
- Three tablespoons sweet white miso paste
- One tablespoon miring rice wine
- 4 cups cooked sushi rice
- Four spring onions
- One tablespoon toasted sesame seeds
- One teaspoon salt
- One tablespoon sugar

Directions: Coat the cucumber slices with the rice wine vinegar, salt and sugar.
Place a plate over the bowl to weigh it down completely.
In a bowl, mix the eggplant, rice wine miring and miso paste. Allow to marinate for half an hour.
Preheat the fryer oven to 400°F.
Place the eggplant slices in the fryer basket. Select Air Fry and set the time to 10 mins.
Fill the bottom of a bowl with the rice and add the eggplant and pickled cucumbers.
Add the spring onions and sesame seeds for garnish.

604. Potatoes and Zucchinis

Prep Time: 10mins
Serving: 4

Cook Time: 45 mins

Ingredients:
- Two potatoes, peeled and cubed
- Four carrots, cut into chunks
- One head broccoli, cut into florets
- Four zucchinis, sliced thickly
- Salt and ground black pepper, to taste
- ¼ cup olive oil
- One tablespoon dry onion powder

Directions: Preheat the air fryer oven to 400°F
In a baking pan, add all the ingredients and combine well.
Select Bake, and set time to 45 mins, ensuring the vegetables are soft and the sides have browned.

605. Mushrooms with Mascarpone

Prep Time: 10mins
Serving: 4

Cook Time: 15 mins

Ingredients:
- Vegetable oil spray
- 4 cups sliced mushrooms
- One medium yellow onion, chopped
- Two cloves garlic, minced
- ¼ cup heavy whipping cream or half-and-half
- 8 ounces (227 g) mascarpone cheese
- One teaspoon dried thyme
- 1/2 teaspoon red pepper flakes
- 4 cups cooked konjac noodles, for serving
- 1/2 cup grated Parmesan cheese
- One teaspoon kosher salt
- One teaspoon black pepper

Directions: Preheat the fryer oven to 350°F. Spray a heat-resistant pan with vegetable oil spray.
In a bowl, combine mushrooms, cream, mascarpone cheese, thyme, onion, garlic, salt, black pepper and red pepper flakes. Stir to combine. Transfer mixture to prepared pan.
Place the skillet in the frying basket. Select Bake, and set time for 15 mins, stirring halfway through cook time.
Spread mushroom mixture evenly over pasta. Sprinkle with Parmesan cheese.

606. Chickpea, Fig, and Arugula Salad

Prep Time: 15 mins
Serving: 4

Cook Time: 20mins

Ingredients:
- *Eight fresh figs halved*
- *11/2 cups cooked chickpeas*
- *One teaspoon crushed roasted cumin seeds*
- *Four tablespoons balsamic vinegar*
- *Two tablespoons olive oil, plus more for greasing*
- *Salt and ground black pepper*
- *3 cups arugula rocket, washed and dried*

Directions: Preheat the air fryer oven to 375ºF.
Cover the fry basket with aluminum foil and grease lightly with oil. Put the figs in the fry basket. Select Air Fry, and set time to 10 mins.
In a bowl, combine the chickpeas and cumin seeds.
Remove the air fried figs from the air fryer oven and replace it with the chickpeas. Air fry for 10 mins. Leave to cool.
In the meantime, prepare the dressing. Mix the balsamic vinegar, olive oil, salt, and pepper.
In a salad bowl, combine the arugula rocket with the cooled figs and chickpeas.
Toss with the sauce.

607. Sriracha Cauliflower

Prep Time: 5mins
Serving: 4

Cook Time: 17 mins

Ingredients:
- *¼ cup butter, melted*
- *¼ cup sriracha sauce*
- *4 cups cauliflower florets*
- *1 cup bread crumbs*
- *One teaspoon salt*

Directions: Preheat the air fryer oven to 375ºF.
Mix the sriracha and butter in a bowl and pour this mixture over the cauliflower, taking care to cover each floret entirely.
In a separate bowl, combine the bread crumbs and salt. Dip the cauliflower florets in the bread crumbs, coating each one well. Transfer to the fry basket.
Select Air Fry, and set time to 17 mins.

608. Roasted Apple Potatoes

Prep Time: 5 mins
Serving: 2

Cook Time: 30 mins

Ingredients:
- *Two potatoes, diced*
- *2 tsp. cinnamon*
- *Two large green apples, diced*
- *2 tbsp. maple syrup*
- *1 tbsp. olive oil*

Directions: In a bowl, add potatoes, oil, cinnamon, and apples and stir well.
Spread potatoes mixture onto the cook pan.
Select bake mode and set the oven to 400º F for 30.
Drizzle with maple syrup.

Nutrition: Cal 352 Fat 7.6 g Carbs 74 g Protein 2.2 g

609. Parmesan Brussels Sprouts

Prep Time: 5 mins
Serving: 4

Cook Time: 12 mins

Ingredients:
- *1 lb. Brussels sprouts cut stems and halved*
- *1/4 cup parmesan cheese, grated*
- *1 1/2 tbsp. olive oil*
- *Pepper*
- *Salt*

Directions: Stir Brussels sprouts, pepper, oil, and salt into the bowl.

Transfer Brussels sprouts into the air fryer basket.

Place air fryer basket into the oven, and select air fry mode; set the oven to 350° F for 12 mins. Stir twice.

Top with parmesan cheese.

Nutrition: Cal 114 Fat 7 g Carbs 10.6 g Protein 5.9 g

610. Garlicky Cauliflower

Prep Time: 5 mins   **Cook Time: 20 mins**
Serving: 4

Ingredients:
- 5 cups cauliflower florets
- Six garlic cloves, chopped
- 1/2 tsp. cumin powder
- 1/2 tsp. coriander powder
- Four tablespoons olive oil
- 1/2 tsp. salt

Directions: Add all ingredients into a bowl and stir well.

Add cauliflower florets into the air fryer basket.

Place air fryer basket into the oven, and select air fry mode. Set the oven to 400° F for 20 mins. Stir twice.

Nutrition: Cal 159 Fat 14.2 g Carbs 8.2 g Protein 2.8 g

611. Green Beans

Prep Time: 5 mins   **Cook Time: 10 mins**
Serving: 2

Ingredients:
- 2 cups green beans
- 1/8 tsp. cayenne pepper
- 1/8 tsp. ground allspice
- 1/4 tsp. ground cinnamon
- 1/2 tsp. dried oregano
- 1/4 tsp. ground coriander
- 1/4 tsp. ground cumin
- 2 tbsp. olive oil
- 1/2 tsp. salt

Directions: Add all ingredients into the mixing bowl and toss well.

Spray air fryer basket with cook spray.

Add bowl mixture into the air fryer basket.

Place air fryer basket into the oven, and select air fry mode; set the oven to 370° F for 10 mins.

Nutrition: Cal 158 Fat 14.3 g Carbs 8.6 g Protein 2.1 g

612. Potato Casserole

Prep Time: 5 mins   **Cook Time: 35 mins**
Serving: 6

Ingredients:
- Five eggs
- 1/2 cup cheddar cheese, shredded
- Two medium potatoes, diced into 1/2-inch cubes
- One green bell pepper, diced
- One onion, chopped
- 1 tbsp. olive oil
- 3/4 tsp. pepper
- 3/4 tsp. salt

Directions: Spray a casserole dish with cook spray and set aside.

Heat olive oil in a skillet over medium heat.

Add the onion and sauté for 1 minute. Add potatoes, peppers, 1/2 teaspoon black pepper and 1.2 teaspoons salt and sauté for an additional 4 mins.

Transfer the sautéed vegetables to the prepared casserole dish and distribute evenly.

In a bowl, whisk the eggs and remaining pepper and salt.

Pour the egg mixture into the casserole dish and sprinkle with cheddar cheese.

Select the baking mode and set the oven to 350° F for 35 mins. Place the casserole in the oven.

Nutrition: Cal 174 Fat 9.2 g Carbs 14.9 g Protein 8.6 g

613. Baked Zucchini Egg

Prep Time: 5 mins
Serving: 4

Cook Time: 30 mins

Ingredients:

- 1 cup zucchini, shredded and squeezed out all liquid
- Six eggs
- 1/2 tsp. dill
- 1/2 tsp. oregano
- 1/2 tsp. basil
- 1/2 tsp. baking powder
- 1/2 cup almond flour
- 1 cup cheddar cheese, shredded
- 1 cup kale, chopped
- One onion, chopped
- 1/2 cup milk
- 1/4 tsp. salt

Directions: Grease a baking dish and set aside.
In a bowl, whisk eggs with milk.
Add remaining ingredients and mix until well combined.
Pour egg mixture into the prepared baking dish.
Select bake mode and set the oven to 375 F for 30 mins.

Nutrition: Cal 269 Fat 18.4 g Carbs 8.9 g Protein 18.3 g

614. Roasted Broccoli

Prep Time: 5 mins
Serving: 12

Cook Time: 15 mins

Ingredients:

- 4 cups broccoli florets
- 2/3 cup parmesan cheese, grated and divided
- Six garlic cloves, minced
- 1/3 cup olive oil
- Pepper
- Salt

Directions: Preheat the oven to 400° F.
Spray a baking dish with cook spray and set aside.
Add broccoli, half cheese, garlic, and olive oil in a bowl and toss well—season with pepper and salt.
Arrange broccoli mixture on a prepared baking dish.
Select bake mode and set the oven to 400° F for 15 mins
Before serving, add remaining cheese and toss well.

Nutrition: Cal 86 Fat 6.9 g Carbs 4.5 g Protein 3.4 g

615. Vegetable Tots

Prep Time: 10 mins
Serving: 2

Cook Time: 10 mins

Ingredients:

- 1 egg
- 1 carrot, grated & squeeze out the liquid
- 1/4 cup breadcrumbs
- 1 zucchini, grated & squeeze out the liquid
- 1/4 cup parmesan cheese, grated
- Pepper
- Salt

Directions: Spray air fryer basket with cook spray.
Add all ingredients into the bowl and stir until well combined.
Make tots from mixture and place into the air fryer basket.
Place air fryer basket into the oven and select air fry mode; set the oven to the 400° F for 15 mins.

Nutrition: Cal 153 Fat 5.8 g Carbs 16.7 g Protein 10 g

616. Delicious Potato Fries

Prep Time: 10 mins
Serving: 2

Cook Time: 20 mins

Ingredients:
- 1 lb potatoes, wash, peel and cut into fries shape
- 1/4 tsp. chili powder
- 1/2 tbsp olive oil
- 1/4 tsp. smoked paprika
- Salt

Directions: Spray air fryer basket with cook spray.
Add potato fries in a large bowl and drizzle with olive oil. Season with paprika, chili powder, and salt.
Add potato fries into the air fryer basket.
Place air fryer basket into the oven and select air fry mode; set the oven to the 370° F for 20 mins. Stir twice.

Nutrition: Cal 188 Fat 3.8 g Carbs 36 g Protein 3.9 g

617. Parmesan Potatoes

Prep Time: 10 mins
Serving: 2

Cook Time: 40 mins

Ingredients:
- 2 potatoes make the thin slices
- 2tbsps. butter, melted
- tbsps. mushrooms, sliced
- 4 tbsps. parmesan cheese, grated
- Pepper
- Salt

Directions: Spray the baking pan with cook spray and set aside.
Slide mushroom slices into each slit.
Place potatoes on baking pan and brush with half-melted butter.
Select air fry mode set oven to the 350° F for 20 mins.
Turn potatoes to the other side and brush with remaining butter and air fry for 20 mins more.
Sprinkle with parmesan cheese.

Nutrition: Cal 345 Fat 18 g Carbs 34.8 g Protein 13.4 g

618. Masala Gallettes

Prep Time: 10 mins
Serving: 4

Cook Time: 35 mins

Ingredients:
- 2 - tbsp. garam masala
- 2 - medium potatoes boiled and mashed
- 1 1/2 - cup coarsely crushed peanuts
- 3 - tsp. ginger finely chopped
- 1 to 2 - tbsp. fresh coriander leaves
- 2 or 3 - green chilies finely chopped
- 1 1/2 - tbsp. lemon juice
- Salt and pepper

Directions: Mix the ingredients in a bowl. Form this mixture into round, flat galettes.
Wet galettes with water. Coat each galette with crushed peanuts.
Preheat the air fryer to 160° F for 5 mins.
Place the galettes in the fryer container and let them cook for another 25 mins. Continue to flip them to cook evenly.
Serve with mint chutney or ketchup.

619. Potato Samosa

Prep Time: 10 mins
Serving: 4

Cook Time: 30mins

Ingredients:

For wrappers:
- 2 - tbsp. unsalted butter
- 1 1/2 - cup all-purpose flour

- A pinch of salt
- Water

For filling:
- 2 to 3 - large potatoes
- ¼ - cup boiled peas
- 1 - tsp. powdered ginger
- 1 or 2 - green chilies

- 1/2 - tsp. cumin
- 1 - tsp. coarsely crushed coriander
- 1 - dry red chili
- A small amount of salt

- 1/2 - tsp. mango powder
- 1/2 - tsp. Red chili powder
- 1 to 2 - tbsp. Coriander

Directions: Mix together the ingredients for the wrapper. Let stand while you prepare the filling.
Cook ingredients in a skillet and blend well to make a thick paste.
Form the dough into balls. Cut them in half and insert the filling.
Preheat the air fryer to 300° F. Place the samosas in the frying pan.
Bake for 20-25 mins. Flip halfway through for even cook.
Serve with tamarind chutney or mint.

620. Veggie Kebab

Prep Time: 10 mins
Serving: 4

Cook Time: 25 mins

Ingredients:
- 2 cups of mixed vegetables
- Three onions chopped
- Five green chilies-roughly chopped
- 1 1/2 tbsp. ginger paste
- 1 1/2 tsp. garlic paste

- 3 tsp. lemon juice
- 2 tsp. garam masala
- 4 tbsp. chopped coriander
- 3 tbsp. cream
- 3 tbsp. chopped capsicum

- Three eggs
- 2 1/2 tbsp. white sesame seeds
- 1 1/2 tsp. salt

Directions: Mix the ingredients except for the egg and form a smooth paste.
Coat the vegetables in the paste. Beat in the eggs and add salt to season.
Dip the vegetables in the egg mix and coat well with sesame seed.
Place the vegetables on skewers.
Preheat the Air fryer to 160° F. Cook for 25 mins.
Turn the sticks over halfway through to cook uniformly.

621. Sago Galette

Prep Time: 10 mins
Serving: 4

Cook Time: 35 mins

Ingredients:
- 2 cup sago, soaked
- 1 1/2 cup coarsely crushed peanuts
- 3 tsp. ginger finely chopped

- 1-2 tbsp. fresh coriander leaves
- 2 or 3 green chilies finely chopped
- 1 1/2 tbsp. lemon juice

- Salt and pepper

Directions: Mix ingredients in a bowl.
Form this mixture into round, flat galettes.
Wet the galettes with a little water. Coat each galette with the crushed peanuts.
Preheat the Air Fryer to 160° F for 5 mins. Place the galettes in the fryer and let them cook for another 25 mins. Continue to flip them over to cook evenly.
Serve with mint chutney or ketchup.

622. Stuffed Peppers Baskets

Prep Time: 10 mins
Serving: 4

Cook Time: 35 mins

Ingredients:

For baskets:
- 3-4 long capsicum
- 1/2 tsp. Salt
- 1/2 tsp. pepper powder

For filling:
- One medium onion
- One green chili
- 2 or 3 large potatoes
- 1 1/2 tbsp. chopped coriander leaves
- 1 tsp. fenugreek
- 1 tsp. dried mango powder
- 1 tsp. cumin powder
- Salt and pepper

For topping:
- 3 tbsp. grated cheese
- 1 tsp. Red chili flakes
- 1/2 tsp. Oregano
- 1/2 tsp. Basil
- 1/2 tsp. parsley

Directions: Mix all of the filling ingredients in a bowl.
Remove the stem, seeds, and top of the capsicum.
Sprinkle some salt and pepper inside the capsicums. Set aside.
Place the filling inside the peppers, leaving a little space at the top.
Mix topping spices and sprinkle ground cheese and seasoning on top.
Preheat the Air Fryer to 140° F for 5 mins.
Put the capsicums in the fry case and cook for 20 mins.

623. Macaroni Samosa

Prep Time: 10 mins
Serving: 4

Cook Time: 25 mins

Ingredients:

For wrappers:
- cup all-purpose flour
- 2- tbsp. unsalted butter
- A pinch of salt to taste
- Take the amount of water sufficient

For filling:
- 3- cups boiled macaroni
- 2- onion
- 2- capsicum
- 2- Carrots
- 2- Cabbage
- 2- tbsp. soy sauce
- 2- tsp. vinegar
- 2- tbsp. ginger
- 2- tbsp. garlic
- 2- tbsp. green chilies
- 2- tbsp. ginger-garlic paste
- Some salt and pepper
- 2- tbsp. olive oil

Directions: Blend the wrapper ingredients until smooth. Set aside while making the filling.
Boil the filling ingredients and blend them to make a thick paste.
Form the batter into balls. Cut them in half and insert the filling.
Preheat the Air Fryer to 300° F. Place the samosas in the fry holder and cook for 20 to 25 mins
Around the midpoint, turn the samosas over for uniform cook.
Serve hot with tamarind or mint chutney.

624. Greek Potato

Prep time: 10 mins
Servings: 4

Cook time: 20 mins

Ingredients:
- 1½ pounds potatoes, peeled and cubed
- Two tbsp. olive oil
- One tbsp. hot paprika
- 2 ounces coconut cream
- Salt and black pepper

Directions: Place potatoes in a bowl and add water to cover. Set them aside for 10 mins.
Drain and mix with half the oil, salt, pepper and paprika and toss.
Place the potatoes in the basket of your air fryer.
Cook at the set temperature of 360 degrees F for 20 mins.
In a bowl, mix the coconut cream with salt, pepper and the rest of the oil and mix well.
Divide the potatoes among the plates.
Add the coconut cream on top.

Nutrition: Cal: 203 Protein: 4 g Fat: 7.1 g Carbs: 32.2 g

625. Mushroom Cakes

Prep time: 10 mins   **Cook time: 2 Hours 8 Mins**
Servings: 8

Ingredients:
- Ounces mushrooms, chopped
- One small yellow onion, chopped
- Salt and black pepper to the taste
- ¼ tsp. nutmeg, ground
- Two tbsp. olive oil
- One tbsp. breadcrumbs
- 14 ounces of coconut milk

Directions: Over medium-high heat, cook and heat half the oil in a skillet. Add the onion and mushrooms.
Stir and cook for 3 mins. Add the coconut milk, salt, nutmeg and pepper and stir.
Remove from heat and set aside for 2 hours.
Mix the rest of the oil in a bowl, with the breadcrumbs and mix well.
Take a tablespoon of the mushroom filling, roll it in the breadcrumbs and place it in the basket of your air fryer.
Repeat with the rest of the mushroom mixture and bake the pies at 400 degrees F for 8 mins.
Divide the mushroom cakes among the plates.

Nutrition: Cal: 46 Protein: 0.64 g Fat: 3.5 g Carbs: 3.3 g

626. Green Salad

Prep time: 10 mins   **Cook time: 10 mins**
Servings: 4

Ingredients:
- One tbsp. lemon juice
- Four red bell peppers
- One lettuce head, cut into strips
- Salt and black pepper to taste
- Three tbsp. coconut cream
- Two tbsp. olive oil
- 1 ounces rocket leaves

Directions: Place the bell bell pepper in the basket of the air fryer.
Cook at a temperature of 400 degrees F for 10 mins.
Transfer to a bowl and set aside to cool.
Peel them, cut them into strips and place them in a bowl.
Add the arugula leaves and lettuce strips and toss to combine.
In a bowl, mix the oil with the lemon juice, coconut cream, salt and pepper and whisk well.
Add on top of the salad, toss to coat and divide between plates.

Nutrition: Cal: 130 Protein: 2.71 g Fat: 11 g Carbs: 7.4 g

627. Tomatoes Salad

Prep time: 10 mins   **Cook time: 20 mins**
Servings: 2

Ingredients:
- Two tomatoes halved
- Cook spray
- Salt and black pepper
- One tsp. parsley, chopped
- One tsp. basil, chopped
- One tsp. oregano, chopped

- *One tsp. rosemary, chopped*
- *One cucumber, chopped*
- *One green onion, chopped*

Directions: Spray tomato halves with cook oil.
Season with salt and pepper. Place them in your air fryer's basket.
Cook for 20 mins at 320 degrees F.
Transfer tomatoes to a bowl. Add parsley, basil, oregano, rosemary, cucumber and onion, and toss.

Nutrition: Cal: 55 Protein: 2.59 g Fat: 0.67 g Carbs: 11.62 g

628. French Mushroom

Prep time: 10 mins   **Cook time: 25 mins**
Servings: 4

Ingredients:
- *2 pounds mushrooms, halved*
- *Two tsp. herbs de Provence*
- *½ tsp. garlic powder*
- *One tbsp. olive oil*

Directions: Over a medium heat, heat a pan with the oil. Add herbs and heat them for 2 mins.
Add mushrooms and garlic powder and stir.
Introduce pan in your air fryer's basket and cook at 360 degrees F for 25 mins.

Nutrition: Cal: 81 Protein: 7.07 g Fat: 4.15 g Carbs: 7.69 g

629. Zucchini and Pumpkin Salad

Prep time: 10 mins   **Cook time: 25 mins**
Servings: 4

Ingredients:
- *Six tsp. olive oil*
- *1 pound zucchinis, cut into half-moons*
- *½ pound carrots, cubed*
- *One yellow squash, cut into chunks*
- *Salt and white pepper to taste*
- *One tbsp. tarragon, chopped*
- *Two tbsp. tomato paste*

Directions: In your air fryer pan, mix oil with zucchinis, carrots, squash, salt, pepper, tarragon and tomato paste.
Cover and then cook at 400 degrees F for 25 mins.
Divide between plates.

Nutrition: Cal: 116 Protein: 4.18 g Fat: 7.4 g Carbs: 10.99 g

630. Squash Stew

Prep time: 10 mins   **Cook time: 30 mins**
Servings: 8

Ingredients:
- *Two carrots, chopped*
- *One yellow onion, chopped*
- *Two celery stalks, chopped*
- *Two green apples, cored, peeled and chopped*
- *Four garlic cloves, minced*
- *2 cups butternut squash, peeled and cubed*
- *6 ounces canned chickpeas, drained*
- *6 ounces canned black beans, drained*
- *7 ounces canned coconut milk*
- *Two tsp. chilli powder*
- *One tsp. oregano, dried*
- *One tbsp. cumin, ground*
- *2 cups veggie stock*
- *Two tbsp. tomato paste*
- *Salt and black pepper*
- *One tbsp. cilantro, chopped*

Directions: In your air fryer, mix carrots with onion, celery, apples, garlic, squash, chickpeas, black beans, coconut milk, chilli powder, oregano, cumin, stock, tomato paste, salt and pepper.
Mix, cover and cook at 370 degrees F for 30 mins. Add cilantro and stir.

Nutrition: Cal: 112 Protein: 3.28 g Fat: 2.37 g

631. Stew of Okra and Eggplant

Prep time: 10 mins   **Cook time: 25 mins**
Servings: 10

Ingredients:
- 2 cups eggplant, cubed
- One butternut squash, peeled and cubed
- 2 cups zucchini, cubed
- 10 ounces tomato sauce
- One carrot, sliced
- One yellow onion, chopped
- ½ cup veggie stock
- 10 ounces okra
- 1/3 cup raisins
- Two garlic cloves, minced
- ½ tsp. turmeric powder
- ½ tsp. cumin, ground
- ½ tsp. red pepper flakes, crushed
- ¼ tsp. sweet paprika
- ¼ tsp. cinnamon powder

Directions: In your air fryer, mix eggplant with squash, zucchini, tomato sauce, carrot, onion, okra, garlic, stock, raisins, turmeric, cumin, pepper flakes, paprika and cinnamon
Stir, cover and cook at 360 degrees for 5 mins.

Nutrition: Cal: 39 Protein: 1.4 g Fat: 1.17 g Carbs: 7 g

632. White Beans Stew

Prep time: 10 mins   **Cook time: 20 mins**
Servings: 10

Ingredients:
- 2 pounds white beans, cooked
- Three celery stalks, chopped
- Two carrots, chopped
- One bay leaf
- One yellow onion, chopped
- Three garlic cloves, minced
- One tsp. rosemary, dried
- One tsp. oregano, dried
- One tsp. thyme, dried
- A drizzle of olive oil
- Salt and black pepper
- 28 ounces canned tomatoes, chopped
- 6 cups chard, chopped

Directions: In your air fryer's pan, mix white beans with celery, carrots, bay leaf, onion, garlic, rosemary, oregano, thyme, oil, salt, pepper, tomatoes and chard. Toss, cover and cook at 365 degrees F for 20 mins.

Nutrition: Cal: 58 kcal Protein: 2.43 g Fat: 1.66 g Carbs: 10.31 g

633. Spinach and Lentils

Prep time: 10 mins   **Cook time: 15 mins**
Servings: 8

Ingredients:
- 10 ounces spinach
- 2 cups canned lentils, drained
- One tbsp. garlic, minced
- 15 ounces canned tomatoes, chopped
- 2 cups cauliflower florets
- One tsp. ginger, grated
- One yellow onion, chopped
- Two tbsp. curry paste
- ½ tsp. cumin, ground
- ½ tsp. coriander, ground
- Two tsp. stevia
- A pinch of salt and black pepper
- ¼ cup cilantro, chopped
- One tbsp. lime juice

Directions: In a baking pan that suites your air fryer, mix spinach with lentils, garlic, curry paste, cumin, tomatoes, cauliflower, ginger, onion, coriander, stevia, salt, pepper and lime juice.
Toss, introduce in the air fryer and cook at 370 degrees F for 15 mins.
Add cilantro and stir.

Nutrition: Cal: 68 Protein: 4.23 g Fat: 1.9 g Carbs: 11.62 g

634. Winter Green Beans

Prep time: 10 mins   **Cook time: 16 mins**
Servings: 4

Ingredients:
- 1 pound green beans, halved
- One small yellow onion, chopped
- One tbsp. olive oil

- Two garlic cloves, minced
- One and ½ cups mushrooms, sliced
- Three tsp. ginger, grated
- 2 cups corn
- 4 cups red cabbage, chopped
- One tbsp. nutritional yeast
- Two tsp. tomato paste
- One tsp. coconut aminos
- One tsp. sriracha sauce
- 4 ounces canned tomatoes, chopped
- Two tsp. oregano, dried
- One jalapeno, chopped
- Salt and pepper
- 1½ tsp. cumin, ground

Directions: Preheat your air fryer at 365 degrees F temperature.
Add oil to the pan; also add all ingredients
Cover and cook for 16 mins.

Nutrition: Cal: 503 Protein: 13.31 g Fat: 15.3 g Carbs: 84.8 g

635. Green Beans Casserole

Prep time: 10 mins
Servings: 4

Cook time: 20 mins

Ingredients:
- 1 cup green beans, trimmed and halved
- One tsp. olive oil
- Two red chillies, dried
- ¼ tsp. fenugreek seeds
- ½ tsp. black mustard seeds
- Ten curry leaves, chopped
- ½ cup red onion, chopped
- Three garlic cloves, minced
- Two tsp. coriander powder
- Two tomatoes, chopped
- 2 cups eggplant, chopped
- ½ tsp. turmeric powder
- ½ cup green bell pepper, chopped
- A pinch of salt and black pepper
- Two tsp. tamarind paste
- One tbsp. cilantro, chopped

Directions: In a baking pan combines the oil with chillies, curry leaves, onion, coriander, tomatoes, eggplant, turmeric, green bell pepper, salt, pepper, fenugreek seeds, black mustard seeds, green beans, tamarind paste and cilantro.
Toss and put in your air fryer.
Cook at 365 degrees F temperature for 20 mins.

Nutrition: Cal: 57 Fat: 1.7 g Carbs: 10.21 g

636. Chinese Cauliflower Rice

Prep time: 10 mins
Servings: 4

Cook time: 20 mins

Ingredients:
- Four tbsp. coconut aminos
- ½ block firm tofu, cubed
- 1 cup carrot, chopped
- ½ cup yellow onion, chopped
- One tsp. turmeric powder
- 3 cups cauliflower, riced
- 1½ tsp. sesame oil
- One tbsp. rice vinegar
- ½ cup broccoli florets, chopped
- One tbsp. ginger, minced
- Two garlic cloves, minced
- ½ cup peas

Directions: In a bowl, mix tofu with two tablespoons coconut aminos, ½ cup onion, turmeric and carrot.
Stir to coat and then transfer to your air fryer.
Bake at 370 degrees F for 10 mins, shaking halfway through.
In a bowl, mix the cauliflower rice with the rest of the coconut aminos, sesame oil, garlic, vinegar, ginger, broccoli and peas. Mix and add to the tofu mix from the fryer.
Stir and bake at 370 degrees F for 10 mins.

Nutrition: Cal: 111 Protein: 6.56 g Fat: 5.44 g Carbs: 11.34 g

637. Artichokes Dish

Prep time: 5 mins
Servings: 4

Cook time: 12 mins

Ingredients:
- Four big artichokes
- Two tbsp. lemon juice
- ¼ cup olive oil
- Two tsp. balsamic vinegar
- One tsp. oregano, dried
- Two garlic cloves, minced
- Salt and black pepper

Directions: Season the artichokes with salt and pepper.

Now rub them with half of the oil and half of the lemon juice.

Then, place them in your air fryer and cook them at 360 degrees for 7 mins.

In a bowl, mix these ingredients the remaining oil, lemon juice, vinegar, salt, pepper, garlic and oregano and mix very well. Divide the artichokes among the plates. Pour the vinaigrette over all.

Nutrition: Cal: 207 Protein: 5.68 g Fat: 13.8 g Carbs: 19.74 g

638. Yellow Lentil

Prep time: 10 mins
Servings: 2

Cook time: 15 mins

Ingredients:

- 1 cup yellow lentils, soaked in water for 1 hour and drained
- One hot chilli pepper, chopped
- The 1-inch ginger piece, grated
- ½ tsp. turmeric powder
- One tsp. garam masala
- Salt and black pepper to taste
- Two tsp. olive oil
- ½ cup cilantro, chopped
- 1½ cup spinach, chopped
- Four garlic cloves, minced
- ¾ cup red onion, chopped

Directions: In a pan that suites your air fryer, mix lentils with chilli pepper, ginger, turmeric, garam masala, salt, pepper, olive oil, cilantro, spinach, onion and garlic.

Stir, introduce in your air fryer.

Cook at 400 degrees F temperature for 15 mins.

Nutrition: Cal: 115 Protein: 5.56 g Fat: 5.01 g Carbs: 15.78 g

639. Vegetables Lasagna

Prep time: 10 mins
Servings: 4

Cook time: 20 mins

Ingredients:

- 0.66 lbs. zucchini
- One carrot
- 0.44 lbs. tomatoes
- 0.44 lbs. tofu
- 0.4 cup water
- Four tsp. soy milk
- One tsp. black pepper
- One tsp. chilli pepper
- One tsp. cilantro
- One tsp. oregano
- One yellow onion

Directions: Remove the skin from the tomatoes.

Take a bowl of hot water and put the tomatoes in it for 1 minute. Then remove the tomatoes from the water and peel them. Slice the tomatoes. Chop the tofu cheese. Peel the carrot and slice it. Peel the onion and chop it very coarsely. Slice the zucchini with the help of a manual slicer.

Preheat the fryer to 380 degrees F.

Take the large bowl and make the lasagna. Put the sliced zucchini on the bottom of the container, and then add the tofu cut little. Then put the layer of tomatoes. Add the chopped onion. Then cover the mixture again with the tofu.

Sprinkle the lasagna with oregano, cilantro, chili and black pepper.

Transfer to the air fryer and bake for 15 mins.

Nutrition: Cal 79 Protein 6.2 g Fat 2.5 g Carbs 10.4 g

640. Onion Pie

Prep time: 10 mins
Servings: 4

Cook time: 35 mins

Ingredients:

- 0.33 lbs. flour
- 0.2 cup almond milk
- One tsp. salt
- 0.2 cup water
- 0.66 lbs. onion
- One tsp. olive oil

- *0.22 lbs. tofu*
- *0.2 cup soy milk*

- *Four tomatoes*

Directions: Peel the onion and then chop it into small pieces. Transfer the chopped onion to the large bowl and sprinkle with salt. Next, shred the tofu cheese and add it to the mixing bowl.

Gently stir until you have a smooth mass. Take small tomatoes for this dish and cut them into two parts. Then leave the mixture with the chopped onion and take another bowl and sift the flour into it. Add the soy milk and the almond milk. Take the hand mixer and mix the mass very carefully.

Preheat the air fryer and set it to 390 F temperature.

Meanwhile, take the cake pan and spray it with olive oil. Work the dough very carefully.

Then place it on the tray and make it flat. Transfer the onion mixture to the dough and add the tomato halves. Take another container and pour water into it.

Transfer the container with water to the air fryer and put the tray with the pie in it.

Set the temperature to 360 F and bake the cake for 20 mins.

Nutrition: Cal 252 Protein 8.5 g Fat 6.1 g Carbs 42.3 g

641. Vegetables Pizza

Prep time: 10 mins
Servings: 4

Cook time: 20 mins

Ingredients:
- *0.44 lbs. flour*
- *0.4 cup water*
- *One tsp. dried yeast*
- *One tsp. sugar*
- *Three tomatoes*

- *0.22 lbs. black olives*
- *One yellow zucchini*
- *0.44 lbs. tofu*
- *0.22 lbs. spinach*
- *Two tsp. dill*

- *Two tsp. parsley*
- *One tsp. tomato paste*
- *One sweet red pepper*
- *One onion*

Directions: First prepare the pizza dough: take the large bowl and combine the warm water with the dry yeast. Mix carefully until the yeast is dissolved. Then sprinkle the mass with the sugar and mix again. Sift the flour and add half of it to the mixture and mix gently. Cover the mass with a towel and leave it in a warm place.

Meanwhile, slice the black olives and shred the tofu cheese. Slice the tomatoes and chop the red bell bell pepper. Then peel the onion and cut it into small pieces. Chop the parsley and dill and combine them in the bowl. Slice the zucchini.

Preheat the air fryer and set to 390 F.

Remove the towel from the dough and gently stir again. Add the other half of the dough and knead it. Then make the circle flat and transfer it to the tray.

Place the tofu cheese on the bottom of the dough. Add the sliced zucchini and onion. Then place the red bell bell pepper and tomatoes.

Sprinkle the pizza with a mixture of chopped parsley and dill.

Transfer the pizza to the air fryer and cook for 18 mins.

Nutrition: Cal 305 Protein 12.7 g Fat 5.8 g Carbs 53 g

642. Vegetable Stew

Prep time: 10 mins
Servings: 4

Cook time: 30 mins

Ingredients:
- *0.66 lbs. tomatoes*
- *0.44 lbs. zucchini*
- *One onion*
- *Two sweet green peppers*

- *One sweet yellow pepper*
- *0.22 lbs. tomato paste*
- *0.4 cup almond milk*
- *One tsp. cilantro*

- *One tsp. chilli pepper*
- *0.22 lbs. leek*
- *0.22 lbs. lentils*
- *1.2 cup vegetables stock*

Directions: Cut the tomatoes into small pieces. Then slice the zucchini and cut it into two parts again.

Remove the seeds from the bell bell pepper and cut it into strips. Cut each strip into two more parts. Chop the leek.

Take the large bowl and combine all the ingredients in it. Stir gently. Then add the lentils and sprinkle the mass with the cilantro, chili and tomato paste. Stir carefully and let stand.

Preheat the air fryer set to 390 degrees F.

Meanwhile, peel the onion and coarsely chop it. Combine the vegetable broth with the almond milk and stir.

Pour the liquid into the air fryer and add the vegetable mass. Stir gently with the help of the wooden spoon. Cook for 20 mins. The lentils should absorb all the water. Then remove the stew, cool it a bit and serve immediately.

Nutrition: Cal 247 Protein 11.2 g Fat 7.1 g Carbs 38 g

643. Spinach Dish

Prep time: 10 mins   **Servings: 4**

Ingredients:
- 0.44 lbs. oatmeal flour
- 0.6 cup water
- ½ tsp. baking soda
- 0.44 lbs. spinach
- 0.22 lbs. oatmeal
- One onion
- One tsp. olive oil
- One tsp. oregano
- One tsp. dill

Directions: Take the bowl put oatmeal flour in it together. Add dill and oregano. Stir it. Take the bowl and pour warm water into it. Add baking soda and stir it till baking soda is dissolved.
Combine oatmeal flour with liquid and knead the dough. Put it in the fridge. Meanwhile, chop the spinach and combine it with oatmeal. Take the tray and spray it with olive oil.
Then take the dough and grate dough on it. Add spinach mass and stir it with the help of hands very gently.
Preheat the air fryer and set at 360 degrees F and transfer the tray with the mixture in it.
Cook it for 15 mins.

Nutrition: Cal 319 Protein 11.7 g Fat 6.3 g Carbs 55.6 g

644. Vegetable Burger

Prep time: 10 mins   **Cook time: 15 mins**
Servings: 4

Ingredients:
- 1/2-pound cauliflower, steamed and diced, rinsed and drained
- Two tsp. coconut oil, melted
- Two tsp. minced garlic
- ¼ cup desiccated coconut
- ½ cup oats
- Three tbsp. flour
- One tbsp. flaxseeds plus three tbsp. water divided
- One tsp. thyme
- Two tsp. parsley
- Two tsp. chives
- Salt and ground black pepper, to taste
- 1 cup bread crumbs

Directions: Preheat and set temperature to 390 degrees F.
Combine cauliflower with all ingredients, except breadcrumbs, incorporating everything well.
Shape eight equal amounts of the mixture into hamburger patties. Coat the patties in the breadcrumbs before placing them in the basket of the air fryer in a single layer.
Place the air fryer basket on the baking sheet. Select Air Fryer and set the time to 12 mins.

Nutrition: Cal: 117 Protein: 4.97 g Fat: 3.65 g Carbs: 21.58 g

645. Potatoes with Zucchini

Prep time: 20 mins   **Cook time: 20 mins**
Servings: 4

Ingredients:
- Two large-sized sweet potatoes, peeled and quartered
- One medium zucchini, sliced
- 1 Serrano pepper, deseeded and thinly sliced
- One bell pepper, deseeded and thinly sliced
- 2 carrots cut into matchsticks
- ¼ cup olive oil
- 1 ½ tbsp. maple syrup
- ½ tsp. porcini powder
- ½ tsp. fennel seeds
- One tbsp. garlic powder
- ½ tsp. fine sea salt
- ¼ tsp. ground black pepper
- Tomato ketchup, for serving

Directions: Preheat the air fryer oven set at 350° F.
Put the sweet potatoes, zucchini, peppers, and carrot into the air fryer basket. Coat with a drizzling of olive oil

Place the air fryer basket on the baking pan and move into rack position2, pick the air fryer and set the time for 15 mins.
In the meantime, prepare the sauce by vigorously combining the other ingredients, except for tomato ketchup, with a whisk
Lightly grease a baking dish
Transfer the cooked vegetable to the baking dish, pour over the sauce and coat the vegetable well
Set the temperature at 390° F and air fry the vegetable for an additional 5 mins
Serve warm with a side of ketchup

Nutrition: Cal: 247 Protein: 3.05 g Fat: 13.84 g Carbs: 29.74 g

646. Ratatouille

Prep time: 20 mins   **Cook time: 25 mins**
Servings: 4

Ingredients:
- One sprig basil
- One sprig flat-leaf parsley
- One sprig mint
- One tbsp. coriander powder
- One tsp. capers
- ½ lemon, juiced
- Salt and ground black pepper, to taste
- Two eggplants sliced crosswise
- Two red onions, chopped
- Four cloves garlic, minced
- Two red peppers sliced crosswise
- One fennel bulb cut crosswise
- Three large zucchinis sliced crosswise
- Five tbsp. olive oil
- Four large tomatoes, chopped
- Two tsp. herbs de Provence

Directions: Blend the cilantro, mint, basil, parsley, lemon juice and capers with a little salt and pepper. Make sure all ingredients are well incorporated.
Preheat and set the temperature to 400 degrees F.
Coat the eggplant, bell pepper, onion, garlic, fennel and zucchini with olive oil.
Transfer the vegetables to the baking dish and top with the tomatoes and herb puree. Sprinkle with more salt and pepper and the Herbes de Provence.
Place the baking dish, cook and set the time to 26 mins.

Nutrition: Cal: 358 Protein: 6.99 g Fat: 19.36 g Carbs: 45.8 g

647. Potato and Broccoli with Tofu Scramble

Prep time: 15 mins   **Cook time: 30 mins**
Servings: 3

Ingredients:
- 2 ½ cups chopped red potato
- Two tbsp. olive oil, divided
- One block tofu, chopped finely
- Two tbsp. tamari
- One tsp. turmeric powder
- ½ tsp. garlic powder
- ½ cup chopped onion
- 4 cups broccoli florets

Directions: Preheat and set temperature to 400 degrees F.
Mix the potatoes and a tablespoon of olive oil, then transfer to a baking pan.
Select the Bake mode and set the time to 15 mins. Stir the potatoes once during baking.
Combine the tofu, remaining tablespoon of olive oil, turmeric, onion powder, tamari and garlic powder, stirring in the onions, followed by the broccoli.
Top the potatoes with the tofu mixture and bake for another 15 mins.

Nutrition: Cal: 220 Protein: 11.88 g Fat: 11.41 g Carbs: 20.77 g

648. Summer Rolls

Prep time: 15 mins   **Cook time: 15 mins**
Servings: 4

Ingredients:
- 1 cup shiitake mushroom, sliced thinly
- One celery stalk, chopped
- One medium carrot, shredded
- ½ tsp. finely chopped ginger
- One tsp. soy sauce
- One tsp. nutritional yeast

- *Eight spring roll sheets*
- *One tsp. corn water*
- *Two tbsp. water*

Directions: Preheat and set the temperature at 400 degrees F.
In a bowl, combine the ginger, soy sauce, carrots, celery, nutritional yeast, mushroom, and sugar.
Mix the cornstarch and water to create an adhesive for the spring rolls.
Scoop a tbsp. full of the vegetable mixture into the middle of the spring roll sheets. Brush the edges of the sheets with the cornstarch adhesive and enclose around the filling to make spring rolls. Arrange the rolls in the air fryer basket.
Place the air fryer basket on the baking pan; choose Air Fry and set the time to 15 mins.

Nutrition: Cal: 250 Protein: 8.99 g Fat: 3.47 g Carbs: 45.4 g

649. Veg Rolls

Prep time: 20 mins
Servings: 6

Cook time: 10 mins

Ingredients:
- *Two potatoes, mashed*
- *¼ cup peas*
- *½ cup mashed carrots*
- *One small cabbage, sliced*
- *¼ cups beans*
- *Two tbsp. sweet corn*
- *One small onion, chopped*
- *½ cup bread crumbs*
- *One packet spring roll sheets*
- *½ cup cornstarch slurry*

Directions: Preheat and set temperature to 390 degrees F
Boil all vegetables in water over low heat. Rinse and allow to dry
Unroll spring roll sheets and pour an equal amount of vegetables in the center of each. Fold into spring instruments and coat each with the slurry and bread crumbs. Transfer to the basket of the air fryer.
Place air fryer basket on baking sheet; choose Air Fry and set time to 10 mins

Nutrition: Cal: 202 Protein: 5.1 g Fat: 0.69 g Carbs: 45.4 g

650. Potatoes with Tofu

Prep time: 15 mins
Servings: 8

Cook time: 35 mins

Ingredients:
- *Eight sweet potatoes, scrubbed*
- *Two tbsp. olive oil*
- *One large onion, chopped*
- *Two green chillies, deseeded and chopped*
- *8 ounces (227 g) tofu, crumbled*
- *Two tbsp. Cajun seasoning*
- *1 cup chopped tomatoes*
- *One can of kidney beans, must drained and rinsed*
- *Salt and ground black pepper, to taste*

Directions: Preheat and set temperature to 400 F.
Using a knife, pierce the skin of the sweet potatoes and transfer them to the basket of the air fryer.
Place the air fryer basket on the baking sheet and slide into the Rack 2 position. Select the air fryer and set the time to 30 mins, or until soft.
Remove from oven, halve each potato and set aside.
Over medium heat, sauté onions and chilies in olive oil in a skillet for 2 mins until fragrant.
Add the tofu and Cajun seasoning and sauté for another 3 mins before incorporating the beans and tomatoes. Sprinkle with salt and pepper to taste.
Top each sweet potato half with a spoonful of the tofu mixture.

Nutrition: Cal: 127 Protein: 5.45 g Fat: 9.16 g Carbs: 7.22 g

651. Rice and Eggplant

Prep time: 15 mins
Servings: 4

Cook time: 10 mins

Ingredients

- One tbsp. mirin rice wine
- Three medium eggplants, sliced
- ¼ cup sliced cucumber
- One tbsp. sugar
- Seven tbsp. Japanese rice vinegar
- Three tbsp. sweet white miso paste
- 4 cups cooked sushi rice
- Four spring onions
- One tbsp. toasted sesame seeds
- One tsp. salt

Directions: Coat cucumber slices with rice wine vinegar, salt and sugar.
Place a plate over the bowl to weigh it down completely.
In a bowl, mix the eggplant, mirin rice wine and miso paste. Allow to marinate for half an hour
Preheat and set temperature to 400 F.
Slice eggplant and place in air fryer basket.
Place the air fryer basket on the baking sheet, select the air fryer and set the time to 10 mins.
Fill the bottom of a bowl with the rice and add the eggplant and pickled cucumbers.
Add the spring onions and sesame seeds for garnish.

Nutrition: Cal: 516 Protein: 20.82 g Fat: 26.8 g Carbs: 88.5 g

652. Mushroom and Pepper Pizza Squares

Prep time: 10 mins
Servings: 10

Cook time: 10 mins

Ingredients:

- One pizza dough, cut into squares
- 1 cup chopped oyster mushrooms
- One shallot, chopped
- ¼ red bell pepper, chopped
- Two tbsp. parsley
- Salt and ground black pepper

Directions: Preheat and set the temperature at 400 F.
In a bowl, combine the oyster mushrooms, shallot, bell pepper and parsley. Sprinkle some salt and pepper as desired
Spread the mixture on top of the pizza squares, and then transfer to a baking pan.
Slide the baking pan, select bake and set time to 10 mins.

Nutrition: Cal: 161 Protein: 7.8 g Fat: 5.28 g Carbs: 20.85 g

653. Green Beans with Shallot

Prep time: 10 mins
Servings: 4

Cook time: 10 mins

Ingredients:

- 1 ½ pound French green beans, stems removed and blanched
- One tbsp. salt
- ½ pound shallots, peeled and cut into quatres
- ½ tsp. ground white pepper
- Two tbsp. olive oil

Directions: Preheat and set the temperature at 400 F.
Coat the vegetables with the rest of the ingredients in a bowl. Transfer to the air fryer basket.
Place the air fryer basket onto baking pan, select air fry and set time 10 mins.

Nutrition: Cal: 166 Protein: 3.91 g Fat: 7.16 g Carbs: 22.4 g

654. Herbed Chips

Prep time: 5 mins
Servings: 4

Cook time: 6 mins

Ingredients:

- Two whole 6-inch pitas, whole grain or white cook spray
- ¼ tsp. dried basil
- ¼ tsp. marjoram
- ¼ tsp. ground oregano
- ¼ tsp. garlic powder
- ¼ tsp. ground thyme
- ¼ tsp. salt

Directions: Preheat and set temperature to 330 degrees F.
Mix all toppings together.
Cut each pita half into four wedges; break wedges at crease.
Drizzle one side of pita wedges with oil. Sprinkle with half of the seasoning mixture.
Turn pita wedges over, spray other side with oil and sprinkle with remaining seasoning. Place pita wedges in baking dish.
Select the bake mode and set the time to 4 mins. Shake the baking sheet halfway through the cook time.

Nutrition: Cal: 485 Protein: 17.9 g Fat: 4.74 g Carbs: 100.36 g

655. Lemony Pear Chips

Prep time: 15 mins
Servings: 4

Cook time: 12 mins

Ingredients:

- Two firm bosc pears, cut crosswise into 1/8-inch-thick slices
- One tbsp. freshly squeezed lemon juice
- ½ tsp. ground cinnamon
- 1/8 tsp. ground cardamom

Directions: Preheat and set temperature to 380 degrees F.
Separate smaller pear slices with stems from large pear slices with seeds. Remove core and seeds from large slices. Sprinkle all slices with lemon juice, cinnamon and cardamom.
Place the smaller slices in the basket of the air fryer.
Place the air fryer basket on the baking sheet; select the air fry and set the time to 5 mins. Shake the basket once during cook. Remove from oven.
Repeat with larger slices, air frying for 6 to 8 mins, or until lightly browned, shaking the basket once during cook
Remove chips from oven, cool and serve or store in an airtight container at room temperature for up to two days

Nutrition: Cal: 62 Protein: 0.36 g Fat: 0.1 g Carbs: 14.99 g

656. Fishless Tacos With Chipotle Cream

Prep time: 10 mins
Servings: 4

Cook time: 20 mins

Ingredients:

For the tacos:
- 6 Gardein fishless filets
- Six soft corn tortillas
- 1 ½ cups chopped green leaf lettuce
- 3 Tbsp. chopped onions
- Two avocados, pit removed and sliced
- Cilantro, chopped (garnish)
- One lime, sliced

For the chipotle cream:
- ½ cup + 1 Tbsp. raw cashews
- ¾ cup of water (plus extra for soaking, if not using a high-speed blender)
- Two chipotle peppers in adobo sauce (from 7 oz. can)
- One tsp. adobo sauce from a can
- One tsp. agave syrup
- ½ tsp. lemon juice
- 1/8 tsp. salt

Directions:

To make the tacos:

Cook Gardein fishless fillets without package directions.

In a prepared skillet, heat the corn tortillas one at a time for about 1 minute on each side over medium heat. If each tortilla has been heated on both sides, move it to a plate and then cover with a clean dish towel.

Once the tenderloins are fully cooked, remove them from the oven and cut them into four bias pieces. Place a sliced fillet in each tortilla and stuff with green leaf lettuce, onions, sliced avocado and a sprinkle of cilantro. Drizzle each taco with the chipotle cream and serve with lime wedges.

To make the chipotle cream:

Soak cashews in water for several hours and then drain.

Place the cashews, ¾ cup water, chipotle peppers, adobo sauce, agave syrup, and lemon juice in a blender. Blend until smooth. For 24 hours, it will be the best.

Nutrition: Cal: 465 Protein: 8.64 g Fat: 33.6 g Carbs: 39.9 g

657. Thai-Style Crab Cakes

Prep time: 10 mins
Servings: 4

Cook time: 15 mins

Ingredients:

- 4 cups diced or about four medium potatoes
- 1 bunch green onions
- One lime, zest & juice
- 1½ inch knob of fresh ginger
- One tbsp. Tamari, or soy sauce
- Four tbsp. Thai Red Curry Paste
- Four sheets nori
- 1 can heart of palm
- ¾ cup canned artichoke hearts
- pepper
- salt
- Two tbsp. oil for pan-frying

Directions: Potatoes are peeled and diced, then added to a pan. Cover with water and simmer, then rinse, mash and set aside. When the potatoes are simmering, add a food processor with the green onions, lime juice, lime zest, ginger, tamari and curry paste. Break the nori sheets into manageable pieces and place them with the other ingredients in the food processor. Process until a paste is obtained. The nori seems to stay a little more shredded than everything else, which is fine.

Drain the hearts of palm and grate or shred them with a fork, then drain the artichokes and coarsely chop them.

When the potatoes are cool enough to handle, add the dough and mix well so it is evenly distributed, then add the shredded hearts of palm and chopped artichokes and mix gently. Form into patties and place them as you go on a tray with baking paper. You can cook them in a pan, in the oven or on a griddle. Since they develop a nice golden crust, it is best to pan fry them.

For pan frying: Heat a couple of tablespoons of oil in a skillet over medium-high heat. Once very hot, carefully add the crab cakes. To allow a thick, golden crust to develop, leave them for about 4 mins, then flip them over and do the same on the other side. To soak up the excess oil, remove them from the pan and place them on some paper towels.

For grilling: Heat your griddle over medium-high heat. When hot, place the crab cakes on the griddle and cook for 4-5 mins on each side.

To bake: Place on a tray on baking paper and bake at 400°F for about 25 mins. Turn halfway through baking.

Nutrition: Cal: 477 Protein: 11.6 g Fat: 8.6 g Carbs: 94.2 g

658. Vegan Spring Rolls

Prep time: 10 mins
Servings: 4

Cook time: 15 mins

Ingredients

- Four cloves of garlic
- One onion
- Two carrots
- Four leaves of cabbage
- ounce or 30 grams soy sprouts
- Two tbsp. tamari or soy sauce
- Eight sheets spring roll pastry
- Extra virgin olive oil
- Water
- Sweet and sour sauce

Directions: In a wok, heat extra virgin olive oil (1 tablespoon is enough), add vegetables (garlic, julienne, carrots, cabbage and soy. sprouts) and tamari sauce. Cook over medium-high heat for about 5 mins.

Simply arrange the wrap like a diamond, place two tablespoons of filling near one corner, roll the wrap tightly, fold over the left side, fold over the right side, paint a little water along the edge and close.

In the wok, heat lots of extra virgin olive oil, and when it's red-hot, add the spring rolls and cook for about 1 minute or until golden brown on both sides.

Nutrition: Cal: 285 Protein: 9.66 g Fat: 4.72 g Carbs: 50.6 g

659. Popcorn (Vegan)

Prep time: 10 mins
Servings: 4

Cook time: 15 mins

Ingredients:
- 2 cups dried soy chunks
- 3 cups vegetable broth
- Two cloves of garlic, mashed
- 1 tsp. salt
- 1-inch cube of ginger, grated
- ½ cup flour
- ½ cup cornstarch
- 1 cup bread crumbs
- 1 tbsp. garlic powder
- 1 tbsp. lemon pepper

For the dip:
- 1 tbsp. chopped fresh dill
- 1/3 Cup sour cream
- dash of salt and pepper

Directions: Combine the soy chunks, ginger, crushed garlic, 1 teaspoon salt and fill the bowl with vegetable broth in a large bowl until the soy chunks are coated. Let soak until the chunks are soft, or about 20 mins.
Heat a saucepan with 1 inch of oil over medium-high heat.
Mix ½ cup flour and ¾ cup vegetable broth from the soaked soy pieces and whisk until no lumps remain - divide between two bowls.
Gently squeeze excess liquid from soy pieces and coat in one of the bowls of the flour mixture until pieces are soft and soaked.
Use 1/2 cup cornstarch to move the pieces to a Ziploc bag. Shake until coated, then move to the second bowl of flour mixture, cover, and then place the garlic powder, bread crumbs, lemon pepper, and salt in another ziploc container.
In batches, fry the pieces in the oil until golden brown. To fry both sides, you may need to move them around because they seem to like to float in one direction. Remove and drain on a sheet of paper towels.
In a food processor, blend the dill, sour cream, salt and pepper to make the sauce.
Serve the fried pieces with the sauce.

Nutrition: Cal: 1676 Protein: 15.79 g Fat: 16.67 g Carbs: 45.24 g

660. Stuffed Eggplant

Prep time: 8 mins
Servings: 4

Cook time: 12 mins

Ingredients:

For the eggplant:
- Eight eggplants rinsed and patted dry
- 2 tsp. olive oil
- For the spice stuffing:
- 1 tsp. Ground cumin
- ¾ tbsp. Coriander powder
- ¾ tbsp. Dry mango powder
- ½ tsp. Ground turmeric
- ½ tsp. Kashmiri red chilli powder
- ½ tsp. garlic powder
- 1 tsp. salt

To Garnish:
- tbsp. cilantro leaves to garnish

Directions: In a bowl, mix all the spices for the filling.
Take the eggplant and leave the stems intact. Cut down the center from the bottom to just above the branch, being careful not to split the eggplant into two pieces.
Now turn the eggplant 90 degrees and add another cut from the center. The eggplant should be in 4 but still held together by the stem.
Mix a tablespoon of oil with the spices, and with a small spoon, fill the spice paste into each slit of the eggplant.
In the air fryer, place the eggplant in a single layer and brush the oil over each eggplant, making sure both sides are coated. Air fry at 360 degrees F for 8-12 mins.
The color will change when they are cooked through. At 8 mins, check the eggplant and cook for additional time if needed.
Garnish with the cilantro.

Nutrition: Cal: 106 Carbs 20 g Protein 3 g Fat 3 g

661. Potato Air Fried Hash Browns

Prep time: 10 mins
Servings: 4

Cook time: 20 mins

Ingredients:
- Four potatoes, peeled
- Two garlic cloves, minced
- 1 tsp. smoked paprika
- 1 tsp. ground cinnamon
- 2 tsp. olive oil
- Salt and pepper

Directions: Grate the potatoes using the larger side of a cheese grater.
Place the potatoes in a bowl of cold water and soak them for 20-25 mins. Soaking the potatoes in cold water will help remove the starch from the potatoes, which will make them crispier.
Drain the potatoes.
Place the potatoes in a dry bowl and then add the olive oil, paprika, garlic, salt and pepper. Stir to combine.
Add the potatoes to the air fryer and cook at 400 degrees F for 10 mins.
Shake the potatoes at this stage and then bake for another 10 mins.

662. Kale Salad Sushi Rolls

Prep time: 70 mins
Servings: 3

Cook time: 10 mins

Ingredients:
- One batch Pressure Cooker sushi rice cooled to room temperature
- ½ a Haas avocado, sliced
- Three sheets of sushi nori
- 1½ cups chopped kale, de-stemmed
- ¾ tsp. soy sauce
- ¾ tsp. toasted sesame oil
- ½ tsp. rice vinegar
- ¼ tsp. ground ginger
- 1/8 tsp. garlic powder
- 1 tbsp. sesame seeds
- ½ cup panko breadcrumbs
- ¼ cup of mayonnaise
- Sriracha sauce

Directions:

To make the cabbage salad: In a large prepared bowl, combine the cabbage, sesame oil, vinegar, garlic powder, ginger and soy sauce. Massage the cabbage until bright green and slightly wilted, then stir in the sesame seeds. Set aside.

To make the Sushi Rolls: Spread a sheet of nori on a clean, dry surface.
With slightly damp fingertips, take a handful of sushi rice and spread it over the nori. Try to get a thin layer of rice to cover almost all of the nori sheet.
Along one edge, leave about ½ inch of bare seaweed; this is the flap that will seal the sushi roll.
On the other end of the seaweed, place 2 - 3 tablespoons of coleslaw and top with a couple of avocado slices.
Starting with the filling, roll up the sushi roll, pressing gently to make a tight roll.
At the end, use the bare part of the seaweed to seal the roll.
If necessary, wet your fingertips and moisten that piece of seaweed to make it stick.
Repeat the above steps to make three more sushi rolls.

To make Sriracha Mayo: In a small bowl, whisk together the mayo with the Sriracha.
Start by adding one teaspoon of Sriracha, and keep adding more, half a teaspoon at a time, until you reach the desired level of spice.

For frying and slicing: Pour the breadcrumbs into a shallow bowl.
Take the first sushi roll and toss it evenly in the Sriracha mayo and then in the breadcrumbs. Repeat for all of the sushi rolls.
Place the rolls in the basket of the air fryer and cook at 390 degrees F for 10 mins, shaking gently after 5 mins so they cook evenly.
When the rolls are cool, take a sharp knife and gently slice them into 6-8 pieces.
Serve with soy sauce for dipping.

Nutrition: Cal: 154 Protein: 2.88 g Fat: 14.36 g Carbs: 5.04 g

663. Jackfruit Taquitos

Prep time: 10 mins
Servings: 4

Cook time: 20 mins

Ingredients:

- *Four 6-inch corn or whole wheat tortillas*
- *1 cup of cooked or canned red kidney beans, drained and rinsed*
- *1 14-oz. can water-packed jackfruit, drained and rinsed*
- *¼ cup of water*
- *½ cup Pico de Gallo sauce*
- *Canola oil cook spray*

Directions: In a saucepan, combine the beans, Pico de Gallo, jackfruit, and water.
Heat the mixture over medium-high heat until it begins to boil.
If cook on the stove, reduce heat, cover and simmer for 20 to 25 mins.
If using a pressure cooker, cover to bring to pressure, cook at low pressure for 3 mins, and then do a natural release.
Mash the cooked jackfruit with a potato masher to break it up into a meaty consistency.
Preheat the air fryer to a temperature of 370 degrees F for 3 mins.
Place a tortilla on a clean, dry work surface and spoon 1/4 cup of the jackfruit mixture onto the tortilla.
Roll tightly, putting back any mixture that falls into the tortilla.
Repeat this process to make four taquitos total.
Coat the fryer basket with cook oil spray. Spray the top of the tortillas as well.
Place the rolled tortillas in the fryer basket and cook for 8 mins.

Nutrition: Cal: 895 Protein: 26.8 g Fat: 26.6 g Carbs: 140.4 g

664. Ginger Tofu Sushi Bowl

Prep time: 10 mins
Servings: 4

Cook time: 40 mins

Ingredients:

- *2-inch piece of fresh ginger*
- *One clove garlic*
- *2 tbsp. real maple syrup*
- *1 tbsp. toasted sesame oil*
- *2 tbsp. soy sauce*
- *1 tsp. rice vinegar*
- *1 tbsp. cornstarch*
- *One block extra firm tofu pressed and cut into 1-inch pieces*

For the Sushi Bowls:

- *One batch Pressure Cooker sushi rice or 3 cups of cooked rice.*
- *One green onion, sliced*
- *¾ cup cucumber sliced into ¼-inch thick half-moons*
- *½ cup carrot sticks*
- *1 Haas avocado, sliced*
- *One 0.16-oz packet roast seaweed snacks cut into thirds*
- *½ cup roasted cashews*
- *¼ cup pickled ginger*

Directions:

To make the tofu: To make the marinade, combine the garlic, ginger, maple syrup, soy sauce, sesame oil and vinegar in a blender or food processor. Puree on high speed until smooth.
In a deep bowl, mix the tofu with the marinade. Set aside and let marinate for 10 mins, then drain off excess marinade.
In the same bowl, mix the marinated tofu with the cornstarch. Pour into the basket of the air fryer and cook at 370 degrees F for 15 mins. After 8 mins of cook, shake to make sure it cooks evenly.

To make the sushi bowls: Divide sushi rice between two bowls.
Add tofu, green onion, avocado, cucumber, carrot, seaweed pieces and pickled ginger.
Sprinkle with cashews and garnish with sliced green onion.

Nutrition: Cal: 597 Protein: 21.45 g Fat: 43.2 g Carbs: 47.6 g

665. Spicy Cauliflower

Prep time: 5 mins
Servings: 4

Cook time: 25 mins

Ingredients:

- *One head cauliflower, cut into florets*
- *Five cloves garlic, finely sliced*
- *¾ cup Spanish onion, thinly sliced*

- 1½ tbsp. tamari
- 1 tbsp. Sriracha

- 1 tbsp. rice vinegar
- ½ tsp. coconut sugar

- Two scallions, sliced

Directions: Preheat the air fryer at temperature of 350 degrees F, place the cauliflower, and cook for 10 mins.

Open the air fryer, remove and shake the insert and slide back into the compartment.

Add the sliced white onion, stir and cook for a further 10 mins.

Attach the garlic, then stir and cook for an additional five mins.

In a small bowl, mix the rice vinegar, soy sauce, coconut sugar, Sriracha hot sauce, salt and pepper.

Add the mixture to the cauliflower in the air fryer and stir—Cook for a further 5 mins. The insert will keep all of the juices inside.

Transfer to a serving bowl and then sprinkle the sliced scallions over the top to garnish.

Nutrition: Cal: 93 Carbs 12 g Fat 3 g Protein 4 g

666. Italian Eggplant Parmesan

Prep time: 10 mins
Servings: 6

Cook time: 20 mins

Ingredients:
- One large eggplant, sliced and de-stemmed
- ½ cup almond milk
- ½ cup flour

- 2 tbsp. Parmesan, grated
- ½ cup bread crumbs
- Garlic powder
- Onion powder

- Salt and pepper

For the Topping:
- 1 cup of Marinara sauce, plus more for serving

- Parmesan, grated
- ½ cup Mozzarella Shreds

To Serve:
- 4 oz. spaghetti, cooked al dente

- Parmesan, grated

- Italian parsley, chopped

Directions: Wash, dry, and stem the eggplant and slice lengthwise.

Season the breadcrumbs with Parmesan cheese, garlic powder, onion powder, salt and pepper.

Dip the sliced eggplant into the flour, then into the almond milk and finally into the seasoned breadcrumbs.

Lightly spray eggplant with cook oil spray and place in the basket of air fryer at 390 degrees F for 15 mins. Check the eggplant halfway through cook, turn it over and lightly spray the second side with cook oil spray.

Nutrition: Cal: 146 Protein: 7.2 g Fat: 3.1 g Carbs: 23.7 g

667. Stuffed Potatoes

Prep time: 10 mins
Servings: 4

Cook time: 90 mins

Ingredients:
- Two large Russet baking potatoes
- 1 - 2 tsp. olive oil
- 1 cup spinach or kale, chopped

- 2 tbsp. nutritional yeast
- ¼ cup unsweetened almond milk
- ¼ cup unsweetened vegan yogurt

- ½ tsp. salt
- ¼ tsp. pepper

For Topping:
- Smoked salt and black pepper

- Chopped chives

- ¼ cup unsweetened vegan yogurt

Directions: Rub the skin of each Russet potato with oil on all sides.

Preheat the air fryer to 390 degrees F unless the brand calls for it.

Once it is hot, add the potatoes to the basket of the air fryer.

Cook the potatoes for 30 mins, and when the time is up, flip the potatoes and cook for another 30 mins. Set them aside to cool.

Cut each potato in half lengthwise and then scoop out the flesh, leaving enough to create a firm shell of potato skin.

Mash the potato flesh, almond milk, vegan yogurt, nutritional yeast, pepper and salt until smooth.

Then mix in the chopped spinach and fill the potato shells.

Bake the stuffed potatoes again at 350 degrees F for 5 mins.

Serve with the topping.

Nutrition: Cal: 211 Protein: 7.64 g Fat: 3.2 g Carbs: 38.7 g

668. Turmeric Cauliflower Steaks

Prep time: 10 mins
Servings: 2

Cook time: 15 mins

Ingredients:

- 1-2 medium heads cauliflower, stems intact
- 2 tbsp. coconut oil
- 1 tsp. ground turmeric
- ¼ tsp. ground ginger
- 1/8 tsp. ground cumin
- 1/8 tsp. salt
- A pinch of black pepper
- Mixed steamed greens
- Tahini
- White Sesame Seeds

Directions: Cut the head off the cauliflower in the middle, leaving the stem intact. Cut off the green leaves.
On either side of the middle, cut 1-inch steaks being careful not to make them too thin. Reserve the fallen florets for later use.
Coat the steaks with coconut oil and rub the spices into all the crevices and interstices of the cauliflower.
Bake at 390 degrees F for about 15 mins, flipping the steaks halfway through cook.
Serve the mixed vegetables on a bed, sprinkled with tahini. Garnish with white sesame seeds.

Nutrition: Cal: 185 Protein: 4.46 g Fat: 14.2 g Carbs: 13.2 g

669. Garlic Beans

Prep time: 5 mins
Servings: 4

Cook time: 6 mins

Ingredients:

- 1 pound green beans, trimmed
- Two tbsp. olive oil
- Three garlic cloves, minced
- Salt and black pepper
- One tbsp. balsamic vinegar

Directions: Place all the ingredients in a prepared bowl, except the vinegar, and mix well.
Put the beans in your air fryer and cook at 400 degrees F for 6 mins.
Divide the green beans between plates and drizzle the vinegar all over.

Nutrition: Cal 101 Fat 3 g Carbs 4 g Protein 2 g

670. Oregano Eggplants

Prep time: 5 mins
Servings: 4

Cook time: 15 mins

Ingredients:

- Four eggplants, roughly cubed
- Two tbsp. lime juice
- Salt and black pepper to taste
- One tsp. oregano, dried
- Two tbsp. olive oil

Directions: Place all ingredients in a pan and toss well.
Put the pan into the fryer and cook at 400 degrees F for 15 mins.

Nutrition: Cal 125 Fat 5 g Carbs 11 g Protein 5 g

671. Garlic Parsnips

Prep time: 5 mins
Servings: 4

Cook time: 15 mins

Ingredients:

- 1 pound parsnips, cut into chunks
- One tbsp. olive oil
- Six garlic cloves, minced
- One tbsp. balsamic vinegar
- Salt and black pepper

Directions: In a bowl, add all ingredients and combine well.
Place them in the air fryer and cook at 380 degrees F for 15 mins.

Nutrition: Cal 121 Fat 3 g Carbs 12 g Protein 6 g

672. Pomegranate and Florets

Prep time: 5 mins
Servings: 4

Cook time: 7 mins

Ingredients:
- One broccoli head, florets separated
- One pomegranate, seeds separated
- A drizzle of olive oil
- Salt and black pepper

Directions: In a bowl, mix the broccoli with the salt, pepper, and oil.
Put the florets in your air fryer and cook at 400 degrees F for 7 mins.
Sprinkle the pomegranate seeds all over.

Nutrition: Cal 141 Fat 3 g Carbs 11 g Protein 4 g

673. Lime Broccoli

Prep time: 5 mins
Servings: 4

Cook time: 6 mins

Ingredients:
- One broccoli head, florets separated
- One tbsp. lime juice
- Salt and black pepper
- Two tbsp. vegan butter, melted

Directions: In a prepared bowl, mix well all the ingredients.
Put the broccoli mixture in your air fryer and cook at 400 degrees F for 6 mins.

Nutrition: Cal 151 Fat 4 g Carbs 12 g Protein 6 g

674. Green Cayenne Cabbage

Prep time: 5 mins
Servings: 4

Cook time: 12 mins

Ingredients:
- One green cabbage head, shredded
- One tbsp. olive oil
- One tsp. cayenne pepper
- A pinch of salt and black pepper
- Two tsp. sweet paprika

Directions: Mix all the ingredients in a baking pan.
Place the pan in the fryer and cook at 320 degrees F for 12 mins.

Nutrition: Cal 124 Fat 6 g Carbs 16 g Protein 7 g

675. Tomato and Balsamic Greens

Prep time: 5 mins
Servings: 4

Cook time: 12 mins

Ingredients:
- One bunch mustard greens, trimmed
- Two tbsp. olive oil
- ½ cup veggies stock
- Two tbsp. tomato puree
- Three garlic cloves, minced
- Salt and black pepper
- One tbsp. balsamic vinegar

Directions: Combine all ingredients in a pan and toss well.
Place the pan in the fryer and cook at 260 degrees F for 12 mins.

Nutrition: Cal 151 Fat 2 g Carbs 14 g Protein 4 g

676. Lime Endives

Prep time: 5 mins   **Cook time: 10 mins**
Servings: 4

Ingredients:
- *Four endives, trimmed and halved*
- *Salt and black pepper*
- *One tbsp. lime juice*
- *One tbsp. olive oil*

Directions: Put the endives in your air fryer, and add the salt, pepper, lemon juice.
Cook at the 360 degrees F for 10 mins.

Nutrition: Cal 100 Fat 3 g Carbs 8 g Protein 4 g

677. Artichokes with Oregano

Prep time: 10 mins   **Cook time: 7 mins**
Servings: 4

Ingredients:
- *Four big artichokes, trimmed*
- *Salt and black pepper to the taste*
- *Two tbsp. lemon juice*
- *¼ cup extra virgin olive oil*
- *Two tsp. balsamic vinegar*
- *One tsp. oregano, dried*
- *2 garlic cloves, minced*

Directions: Season the artichokes with salt and pepper, fry them with half the oil and half the lemon juice, place them in the air fryer and cook for 7 mins at 360 degrees F.
Meanwhile, in a bowl, mix the rest of the lemon juice with the remaining oil, vinegar, salt, pepper, garlic and oregano and stir very well.
Arrange artichokes on a platter, drizzle the balsamic vinaigrette over them.

Nutrition: Cal 200 Fat 3 g Carbs 12 g Protein 4 g

678. Green Veggies

Prep time: 10 mins   **Cook time: 15 mins**
Servings: 4

Ingredients:
- *1-pint cherry tomatoes*
- *1 pound green beans*
- *Two tbsp. olive oil*
- *Salt and black pepper*

Directions:
In a bowl, mix cherry tomatoes with green beans, olive oil, salt and pepper, toss, transfer to your air fryer and cook at 400 degrees F for 15 mins.

Nutrition: Cal 162 Fat 6g Carbs 8g Protein 9g

679. Flavored Green Beans

Prep time: 10 mins
Servings: 4

Cook time: 15 mins

Ingredients:
- *1 pound red potatoes cut into wedges*
- *1 pound green beans*
- *Two garlic cloves, minced*
- *Two tbsp. olive oil*
- *Salt and black pepper to the taste*
- *½ tsp. oregano, dried*

Directions: In a pan combine potatoes with green beans, garlic, oil, salt, pepper and oregano, toss, introduce in your air fryer and cook at 380 degrees F for 15 mins.

Nutrition: Cal 211 Fat 6 g Carbs 8 g Protein 5 g

680. Herbed Eggplant and Zucchini

Prep time: 5 mins
Servings: 4

Cook time: 13 mins

Ingredients:
- *One eggplant, cubed*
- *Three zucchinis, cubed*
- *2 tbsp. lemon juice*
- *Salt and black pepper*
- *1 tbsp. dried thyme*
- *1 tbsp. dried oregano*
- *3 tbsp. olive oil*

Directions: Get a bowl, put in zucchinis, lemon juice, thyme pepper, salt, olive oil and oregano. Toss, put into the air fryer and cook at 360°F for 8 mins.

Nutrition: Cal: 133 Protein: 1.79 g Fat: 10.47 g Carbs: 10.1 g

681. Okra and Corn Salad

Prep time: 5 mins
Servings: 6

Cook time: 17 mins

Ingredients:
- *1-pound okra*
- *Six scallions*
- *Three green bell peppers,*
- *Salt and black pepper*
- *2 tbsp. olive oil*
- *1 tbsp. sugar*
- *28 oz. canned tomatoes*
- *1 cup of corn*

Directions: Heat oil over medium heat in the pan, put bell peppers and scallion, turn and cook for 5 mins.
Get in okra, pepper, salt, tomatoes, sugar and corn, stir, then put into the air fryer—Cook at 360° F for 7 mins.
Share okra blend on plates.

Nutrition: Cal: 209 Protein: 5.95 g Fat: 6.38 g Carbs: 36.07 g

682. Chard Salad

Prep time: 5 mins
Servings: 4

Cook time: 18 mins

Ingredients:
- *One bunch Swiss chard*
- *2 tbsp. olive oil*
- *One small yellow onion*
- *A pinch of red pepper flakes*
- *¼ cup pine nuts*
- *¼ cup raisins*
- *1 tbsp. balsamic vinegar*
- *Salt and black pepper*

Directions: Heat pan and put olive oil over medium heat, put onions and chard, stir. Cook for 5 mins.
Put pepper flakes, salt, pepper, raisins, vinegar and pine nuts, stir, bring into air fryer—Cook at 350° F for 8 mins.

Nutrition: Cal: 136 Protein: 1.76 g Fat: 12.6 g Carbs: 5.62 g

683. Garlic Tomatoes

Prep time: 5 mins
Servings: 4

Cook time: 20 mins

Ingredients:
- Four garlic cloves
- 1 pound mixed cherry tomatoes
- Three thyme springs
- Salt and black pepper
- ¼ cup olive oil

Directions: Mix in tomatoes with salt, garlic, black pepper, thyme and olive oil in a bowl. Toss to coat, bring into the air fryer. Cook at 360°F for 15 mins.

Nutrition: Cal: 200 Protein: 1.56 g Fat: 13.78 g Carbs: 20.26 g

684. Eggplant and Garlic Sauce

Prep time: 5 mins
Servings: 4

Cook time: 15 mins

Ingredients:
- 2 tbsp. olive oil
- Two garlic cloves
- Three eggplants
- One red chilli pepper
- One green onion stalk
- 1 tbsp. ginger
- 1 tbsp. soy sauce
- 1 tbsp. balsamic vinegar

Directions: Add eggplant slices to heated oil in the pan over medium heat and cook for 2 mins.
Put in garlic, chilli pepper, green onions, soy sauce, ginger and Vinegar. Get into an air fryer and cook at 320° F for 7 mins.

Nutrition: Cal: 186 Protein: 4.71 g Fat: 8.27 g Carbs: 27.84 g

685. Stuffed Peppers

Prep time: 5 mins
Servings: 4

Cook time: 11 mins

Ingredients:
- 12 baby bell peppers
- ¼ tbsp. red pepper flakes
- 6 tbsp. jarred basil pesto
- Salt and black pepper
- 1 tbsp. lemon juice
- 1 tbsp. olive oil
- Handful of parsley

Directions: Mix in the pesto, salt, lemon juice, pepper flakes, black pepper, parsley and oil, beat properly and infuse bell pepper halves with the mix.
Put into the air fryer and then cook at 320° F for 6 mins.

Nutrition: Cal: 188 Protein: 25.6 g Fat: 4.3 g Carbs: 14.5 g

686. Green Beans and Tomatoes

Prep time: 5 mins
Servings: 4

Cook time: 20 mins

Ingredients:
- 1-pint cherry tomatoes
- 1 lb. green beans
- 2 tbsp. Olive oil
- Salt and black pepper

Directions: Mix green beans with cherry potatoes, olive oil, pepper and salt. Toss, put into the air fryer and cook at 400° F for 15 mins.

Nutrition: Cal: 91 Protein: 1.46 g Fat: 7.3 g Carbs: 6.4 g

687. Pumpkin Oatmeal

Prep time: 5 mins
Servings: 4

Cook time: 20 mins

Ingredients:
- *1.5 cups Water*
- *5 cup Pumpkin puree*
- *3 tbsp. Stevia*
- *1 tsp. Pumpkin pie spice*
- *5 cup Steel-cut oats*

Directions: Preheat the Air Fryer at 360° F.
Toss in and mix the fixings into the pan of the Air Fryer.
Set the timer for 20 mins.
When the time has elapsed, portion the oatmeal into bowls.

Nutrition: Cal 211 Protein 3 g Carbs 1 g Fat 4 g

688. Yellow Squash, Zucchini and Carrots

Prep time: 5 mins
Servings: 4

Cook time: 30 mins

Ingredients:
- *Carrots (.5 lb.)*
- *Olive oil (6 tsp. - divided)*
- *Lime (1 sliced into wedges)*
- *Zucchini (1 lb. sliced into .75-inch semi-circles)*
- *Yellow squash (1 lb.)*
- *Tarragon leaves (1 tbsp.)*
- *White pepper (.5 tsp.)*
- *Sea salt (1 tsp.)*

Directions: Set the Air Fryer at 400° F.
Trim the stem and roots from the squash and zucchini.
Dice and add the carrots into a bowl with two teaspoons of oil. Toss the carrots into the fryer basket. Prepare for 5 mins. Mix in the zucchini, oil, salt, and pepper in the bowl.
When the carrots are done, fold in the mixture. Cook 30 mins.
Stir the mixture occasionally. Chop the tarragon and garnish using and lime wedges.

Nutrition: Cal: 256 Protein: 7.4 g Carbs: 8.6 g Fat: 9.4 g

689. Hasselback Potatoes

Prep Time: 10 Mins
Servings: 4

Cook Time: 45 mins

Ingredients:
- *4 potatoes wash and dry*
- *1 tablespoon. dried thyme*
- *1 tablespoon. dried rosemary*
- *1 tablespoon. dried parsley*
- *½ cup butter, melted*
- *Pepper*
- *Salt*

Directions: Place potato in Hassel back slicer and slice potato using a sharp knife.
In a small bowl, mix together thyme, melted butter, rosemary, parsley, pepper, and salt.
Rub melted butter mixture over potatoes and arrange potatoes on air fryer oven.
Bake potatoes at 350 F for 25 mins.

Nutrition: Cal: 356 Fat: 23.4 g Carbs: 34.5 g Protein: 0 g

690. Sriracha Honey Brussels Sprouts

Prep Time: 10 Mins
Servings: 4

Cook Time: 15 mins

Ingredients:
- *½ lb. Brussels sprouts, cut stems then cut each in half*
- *1 tablespoon. olive oil*
- *½ teaspoon salt*

For sauce:

- *1 tablespoon. sriracha sauce*
- *1 tablespoon. vinegar*
- *1 tablespoon. lemon juice*
- *2 teaspoon sugar*
- *1 tablespoon. honey*
- *1 teaspoon garlic, minced*
- *½ teaspoon olive oil*

Directions: Add all sauce ingredients to a saucepan and heat over low heat for 2-3 mins or until thickened. Set aside.
Add the Brussels sprouts, oil and salt to a ziplock bag and shake well.
Transfer the Brussels sprouts to the air fryer and fry at 390 F for 15 mins. Shake halfway through.
Transfer the Brussels sprouts to the mixing bowl. Drizzle with prepared sauce and toss until well coated.

Nutrition: Cal: 86 Fat: 4.3 g Carbs: 11.8 g Protein: 2 g

691. Roasted Carrots

Prep Time: 10 Mins
Servings: 6

Cook Time: 20 mins

Ingredients:

- *2 lbs. carrots, peeled, slice in half again slice half*
- *2 ½ tablespoon. dried parsley*
- *1 teaspoon dried oregano*
- *1 teaspoon dried thyme*
- *3 tablespoon. olive oil*
- *Pepper*
- *Salt*

Directions: Add carrots in a mixing bowl. Add remaining ingredients on top of carrots and toss well.
Arrange carrots on air fryer oven pan and roast at 400 F for 10 mins.
After 10 mins turn carrots slices to the other side and roast for 10 mins more

Nutrition: Cal: 124 Fat: 7.1 g Carbs: 15.3 g Protein: 0 g

692. Parmesan Broccoli Florets

Prep Time: 10 Mins
Servings: 4

Cook Time: 5 mins

Ingredients:

- *1 lb. broccoli florets*
- *¼ cup parmesan cheese, grated*
- *1 tablespoon. garlic, minced*
- *2 tablespoon. olive oil*
- *Pepper*
- *Salt*

Directions: Add broccoli florets into the mixing bowl.
Add cheese, garlic, oil, pepper, and salt on top of broccoli florets and toss well.
Arrange broccoli florets on air fryer oven pan and bake at 350 F for 4 mins.
Turn broccoli florets to other side and cook for 2 mins more.

Nutrition: Cal: 252 Fat: 16.4 g Carbs: 8.2 g Protein: 15.3 g

693. Baked Potatoes

Prep Time: 10 Mins
Servings: 4

Cook Time: 40 mins

Ingredients:

- *4 potatoes, scrubbed and washed*
- *¾ teaspoon garlic powder*
- *½ teaspoon Italian seasoning*
- *½ tablespoon. butter, melted*
- *½ teaspoon sea salt*

Directions: Prick potatoes using a fork.
Rub potatoes with melted butter and sprinkle with garlic powder, Italian seasoning, and sea salt.
Arrange potatoes on instant vortex air fryer oven drip pan and bake at 400 F for 40 mins.

Nutrition: Cal: 163 Fat: 1.8 g Carbs: 33.9 g Protein: 3.7 g

694. Parmesan Green Beans

Prep Time: 10 Mins
Servings: 6

Cook Time: 5 mins

Ingredients:
- *1 lb. fresh green beans*
- *½ cup flour*
- *2 eggs, lightly beaten*
- *¾ tablespoon. garlic powder*
- *½ cup parmesan cheese, grated*
- *1 cup breadcrumbs*

Directions: In a dish, add the flour.
In a second dish, add the eggs.
In a third dish, mix together bread crumbs, garlic powder and cheese.
Top the beans with the flour, then the eggs, and finally the breadcrumbs.
Place the coated beans on the skillet of the air fryer and fry at 390 F for 5 mins.

Nutrition: Cal: 257 Fat: 8.6 g Carbs: 27.2 g Protein: 14.9 g

695. Roasted Asparagus

Prep Time: 10 Mins
Servings: 4

Cook Time: 9 mins

Ingredients:
- *1 lb. asparagus cut the ends*
- *1 teaspoon olive oil*
- *Pepper*
- *Salt*

Directions: Arrange asparagus on the oven pan. Season with oil, pepper and salt.
Place pan in the instant vortex and bake asparagus at 370 F for 7-9 mins. Turn asparagus halfway through.

Nutrition: Cal: 33 Fat: 1.3 g Carbs: 4.4 g Protein: 2.5 g

696. Healthy Veggies

Prep Time: 10 Mins
Servings: 4

Cook Time: 18 mins

Ingredients:
- *1 cup carrots, sliced*
- *1 cup cauliflower, cut into florets*
- *1 cup broccoli florets*
- *1 tablespoon. olive oil*
- *Pepper*
- *Salt*

Directions: Add all vegetables in a mixing bowl. Drizzle with olive oil and season with pepper and salt. Toss well.
Add vegetables to the basket and air fry at 380 F for 18 mins.

Nutrition: Cal: 55 Fat: 3.6 g Carbs: 5.6 g Protein: 1.4 g

697. Parmesan Breaded with Zucchini Chips

Prep Time: 10 Mins
Servings: 5

Cook Time: 20 mins

Ingredients:

For the zucchini chips:
- *2 medium zucchini*
- *2 eggs*
- *1/3 Cup bread crumbs*
- *1/3 Cup grated Parmesan cheese*
- *Salt*
- *Pepper*
- *Cook oil*

For the lemon aioli:
- ½ cup mayonnaise
- ½ tablespoon olive oil
- Juice of ½ lemons
- 1 teaspoon minced garlic
- Salt
- Pepper

Directions:

To make the zucchini chips: Slice zucchini into thin chips (about 1/8 inch thick) using a knife or mandoline.

In a small bowl, beat the eggs. In another bowl, combine the bread crumbs, Parmesan cheese, salt and pepper to taste.

Spray the air fryer basket with cook oil.

Dip the zucchini slices one at a time into the eggs and then into the breadcrumb mixture. You can also spread the breadcrumbs over the zucchini slices with a spoon.

Place the zucchini chips in the basket of the air fryer, but do not stack.

Pour into oven basket. Bake in batches. Spray chips with cook oil from a distance. Bake for 10 mins.

Remove the cooked zucchini chips from the Air Fryer, and then repeat with the remaining zucchini chips.

To make the lemon aioli: While the zucchini is cook, combine the mayonnaise, olive oil, lemon juice, and garlic in a small bowl, adding salt and pepper to taste. Mix well until fully combined.

Cool the zucchini and serve alongside the aioli.

Nutrition: Cal: 192 Fat: 13 g Carbs: 0 g Protein: 6 g

698. Spicy Potato Fries

Prep Time: 10 Mins
Servings: 4

Cook Time: 37 mins

Ingredients:
- 2 tablespoon. sweet potato fry seasoning mix
- 2 tablespoon. olive oil
- 2 sweet potatoes

Seasoning Mix:
- 2 tablespoon. salt
- 1 tablespoon. cayenne pepper
- 1 tablespoon. dried oregano
- 1 tablespoon. fennel
- 2 tablespoon. coriander

Directions: Cut off both ends of the sweet potatoes and peel them. Cut in half lengthwise and again crosswise to make four pieces from each potato. Cut each piece of potato into 2-3 slices, and then slice into chips.

Grind together all the ingredients in the seasoning mix and add the salt.

Make sure your air fryer oven is preheated to 350 degrees.

Dip potato pieces in olive oil, sprinkle with seasoning mix and mix well to coat completely.

Add the chips to the basket of the air fryer. Set the temperature to 350°F and set the time to 27 mins.

Remove the basket and turn the fries over. Turn off the fryer and let it cook 10-12 mins until the fries are golden brown.

Nutrition: Cal: 89 Fat: 14 g Carbs: 0 g Protein: 8 g

699. Vegetarian Frittata

Prep Time: 10 Mins
Servings: 4

Cook Time: 30 mins

Ingredients:
- 1 leek, peeled and thinly sliced into rings
- 2 cloves garlic, finely minced
- 3 medium-sized carrots, finely chopped
- 2 tablespoons olive oil
- 6 large-sized eggs
- Sea salt and ground black pepper, to taste
- 1/2 teaspoon dried marjoram, finely minced
- 1/2 cup yellow cheese of choice

Directions: Sauté leek, garlic and carrot in hot olive oil until tender and fragrant.

Meanwhile, preheat the oven of the air fryer to 330 degrees F.

In a bowl, beat the eggs with the salt, ground black pepper and marjoram.

Then, grease the inside of the baking dish with nonstick cook spray. Pour the beaten eggs into the baking dish. Stir in the sautéed carrot mixture. Add the cheese pieces. Place the baking dish in the baking basket of the oven. Bake about 30 mins.

Nutrition: Cal: 153 Fat: 10.9 g Carbs: 3.7 g Protein: 6.7 g

700. Paprika Onion

Prep Time: 10 Mins
Servings: 4

Ingredients:
- 2 pounds cipollini onions, cut into flowers
- Olive oil as needed
- 1 teaspoon cayenne pepper
- 1 teaspoon garlic powder
- 2 cups flour
- 1 tablespoon pepper
- 1 tablespoon paprika
- 1 tablespoon salt
- ¼ cup mayonnaise
- 1 tablespoon ketchup
- ¼ cup mayonnaise
- ¼ cup sour cream

Directions: In a bowl, mix salt, pepper, paprika, flour, garlic powder, and cayenne pepper. Add mayonnaise, ketchup, sour cream to the mixture and stir.
Coat the onions with the prepared mixture and spray with oil.
Preheat your Air Fryer Vortex to 360 F.
Add the coated onions to the basket and cook for 15 mins.

Nutrition: Cal 156.1, Fat 3.8 g, Carbs 24.7 g, Protein 5 g

701. Parsnip & Potato Bake with Parmesan

Prep Time: 10 Mins
Servings: 8

Cook Time: 25 mins

Ingredients:
- 28 oz potato, cubed
- 3 tablespoon pine nuts
- 28 oz parsnips, chopped
- 1 ¾ oz Parmesan cheese, shredded
- 6 ¾ oz crème Fraiche
- 1 slice bread
- 2 tablespoon sage
- 4 tablespoon butter
- 4 teaspoon mustard

Directions: Preheat the Vortex to 360 F, and boil salted water in a pot over medium heat. Add the potatoes and parsnips. Bring to a boil.
In a bowl, mix the mustard, crème fraiche, sage, salt and pepper. Drain the potatoes and parsnips and mash them with the butter using a potato masher. Add the mustard mixture, bread, cheese and nuts to the mashed potatoes and mix.
Add the butter to your baking tray and bake for 25 mins.

Nutrition: Cal 226.4 Fat 6.1 g Carbs 34.9 g Fiber 4.4 g, Protein 4.0 g

702. Spicy Cheese Lings

Prep Time: 10 Mins
Servings: 4

Cook Time: 15 mins

Ingredients:
- 4 cups grated cheese, any
- 1 cup all-purpose flour
- 1 tablespoon butter
- 1 tablespoon baking powder
- ¼ teaspoon chili powder
- ¼ teaspoon salt, to taste
- 2 tablespoon water

Directions: Preheat the oven to 360° F, and boil salted water in a pot over medium heat. Add the potatoes and parsnips. Bring to a boil.
In a bowl, mix the mustard, crème fraiche, sage, salt and pepper. Drain the potatoes and parsnips and mash them with the butter using a potato masher. Add the mustard mixture, bread, cheese and nuts to the mashed potatoes and mix.
Add the butter to the baking dish and bake for 25 mins.

Nutrition: Cal 564 Fat 22.3 Carbs 55.1 g, Protein 24.3 g

703. Green Paneer Ginger Cheese Balls

Prep Time: 10 Mins
Servings: 2

Cook Time: 12 mins

Ingredients:
- 2 oz paneer cheese
- 2 tablespoon flour
- 2 medium onions, chopped
- 1 tablespoon cornflour
- 1 green chili, chopped
- The 1-inch ginger piece, chopped
- 1 teaspoon red chili powder
- A few leaves of cilantro, chopped
- Salt

Directions: Mix all ingredients, except the oil and cheese. Take a small part of the mixture, roll it up, and slowly press it to flatten. Stuff in 1 cube of cheese and seal the edges. Repeat with the rest of the mixture. Fry the balls in the fryer for 12 mins and at 370 F. Serve hot with ketchup.

Nutrition: Cal 399 Fat 34 g Carbs 9 g Protein 18 g

704. Beets with Rosemary and Balsamic Vinegar

Prep Time: 10 Mins
Servings: 2

Cook Time: 10 mins

Ingredients:
- 4 beets, cubed
- 1/3 cup balsamic vinegar
- 1 tablespoon olive oil
- 1 tablespoon honey
- Salt and black pepper to taste
- 2 springs rosemary

Directions: In a bowl, mix rosemary, pepper, salt, vinegar, and honey. Cover beets with the prepared sauce and then coat with oil. Preheat your Air Fryer to 400 F, and cook the beets for 10 mins.
Meanwhile, pour the balsamic vinegar in a pan over medium heat; bring to a boil and cook until reduced by half. Drizzle the beets with balsamic glaze, to serve.

Nutrition: Cal 76 Fat 1 g Protein 2 g

705. Coconut & Spinach Chickpeas

Prep Time: 10 Mins
Servings: 4

Cook Time: 15 mins

Ingredients:
- 2 tablespoon olive oil
- 1 tablespoon pepper
- 1 onion, chopped
- 1 teaspoon salt
- 4 garlic cloves, minced
- 1 can coconut milk
- 1 tablespoon ginger, minced
- 1 pound spinach
- ½ cup dried tomatoes, chopped
- 1 can chickpeas
- 1 lemon, juiced
- 1 hot pepper

Directions: Preheat your Air Fryer to 370 F, and in a bowl, mix lemon juice, tomatoes, pepper, ginger, coconut milk, garlic, salt, hot pepper, and onion. Rinse chickpeas under running water to get rid of all the gunk. Put them in a large bowl. Cover with spinach. Pour the sauce over, and stir in oil. Cook in the Vortex for 15 mins.

Nutrition: Cal 240.7 Fat 7.8 g Carbs 35.1 g Protein 10.4 g

706. Cauliflower, Olives, and Chickpeas

Prep Time: 10 Mins
Servings: 3

Cook Time: 24 mins

Ingredients:
- 3 c. cauliflower florets
- 4 chopped garlic cloves
- ½ c. Spanish green olives
- 15 oz. chickpeas, rinsed and drained
- ¼ teaspoon crushed red pepper
- 1 ½ tablespoon. olive oil
- 1 ½ tablespoon. parsley
- Salt to taste

Directions: Place the cauliflower florets, garlic, Spanish green olives, chickpeas, crushed red pepper, parsley, and salt in a large bowl.

Pour oil over the ingredients, then let it stand for about 2 to 3 mins.

Toss until all the ingredients are well coated in the olive oil.

Place the olive oil coated ingredients at the bottom of a lined pan in a single even layer. Cook for about 22 to 24 mins.

Nutrition: Cal: 176 Fat: 10.1 g Protein: 4.2 g Carbs: 17.6 g

707. Fruit and Vegetable Skewers

Prep Time: 10 Mins
Servings: 4

Cook Time: 20 mins

Ingredients:
- 4 tablespoon virgin olive oil
- 3 tablespoon. lemon juice
- 1 garlic clove, minced
- 2 tablespoon. chopped parsley
- ½ teaspoon. salt
- ½ teaspoon. black pepper
- 1 sliced zucchini
- 1 sliced yellow squash
- ½ red bell pepper
- ½ c. cherry tomatoes
- ½ c. pineapple chunks
- 4 wooden skewers

Directions: In a bowl combine olive oil, garlic, parsley, lemon juice, pepper and salt. Pour into large resealable plastic bag. Add the zucchini, squash, bell pepper and tomatoes. Seal the bag, shake to coat the vegetables and refrigerate for a minimum of 1 hour.

Remove vegetables from marinade and thread onto skewers, along with pineapple, alternating each item.

Place the skewers on the 4-inch grill. Bake on high power (350 degrees) for 8 mins.

Flip the skewers over and cook for another 6-8 mins until the vegetables reach the desired cook level.

Nutrition: Cal: 173 Fat: 2.8 g Carbs: 36.5 g Protein: 5 g

708. Roasted Potatoes with Rosemary

Prep Time: 10 Mins
Servings: 4

Cook Time: 12 mins

Ingredients:
- 1 ½ pound sweet potatoes, cubed
- 1 teaspoon. olive oil
- 1 dash chopped rosemary
- 1 dash lemon juice

Directions: In a bowl, toss sweet potatoes with oil. Evenly spread on the 10-inch baking sheet, sprinkle with rosemary. Place on 1-inch rack and back on 350 degrees F for 12 mins. Flip sweet potatoes over and cook an additional 10 mins.

Drizzle with lemon juice.

Nutrition: Cal: 114 Fat: 0 g Carbs: 27 g Protein: 2 g

709. Spicy Broccoli with Garlic

Prep Time: 10 Mins
Servings: 4

Cook Time: 15 mins

Ingredients:
- 1 broccoli head
- 3 garlic cloves, minced
- 2 teaspoon. virgin olive oil
- 1 teaspoon. sea salt
- ½ teaspoon. black pepper
- ½ teaspoon. lemon juice

Directions: In a mixing bowl, add oil, salt, garlic, and black pepper. Add broccoli. Mix to coat. Evenly scatter broccoli on the 10-inch baking sheet.

Place on1-inch rack and roast on 350 degrees F for about 10 mins. Flip florets and cook another 5-7 mins or until fork-tender.

Plate and drizzle lemon juice. Serve at once.

Nutrition: Cal: 141 Carbs: 10 g Fat: 10 g Protein: 5 g

710. Roasted Carrots with Garlic

Prep Time: 10 Mins   **Cook Time: 20 mins**
Servings: 2

Ingredients:
- 3 tablespoon. olive oil
- 2 minced garlic cloves
- Sea salt, to taste
- 1 pound baby carrots

Directions: In a medium bowl, mix carrots with olive oil, salt, and garlic. Spread carrots in a single layer on a parchment or foil-lined baking sheet.
Place on 1-inch rack and cook on 350 F for 15-20 mins until carrots are tender.

Nutrition: Cal: 95 Fat: 6.9 g Carbs: 7.6 g Protein: 1 g

711. Roasted Balsamic Vegetables

Prep Time: 10 Mins   **Cook Time: 30 mins**
Servings: 4

Ingredients:
- 1½ c. cubed butternut squash
- 1 c. chopped broccoli florets
- ½ chopped red onion
- 1 chopped zucchini
- 1 minced garlic clove
- 2 tablespoon. virgin olive oil
- 1½ teaspoon. rosemary
- A pinch of salt, to taste
- 1 tablespoon. balsamic vinegar

Directions: In a mixing bowl, add oil, rosemary, vinegar, pepper, and salt; mix to blend. Mix in the vegetables, mix to coat evenly. Evenly spread on a parchment-lined baking sheet. Place on 1-inch rack and cook on 350 degrees F for about 15 mins. Flip vegetables and cook for another 15 mins or until squash is just softened.

Nutrition: Cal: 148 Fat: 4.6 g Carbs: 25 g Protein: 7 g

712. Pesto Tomatoes

Prep Time: 10 Mins   **Cook Time: 14 mins**
Servings: 4

Ingredients:
- 3 large heirloom tomatoes, cut into ½ inch thick slices.
- 1 cup pesto
- 8 oz. feta cheese, cut into ½ inch thick slices.
- ½ cup red onions, sliced thinly
- 1 tablespoon olive oil

Directions: Spread some pesto on each slice of tomato.
Top each tomato slice with a feta slice and onion and drizzle with oil.
Select the "Air Fry" mode and cook to 14 mins. Set the temperature at 390 degrees F.
Arrange the tomatoes in a greased "Air Fry Basket" and insert them in the oven.

Nutrition: Cal 480 Fat 41.9 g Carbs 13 g Protein 15.4 g

713. Stuffed Tomatoes

Prep Time: 10 Mins   **Cook Time: 15 mins**
Servings: 2

Ingredients:
- 2 large tomatoes
- ½ cup broccoli, chopped finely
- ½ cup Cheddar cheese, shredded
- Salt and ground black pepper, as required
- 1 tablespoon unsalted butter, melted
- ½ teaspoon dried thyme, crushed

Directions: Cut off the top of each tomato and remove the pulp and seeds.

In a bowl, mix the chopped broccoli, cheese, salt and black pepper.
Fill each tomato evenly with the broccoli mixture.
Select the "Air Fry" mode. Press the "Time" button to set the cook time to 15 mins. Set the temperature to 355 degrees F. Place the tomatoes in a greased "Air Fry Basket" and place in the oven.
Serve hot with the thyme garnish.

Nutrition: Cal 206 Fat 15.6 g Carbs 9 g

714. Parmesan Asparagus

Prep Time: 10 Mins
Servings: 3

Cook Time: 10 mins

Ingredients:
- 1 lb. fresh asparagus, trimmed
- 1 tablespoon Parmesan cheese, grated
- 1 tablespoon butter, melted
- 1 teaspoon garlic powder
- Salt and ground black pepper, as required

Directions: In a bowl, mix asparagus, cheese, butter, garlic powder, salt and black pepper.
Select the "Air Fry" mode and press the "Time" button to set the cook time to 10 mins.
Set the temperature to 400 degrees F.
Place the vegetable mixture in a greased "Air Fry Basket" and place it in the oven.

Nutrition: Cal 73 Fat 4.4 g Carbs 6.6 g Protein 4.2 g

715. Spicy Butternut Squash

Prep Time: 10 Mins
Servings: 4

Cook Time: 20 mins

Ingredients:
- 1 medium butternut squash, peeled, seeded and cut into chunk
- 2 teaspoons cumin seeds
- 1/8 teaspoon garlic powder
- 1/8 teaspoon chili flakes, crushed
- Salt and ground black pepper, as required
- 1 tablespoon olive oil
- 2 tablespoons pine nuts
- 2 tablespoons fresh cilantro, chopped

Directions: In a bowl, mix the squash, spices, and oil.
Select the "Air Fry" mode and press the time button to set the cook time to 20 mins. Set the temperature at 375 degrees F. Arrange the squash chunks in a greased "Air Fry Basket" and insert it in the oven.
Serve hot with the garnishing of pine nuts and cilantro.

Nutrition: Cal 191 Fat 7 g Carbs 34.3 g Protein 3.7 g

716. Sweet & Spicy Parsnips

Prep Time: 10 Mins
Servings: 5

Cook Time: 44 mins

Ingredients:
- 1½ lbs. parsnip, peeled and cut into 1-inch chunks
- 1 tablespoon butter, melted
- 2 tablespoons honey
- 1 tablespoon dried parsley flakes, crushed
- ¼ teaspoon red pepper flakes, crushed
- Salt and ground black pepper, as required

Directions: In a large bowl, mix the parsnips and butter.
Select the "Air Fry" mode and press the time button to set the cook time to 44 mins. Set the temperature at 355 degrees F. Arrange the squash chunks in a greased "Air Fry Basket" and insert it in the oven.
Meanwhile, in another bowl, mix the remaining ingredients.
Transfer the parsnips chunks into the bowl of honey mixture and toss to coat well.
Again, arrange the parsnip chunks in "Air Fry Basket" and insert it in the oven.

Nutrition: Cal 149 Fat 2.7 g Carbs 31.5 g Protein 1.7 g

SOUPS

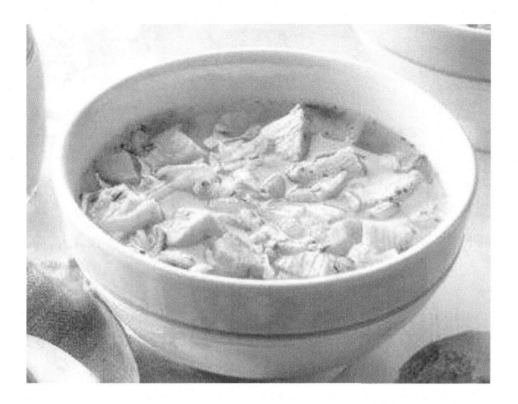

717. Chicken Soup

Prep Time: 35 mins
Servings: 4

Cook Time: 30 mins

Ingredients:

- *Four chicken breasts*
- *One carrot, chopped*
- *1 cup zucchini, peeled and chopped*
- *2 cups cauliflower, broken into florets*
- *One celery rib Chopped*
- *One small onion, chopped*
- *5 cups of water*
- *½ teaspoon. Black pepper*

Directions: Place chicken breasts, onion, carrot, celery, cauliflower, and zucchini in a deep soup pot. Add in salt, black pepper, and 5 cups of water.
Stir and bring to a boil. Simmer for 30 mins, then remove chicken from the pot and let it cool slightly. Blend the soup until completely smooth.
Shred or dice the chicken meat, return it to the pot, stir and serve.

718. Leek, Rice, and Potato Soup

Prep Time: 35 mins
Servings: 4

Cook Time: 30 mins

Ingredients:

- *Three potatoes, peeled and diced*
- *Two leeks, finely chopped*
- *¼ cup brown rice*
- *5 cups of water*
- *3 tablespoon. Extra virgin olive oil*
- *Lemon juice, to taste.*

Directions: Heat olive oil in a deep soup pot and sauté leeks for 3-4 mins.
Add in potatoes and cook for a minute more. Stir in water; bring to a boil, and the brown rice. Reduce heat and simmer for 30 mins.
Add lemon juice.

719. Mushroom and Kale Soup

Prep Time: 35 mins
Servings: 4

Cook Time: 20 mins

Ingredients:

- One onion, chopped
- One carrot, chopped
- One zucchini, peeled and diced
- One potato, peeled and diced
- Ten white mushrooms, chopped
- One bunch kale (10 oz.), stemmed and coarsely chopped
- 3 cups vegetable broth
- 4 tablespoon. Olive oil
- salt and black pepper

Directions: Heat olive oil in a large soup pot.
Add in onions, carrot, and mushrooms and cook until vegetables are tender.
Stir in the zucchini, kale, and vegetable broth—season to taste with salt and pepper and simmer for 20 mins.

720. Italian Chicken Soup

Prep Time: 35 mins
Servings: 4

Cook Time: 30 mins

Ingredients:

- Three chicken breasts, one carrot, chopped
- One small zucchini, peeled and chopped
- One celery stalk, chopped
- One small onion, chopped
- One bay leaf
- 5 cups water; 6-7 black olives, pitted and halved
- ½ teaspoon. Salt; 1 teaspoon. Dried basil
- black pepper, fresh parsley, lemon juice, to serve

Directions: Place chicken breasts, onion, carrot, celery, and bay leaf in a deep soup pot. Add in salt, black pepper, basil, and water.
Stir well and bring to a boil. Add zucchini and olives and reduce heat.
Simmer for 30 mins. Set aside to cool. Serve with lemon juice and sprinkled with parsley.

721. Chicken and Broccoli Soup

Prep Time: 35 mins
Servings: 4

Cook Time: 30 mins

Ingredients:

- Four boneless chicken thighs, diced
- One small carrot, chopped
- One broccoli head, broken into florets
- One garlic clove, chopped
- One small onion, chopped
- 4 cups of water
- 3 tablespoon. Olive oil
- ½ teaspoon. Salt, black pepper

Directions: In a deep soup pot, heat olive oil and gently sauté broccoli for 2-3 mins, stirring occasionally. Add in chicken, onion, carrot, and cook, stirring, for 2-3 mins. Stir in salt, black pepper, and water. Bring to a boil.
Simmer for 30 mins, then remove from heat and set aside to cool. In a blender or food processor, blend soup until completely smooth.

722. Vegetable and Beef Soup

Prep Time: 35 mins
Servings: 4

Cook Time: 30 mins

Ingredients:

- Two slices bacon, chopped
- 1 lb. lean ground beef
- One carrot, chopped
- Two cloves garlic, finely chopped
- One small onion, chopped
- One celery stalk, chopped
- One bay leaf; 1 teaspoon. Dried basil
- 1 cup canned tomatoes, diced and drained
- 4 cups beef broth
- ½ cup canned chickpeas
- ½ cup vermicelli

Directions: In a large soup pot, cook bacon and ground beef until well done, breaking up the meat as it cooks. Drain off the fat and add in onion, garlic, carrot, and celery.

Cook for 3-4 mins until fragrant. Stir in the bay leaf, basil, tomatoes, and beef broth. Bring to a boil, then reduce heat and simmer for about 20 mins.

Add the chickpeas and vermicelli. Cook, uncovered, for about 5 mins more and serves.

723. Beef Soup

Prep Time: 35 mins   **Cook Time: 30 mins**
Servings: 4

Ingredients:

- 12 oz. beef stew meat, cut into
- inch cubes one medium leek, chopped
- garlic cloves, chopped
- bay leaves

- can tomatoes (15 oz.), diced and drained
- ½ cup barley
- 1 cup of frozen mixed vegetables
- cups beef broth

- Tablespoon. Extra virgin olive oil
- 1 teaspoon. Paprika

Directions: Heat oil in a large saucepan over medium-high heat. Sauté beef until well browned. Add in leeks and garlic and sauté until fragrant.

Add paprika, beef broth, and bay leaves; season with salt and pepper.

Cover and bring to a boil, then reduce heat and simmer for 60 mins. Stir in frozen vegetables, tomatoes, and barley.

Return to boiling, reduce heat, and simmer, covered, about 15 mins more or until meat and vegetables are tender. Discard bay leaves and serve.

724. Bean Soup

Prep Time: 35 mins   **Cook Time: 30 mins**
Servings: 4

Ingredients:

- One onion, chopped
- One large carrot, chopped
- Two garlic cloves, minced
- 15 oz. can white beans, rinsed and drained

- 1 cup spinach leaves, trimmed and washed
- cups chicken broth
- 1 tablespoon. Paprika
- 1 tablespoon. Dried mint

- Tablespoon. Extra virgin olive oil
- salt and black pepper, to taste

Directions: Heat the olive oil over medium heat and gently sauté the onion, garlic, and carrot.

Add in beans, broth, salt, and pepper and bring to a boil.

Reduce heat and cook for 10 mins, or until the carrots are tender. Stir in spinach, and simmer for about 5 mins, until spinach is wilted.

DESSERTS

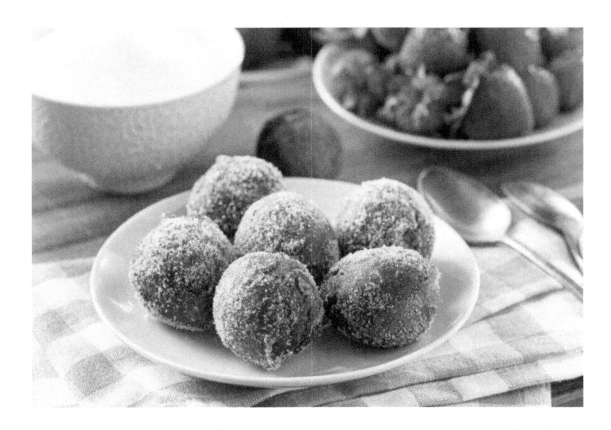

725. Banana Split

Prep Time: 15 mins
Servings: 8

Cook Time: 14 mins

Ingredients:
- *Three tablespoons coconut oil*
- *1 cup panko breadcrumbs*
- *½ cup of corn flour*
- *Two eggs*

- *Four bananas, peeled and halved lengthwise*
- *Three tablespoons sugar*
- *¼ teaspoon ground cinnamon*

- *Two tablespoons walnuts, chopped*

Directions: In a skillet, melt the coconut oil over medium heat and cook the breadcrumbs for about 4 mins or until golden brown and crumbly, stirring constantly.
Transfer the breadcrumbs to a shallow bowl and set aside to cool.
In a second bowl, place the cornmeal.
In a third bowl, beat the eggs.
Coat the banana slices with the flour, dip them in the eggs and finally coat them evenly with the breadcrumbs.
In a small bowl, mix the sugar and cinnamon.
Select "Air Fry" mode. Set the cook time to 10 mins and set the temperature to 280 degrees F.
Arrange banana slices in "Air Fry Basket" and sprinkle with cinnamon sugar. Insert the basket into the oven.
Transfer banana slices to plates to cool slightly.
Sprinkle with chopped walnuts.

Nutrition: Cal 216 Fat 8.8 g Carbs 26 g Protein 3.4 g

726. Sugar-Free Chocolate Soufflé

Prep Time: 15 mins
Servings: 2

Cook Time: 15 mins

Ingredients
- Milk: 1/3 cup
- Butter soft to melted: 2 tbsp.
- Flour: 1 tbsp.
- Splenda: 2 tbsp.
- one Egg Yolk
- Sugar-Free Chocolate Chips: 1/4 cup
- Two egg whites
- Half teaspoon of cream of tartar
- Half teaspoon of Vanilla Extract

Directions: Grease the ramekins with spray oil or softened butter.
Sprinkle with any sugar alternative, make sure to cover them.
Let the air fryer preheat to 325-330 F
Melt the chocolate in a microwave-safe bowl. Mix every 30 seconds until fully melted.
Or use a double boiler method.
Melt the one and a half tablespoons of butter over low-medium heat. In a small-sized skillet.
Once the butter has melted, then whisk in the flour. Keep whisking until thickened. Then turn thc heat off.
Add the egg whites with cream of tartar, with the whisk attachment, in a stand mixer, mix until peaks forms.
Meanwhile, combine the ingredients in a melted chocolate bowl, add the flour mixture and melted butter to chocolate, and blend.
Add in the vanilla extract, egg yolks, remaining sugar alternative.
Fold the egg white peaks gently with the ingredients into the bowl.
Add the mix into ramekins about 3/4 full of five-ounce ramekins
Let it bake for 12-14 mins, or until done.

Nutrition: Cal: 288 Carbs: 5 g Protein: 6 g Fat: 24 g

727. Sugar-Free Air Fried Carrot Cake

Prep Time: 15 mins
Servings: 8

Cook Time: 40 mins

Ingredients
- All-Purpose Flour: 1 ¼ cups
- Pumpkin Pie Spice: 1 tsp
- Baking Powder: one teaspoon
- Splenda: 3/4 cup
- Carrots: 2 cups–grated
- 2 Eggs
- Baking Soda: half teaspoon
- Canola Oil: ¾ cup

Directions: Let the air fryer preheat to 350 F. spray the cake pan with oil spray. And add flour over that.
In a bowl, combine the baking powder, pumpkin pie spice, flour, and baking soda.
In another bowl, mix the eggs, oil, and sugar alternative. Now combine the dry to wet ingredients. Add half of the dry ingredients first mix and the other half of the dry mixture. Add in the grated carrots. Add the cake batter to the greased cake pan.
Place the cake pan in the basket of the air fryer. Let it Air fry for half an hour, but do not let the top too brown.
If the top is browning, add a piece of foil over the top of the cake.
Air fry it until a toothpick comes out clean, 35-40 mins in total.
Let the cake cool down before serving.

Nutrition: Cal 287 Carbs: 19 g Protein: 4 g Fat: 22 g

728. Sugar-Free Low Carb Cheesecake Muffins

Prep Time: 20 mins
Servings: 18

Cook Time: 28 mins

Ingredients
- Splenda: half cup
- One and a half Cream Cheese
- Two Eggs
- Vanilla Extract: 1 tsp

Directions: Let the oven preheat to 300 F.
Spray the muffin pan with oil.
In a bowl, add the sugar alternative, vanilla extract, and cream cheese. Mix well. Add-in the eggs gently, one at a time. Do not over mix the batter. Let it bake for 25 to 30 mins, or until cooked.
Take out from the air fryer and let them cool before adding frosting.

Nutrition: Cal: 93 Carbs: 1 g Protein: 2 g Fat: 9 g

729. Sugar-Free Chocolate Donut Holes

Prep Time: 15 mins
Servings: 32

Cook Time: 15 mins

Ingredients
- 6 tbsp. Splenda
- 1 Cup any flour
- Baking Soda: half tsp.
- 6 tbsp. Unsweetened Cocoa Powder
- 3 tbsp. of Butter
- 1 Egg
- Baking Powder: half tsp.
- 2 tbsp. of Unsweetened Chocolate chopped
- 1/4 cup Plain Yogurt

Directions: In a mixing bowl, combine the baking powder, baking soda, and flour.
Then add in the cocoa powder and sugar alternative.
In a mug or microwave-safe bowl, melt the butter and the unsweetened chocolate.
Mix every 15 seconds and make sure they melt together and combine well.
Set it aside to cool it down.
In that big mixing bowl from before, add in the yogurt and the egg. Add in the melted butter and chocolate mixture.
Cover the bowl with wrap and let it chill in the refrigerator for 30 mins.
To make the donut balls, take out the batter from the fridge.
With the help of a tablespoon, scoop out sufficient batter so a donut ball will form with your hands.
You can use oil on your hands if the dough is too sticky.
Spray the oil on the air fryer basket and sprinkle with flour and let it preheat to 350 F.
Work in batches and add the balls in one single layer.
Let it bake for 10-12 mins until they are done. To check doneness, try a toothpick if it comes out clean.
Take out from air fryer, let it cool and serve hot or cold.

Nutrition: Cal 22 Carbs: 1 g Protein: 1 g Fat: 2 g

730. Low Carb Peanut Butter Cookies

Prep Time: 20nmins
Servings: 23

Cook Time: 9 mins

Ingredients:
- All-natural 100% peanut butter: 1 cup
- One whisked egg
- Liquid stevia drops: 1 teaspoon
- Sugar alternative: 1 cup

Directions: Mix all the ingredients into a dough. Make 24 balls with your hands from the combined dough.
On a cookie sheet or cutting board, press the dough balls with the help of a fork to form a crisscross pattern.
Add six cookies to the basket of air fryer in a single layer. Cook in batches.
Let them Air Fry, for 8-10 mins, at 325. Take the basket out from the air fryer.
Let the cookies cool for one minute, then with care, take the cookies out.
Keep baking the rest of the peanut butter cookies in batches.
Let them cool completely and serve.

Nutrition: Cal: 198 Carbs: 7 g Protein: 9 g Fat: 17 g

731. Air Fryer Blueberry Muffins Recipe

Prep Time: 10 mins
Servings: 8

Cook Time: 12-14 mins

Ingredients:
- Half cup of sugar alternative
- One and 1/3 cup of flour
- 1/3 cup of oil
- Two teaspoons of baking powder
- 1/4 teaspoon of salt
- One egg
- Half cup of milk
- Eight muffin cups (foil) with paper liners
- Or silicone baking cups
- 2/3 cup of frozen and thawed blueberries, or fresh

Directions: Let the air fryer preheat to 330 F.
In a large bowl, sift together baking powder, sugar, salt,and flour. Mix well
In another bowl, add milk, oil, and egg mix it well.

To the dry ingredients to the egg mix, mix until combined but do not over mix
Add the blueberries carefully. Pour the mixture into muffin paper cups or muffin baking tray
Put four muffin cups in the air fryer basket or add more if your basket's size is big.
Cook for 12-14 mins, at 330 F, or until when touch lightly the tops, it should spring back.
Cook the remaining muffins accordingly.
Take out from the air fryer and let them cool before serving.

Nutrition: Cal 213 Fat 10 g Carbs 13.2 g Protein 9.7 g

732. Air Fryer Lemon Slice & Bake Cookies

Prep Time: 5 mins   **Cook Time: 5 mins**
Servings: 24

Ingredients:
- *Half teaspoon of salt*
- *Half cup of coconut flour*
- *Half cup of unsalted butter softened*
- *Half teaspoon of liquid vanilla stevia*
- *Half cup of swerve granular sweetener*
- *One tablespoon lemon juice*
- *Lemon extract: 1/4 tsp, it is optional*
- *Two egg yolks*
- *For icing*
- *Three tsp of lemon juice*
- *2/3 cup of Swerve confectioner's sweetener*

Directions: In a stand mixer bowl, add baking soda, coconut flour, salt and Swerve, mix until well combined
Then add the butter (softened) to the dry ingredients, mix well. Add all the remaining ingredients but do not add in the yolks yet.
Adjust the seasoning of lemon flavor and sweetness to your liking, add more if needed.
Add the yolk and combine well.
Lay a big piece of plastic wrap on a flat surface, put the batter in the center, roll around the dough and make it into a
log form, for almost 12 inches. Keep this log in the fridge for 2-3 hours or overnight, if possible.
Let the oven preheat to 325 F. generously spray the air fryer basket, take the log out from plastic wrap only unwrap how much you
want to use it, and keep the rest in the fridge.
Cut in 1/4 inch cookies, place as many cookies in the air fryer basket in one single, do not overcrowd the basket.
Bake for 3-five mins, or until the cookies' edges become brown. Let it cool in the basket for two mins, then take out from the basket.
And let them cool on a wire rack.
Once all cookies are baked, pour the icing over.

Nutrition: Cal 66 Fat 6 g Carbs 2 g Protein 1 g

733. Brownies

Prep Time: 10 mins   **Cook Time: 10 mins**
Servings: 2

Ingredients
- *2 tbsp. of Baking Chips*
- *1/3 cup of Almond Flour*
- *One Egg*
- *Half teaspoon of Baking Powder*
- *3 tbsp. of Powdered Sweetener (sugar alternative)*
- *2 tbsp. of Cocoa Powder (Unsweetened)*
- *2 tbsp. of chopped Pecans*
- *4 tbsp. of melted Butter*

Directions: Let the air fryer preheat to 350 F.
In a large bowl, add cocoa powder, almond flour, Swerve sugar substitute, and baking powder, give it a good mix.
Add melted butter and crack in the egg in the dry ingredients.
Mix well until combined and smooth.
Fold in the chopped pecans and baking chips.
Take two ramekins to grease them well with softened butter. Add the batter to them.
Bake for ten mins. Make sure to place them as far from the heat source from the top in the air fryer.
Take the brownies out from the air fryer and let them cool for five mins.
Serve with your favorite toppings and enjoy.

Nutrition: Cal 201 Fat 10.2 g Protein 8.7 g Carbs 14.1 g

734. Air Fryer Cookies

Prep Time: 15 mins
Servings: 10

Cook Time: 10 mins

Ingredients
- One teaspoon of baking powder
- One cup of almond flour
- Three tablespoons of natural low-calorie sweetener
- One large egg
- Three and a half tablespoons raspberry (reduced-sugar) preserves
- Four tablespoons of softened cream cheese

Directions: In a bowl, add egg, baking powder, flour, sweetener, and cream cheese, mix well until a dough (wet) forms.
Chill the dough in the fridge for almost 20 mins, until dough is cool enough.
And then form into balls.
Let the air fryer preheat to 400 F, add the parchment paper to the air fryer basket.
Make ten balls from the dough and put them in the prepared air fryer basket.
With your clean hands, make an indentation from your thumb in the center of every cookie. Add one teaspoon of the raspberry preserve in the thumb hole.
Bake in the air fryer for seven mins, or until light golden brown to your liking.
Let the cookies cool completely in the parchment paper for almost 15 mins, or they will fall apart.

Nutrition: 111.6 Cal Protein 3.7 g Carbs 9.1 g Fat 8.6 g

735. Air Fryer Apple Fritter

Prep Time: 10 mins
Servings: 3

Cook Time: 10 mins

Ingredients
- Half apple (Pink Lady Apple or Honey crisp) peeled, finely chopped
- Half cup of All-Purpose Flour
- One teaspoon of Baking Powder
- 1/4 teaspoon of Kosher Salt
- Half teaspoon of Ground Cinnamon
- 2 Tbsp. of Brown Sugar or sugar alternative
- 1/8 teaspoon of Ground Nutmeg
- 3 Tbsp. of Greek Yogurt (Fat-Free)
- One tablespoon of Butter

For the glaze
- Two Tbsp. Of Powdered Sugar
- Half tablespoon of Water

Directions: In a mixing bowl, add baking powder, nutmeg, brown sugar (or alternative), flour, cinnamon, and salt. Mix it well.
With the help of a fork or cutter, slice the butter until crumbly. It should look like wet sand.
Add the chopped apple and coat well, then add fat-free Greek yogurt.
keep stirring or tossing until everything together, and a crumbly dough forms.
Put the dough on a clean surface and with your hands, knead it into a ball form.
Flatten the dough in an oval shape about a half-inch thick. It is okay, even if it's not the perfect size or shape.
Spray the basket of the air fryer with cook spray generously. Put the dough in the air fry for 12-14 mins at 375ºF cook until light golden brown.
For making the glaze mix, the ingredients, and with the help of a brush, pour over the apple fritter when it comes out from the air fryer.
Slice and serve after cooling for 5 mins.

Nutrition: Cal 200 Fat 12 g Protein 9.8 g Carbs 14 g

736. Berry Cheesecake

Prep Time: 10 mins
Servings: 8

Cook Time: 50 mins

Ingredients
- Half cup raspberries
- Two blocks of softened cream cheese, 8 ounce
- Raspberry or vanilla extract: 1 teaspoon
- 1/4 cup of strawberries
- Two eggs
- 1/4 cup of blackberries
- One cup and 2 tbsp. of sugar alternative of confectioner sweetener

Directions: In a big mixing bowl, whip the sugar-alternative confectioner sweetener and cream cheese, mix whip until smooth and creamy.

Then add in the raspberry or vanilla extract and eggs, again mix well.

In a food processor, pulse the berries and fold into the cream cheese mix with two extra tbsp. of sweetener.

Take a springform pan and spray the oil generously, pour in the mixture.

Put the pan in the air fryer, let it air fryer, and cook for ten mins at 300F. Lower the temperature to 400 °F and cook for 40 mins.

To check if it's done, shake it lightly. If everything is set and the middle part is jiggly, it is done.

Take out from the air fryer and cool a bit before chilling in the fridge.

Keep in the fridge for 2-4 hours or as long as you have time.

Slice and serve.

Nutrition: Cal 225 Fat 17 g Carbs 18 g Protein 12 g

737. Grain-Free Cakes

Prep Time: 5 mins   **Cook Time: 10 mins**
Servings: 2

Ingredients

- *Two large eggs*
- *Half cup of chocolate chips, you can use dark chocolate*
- *2 tbsp. of coconut flour*
- *Two tablespoons of honey as a sugar substitute*
- *A dash of sea salt*
- *Half teaspoon of baking soda*
- *Butter and cocoa powder for (two small ramekins)*
- *1/4 cup of butter or grass-fed butter*

Directions: Let the air fryer preheat to 370 degrees F.

Grease the ramekins with soft butter and sprinkle with cocoa powder. It will stick to the butter. Turn the ramekins upside down, so excess cocoa powder will fall out. Set it aside.

In a double boiler or microwave, safe bowl, melt the butter and chocolate chips together, stir every 15 seconds. Make sure to mix well to combine.

In a large bowl, crack the eggs and whisk with either honey or sugar, mix well. Add in the sea salt, baking soda, and coconut flour. Gently fold everything.

Then add the melted chocolate chip and butter mixture to the egg, flour, and honey mixture. Mix well, so everything combines.

Pour the batter in those two prepared ramekins.

Let them air fry for ten mins. Then take them out from the air fryer and let it cool for 3,4 mins.

When cool enough to handle, run a knife along the edges so the cake will out easier.

After flipping them upside down on a serving plate.

Top with mint leaves and coconut cream, raspberries, if you want. Serve right away and enjoy.

Nutrition: Cal 217 Fat 12 g Protein 9.9 g Carbs 14 g

738. Tahini Oatmeal Chocolate Chunk Cookies

Prep Time: 10 mins   **Cook Time: 5 mins**
Servings: 8

Ingredients

- *1/3 cup of tahini*
- *1/4 cup of walnuts*
- *1/4 cup of maple syrup*
- *1/4 cup of Chocolate chunks*
- *1/4 tsp of sea salt*
- *Two tablespoons of almond flour*
- *One teaspoon of vanilla*
- *1 cup of gluten-free oat flakes*
- *One teaspoon of cinnamon*

Directions: Let the air fryer Preheat to 350 F.

In a big bowl, add the maple syrup, cinnamon (if used), the tahini, salt, and vanilla (if used). Mix well, then add in the walnuts, oat flakes, and almond meal. Then fold the chocolate chips gently.

Now the mix is ready, take a full tablespoon of mixture, separate into eight amounts. Wet clean damp hands, press them on a baking tray or with a spatula.

Place four cookies, or more depending on your air fryer size, line the air fryer basket with parchment paper in one single layer.

Let them cook for 5-6 mins at 350 F, air fry for more mins if you like them crispy.

Nutrition: Cal: 185.5 Fat: 11.2 g Carbs: 18.5 g Protein 12 g

739. Eggless & Vegan Cake

Prep Time: 5 mins
Servings: 8

Cook Time: 15 mins

Ingredients
- Olive Oil: 2 Tbsp.
- All-Purpose Flour: 1/4 Cup
- Cocoa Powder: 2 Tbsp.
- Baking Soda: 1/8 Tsp
- Sugar: 3 Tbsp.
- One tablespoon of Warm Water
- Milk: 3 Tbsp.
- Two Drops of Vanilla Extract
- 4 Raw Almonds for decoration – roughly chopped
- A Pinch of Salt

Directions: Let the air fryer preheat to 390°F for at least two mins.
In a large bowl, add sugar, milk, water, and oil. Whisk until a smooth batter forms.
Now add salt, all-purpose flour, cocoa powder, and baking soda, sift them into wet ingredients, mix to form a paste
Spray the four-inch baking pan with oil and pour the batter into it. Then add in the chopped up almonds on top of it.
Put the baking pan in the preheated air fryer. And cook for ten mins.
Check the doneness with a toothpick. If it comes out clean, they are done but may need another minute.
Take out from the air fryer.
Let it cool completely before slicing.

Nutrition: Cal 120 Fat: 8 g Carbs 18 g Protein: 2 g

740. Banana Muffins in Air Fryer

Prep Time: 10 mins
Servings: 8

Cook Time: 10 mins

Wet Mix
- 3 tbsp. of milk
- One teaspoon of Nutella (it is optional)
- Four Cavendish size, ripe bananas
- Half cup sugar alternative
- One teaspoon of vanilla essence
- Two large eggs

Dry Mix
- One teaspoon of baking powder
- One and a 1/4 cup of whole wheat flour
- One teaspoon of baking soda
- One teaspoon of cinnamon
- 2 tbsp. of cocoa powder (it is optional)
- One teaspoon of salt

Optional
- Chopped walnuts: 1 handful
- Fruits, Dried slices
- Chocolate sprinkles

Directions: With the fork, in a bowl, mash up the bananas, add all the wet ingredients to it, and mix well.
Sift all the dry ingredients so they combine well. Add into the wet ingredients. Carefully fold both ingredients together. Do not over mix.
Then add in the diced walnuts, slices of dried up fruits, and chocolate sprinkles.
Let the air fryer preheat to 250°F.
Add the batter into muffin cups before that, spray them with oil generously.
Air fryer them for at least half an hour, or until a toothpick comes out clean.
Take out from the air fryer and let them cool down before serving.

Nutrition: Cal 210 Fat 13 g Protein 12 g Carbs 18 g

741. Apple Cider Vinegar Donuts

Prep Time: 10 mins
Servings: 8

Cook Time: 10 mins

Ingredients:

For Muffins
- Coconut flour: 1 cup
- Four eggs, large
- Coconut oil: 4 tbsp., melted
- Baking soda: 1 tsp
- Apple cider vinegar: 2/3 cup
- Cinnamon: 1 tsp
- Honey: 3 tbsp.
- A pinch of salt

For Drizzle
- *Coffee Syrup (Turmeric Pumpkin Spice)*

Directions: Let the air fryer pre-heat to 350 F. spray oil on a baking tray, spray a generous amount of grease with melted coconut oil

In a large bowl, add apple cider vinegar, honey, melted coconut oil, salt mix well, then crack the eggs and whisk it all together.

In another bowl, sift the coconut flour, baking soda, and cinnamon so that the dry ingredients will combine well.

Add the wet ingredients to dry ingredients until completely combined. Do not worry if the batter is kind of wet.

Pour the batter into the prepared donut baking pan. And add the batter into cavities. With the help of your hands, spread the batter in the cavity evenly.

Let it bake for ten mins or 8 mins at 350 F, or until light golden brown.

Make sure halfway cook if they are not getting too brown, with a toothpick check to see if the donuts are cooked, and a toothpick comes out clean.

Take out from the oven and let them cool for at least ten mins to harden up, then remove otherwise. They will fall apart since they are very tender.

Before serving, drizzle with coffee syrup (turmeric pumpkin spice).

Serve right away and enjoy.

Nutrition: Cal 179 Fat 11.2 Carbs 9 g Protein 5 g

742. Banana Slices

Prep Time: 15 mins
Servings: 8

Cook Time: 15 mins

Ingredients:
- Four medium ripe bananas, peeled
- 1/3 cup rice flour, divided
- Two tablespoons all-purpose flour
- Two tablespoons corn flour
- Two tablespoons desiccated coconut
- ½ teaspoon baking powder
- ½ teaspoon ground cardamom
- Pinch of salt
- Water, as required
- ¼ cup sesame seeds

Directions: In a bowl, mix two tablespoons rice flour, all-purpose flour, cornmeal, coconut, baking powder, cardamom and salt.

Add the water and mix until a thick, smooth dough forms.

In another bowl, place the remaining rice flour.

In a third bowl, add the sesame seeds.

Cut each banana in half and then cut each half into two pieces lengthwise.

Dip the banana into the coconut mixture and then top with the remaining rice flour, followed by the sesame seeds.

Select the "Air Fry" mode and set the cook time to 15 mins. Set the temperature to 390 degrees F.

Arrange banana slices in "Air Fry Basket" and place in oven.

Transfer banana slices to plates to cool slightly.

Nutrition: Cal 121 Fat 3 g Carbs 23.1 g Protein 2.2 g

743. Pineapple Bites

Prep Time: 10 mins
Servings: 4

Cook Time: 10 mins

Ingredients:
- ½ of pineapple
- ¼ cup desiccated coconut
- One tablespoon fresh mint leaves, minced
- 1 cup vanilla yogurt

Directions: Remove the outer skin of the pineapple and cut into long 1-2 inch thick sticks.

In a dish, place the coconut.

Coat the pineapple sticks with coconut evenly.

Select the "Air Fry" and set the cook time to 10 mins. Set the temperature at 390 degrees F.

Arrange the pineapple sticks in a lightly greased "Air Fry Basket" and insert it in the oven.

Meanwhile, for a dip in a bowl, mix mint and yogurt. Serve pineapple sticks with yogurt dip.

Nutrition: Cal 124 Fat 2.6 g Carbs 21.6 g Protein 4.4 g

744. Cheesecake Bites

Prep Time: 20 mins
Servings: 12

Cook Time: 2 mins

Ingredients:
- 8 oz. cream cheese, softened
- ½ cup plus two tablespoons sugar, divided
- Four tablespoons heavy cream, divided
- ½ teaspoon vanilla extract
- ½ cup almond flour

Directions: In a stand mixer fitted with the paddle attachment, add cream cheese, ½ cup sugar, two tablespoons heavy cream, and vanilla extract and beat until smooth.
Using a paddle attachment, pour the mixture onto a baking sheet lined with baking paper.
Freeze for about 30 mins.
In a small bowl, place the remaining cream.
In another bowl, add the almond flour and remaining sugar and mix well.
Dip each cheesecake bite into the cream and then top with the flour mixture.
Select the "Air Fry" mode and set the baking time to 2 mins on your oven.
Set the temperature to 300 degrees F.
Place pan in "Air Fry Basket" and place in the oven.

Nutrition: Cal 149 Fat 10.7 g Carbs 11.7 g Protein 2.5 g

745. Chocolate Bites

Prep Time: 15 mins
Servings: 8

Cook Time: 13 mins

Ingredients:
- 2 cups plain flour
- Two tablespoons cocoa powder
- ½ cup icing sugar
- Pinch of ground cinnamon
- One teaspoon vanilla extract
- ¾ cup chilled butter
- ¼ cup chocolate, chopped into eight chunks

Directions: In a bowl, mix the flour, icing sugar, cocoa powder, cinnamon, and vanilla extract.
Cut the butter and mix till a smooth dough forms.
Divide the dough into eight equal-sized balls.
Press one chocolate chunk in the center of each ball and cover with the dough thoroughly.
Place the balls into the baking pan. Select the "Air Fry" mode and set the cook time to 8 mins. Set the temperature at 355 degrees F.
Arrange the pan in "Air Fry Basket" and insert it in the oven.
After 8 mins of cook, set the temperature at 320 degrees F for 5 mins.
Place the baking pan onto the wire rack to cool before serving.

Nutrition: Cal 328 Fat 19.3 g Carbs 35.3 g Protein 4.1 g

746. Blueberry Tacos

Prep Time: 15 mins
Servings: 2

Cook Time: 5 mins

Ingredients:
- Two soft shell tortillas
- Four tablespoons strawberry jelly
- ¼ cup fresh blueberries
- ¼ cup fresh raspberries
- Two tablespoons powdered sugar

Directions: Spread two tablespoons of strawberry jelly over each tortilla. Top each with berries evenly and sprinkle with powdered sugar.
Select the "Air Fry" mode and set the cook time to 5 mins. Set the temperature at 300 degrees F.
Arrange the tortillas in "Air Fry Basket" and insert it in the oven.

Nutrition: Cal 216 Fat 0.8 g Carbs 53.2 g Protein 1.7 g

747. Shortbread Sticks

Prep Time: 15 mins
Servings: 10

Cook Time: 12 mins

Ingredients:

- *1/3 cup caster sugar*
- *1 2/3 cups plain flour*
- *¾ cup butter*

Directions: In a bowl, mix the sugar and flour. Add the butter and mix until a smooth dough forms. Cut the dough into ten equal-sized sticks. With a fork, lightly prick the sticks.
Place the sticks into the lightly greased baking pan.
Select the "Air Fry" mode and set the cook time to 12 mins. Set the temperature at 355 degrees F.
Arrange the pan in "Air Fry Basket" and insert it in the oven.
Place the baking pan to cool for about 5-10 mins.
Now, invert the shortbread sticks onto a wire rack to completely cool.

Nutrition: Cal 223 Fat 14 g Carbs 22.6 g Protein 2.3 g

748. Apple Pastries

Prep Time: 15 mins
Servings: 6

Cook Time: 10 mins

Ingredients:

- *½ of a large apple, peeled, cored, and chopped*
- *One teaspoon fresh orange zest, grated finely*
- *½ tablespoon white sugar*
- *½ teaspoon ground cinnamon*
- *7.05oz. prepared frozen puff pastry*

Directions: In a bowl, mix all ingredients except puff pastry. Cut the pastry into 16 squares.
Place a teaspoon of the apple mixture in the center of each square.
Fold each square into a triangle and press the edges slightly. Then with a fork, press the edges firmly.
Select the "Air Fry" mode and set the cook time to 10 mins. Set the temperature at 390 degrees F.
Arrange the pastries in a greased "Air Fry Basket" and insert it in the oven.

Nutrition: Cal 198 Fat 12.7 g Carbs 18.8 g Protein 2.5 g

749. Cinnamon Toast

Prep Time: 10 mins
Servings: 6

Cook time: 5 mins

Ingredients:

- *2 tsp. pepper*
- *11/2 tsp. vanilla extract*
- *11/2 tsp. cinnamon*
- *½ C. sweetener of choice*
- *1C. coconut oil*
- *12 slices whole-wheat bread*

Directions: Melt coconut oil and mix with sweetener until dissolved. Mix in remaining ingredients minus bread till incorporated.
Spread mixture onto bread, covering all areas.
Pour the coated pieces of bread into the oven basket. Set temperature to 400°F, and set time to 5 mins.
Remove and cut diagonally.

Nutrition: Cal: 124; Fat: 2 g; Protein: 0 g

750. Chocolate Mug Cake

Prep Time: 5 mins
Servings: 3

Cook time: 15 mins

Ingredients:

- *½ cup cocoa powder*
- *½ cup stevia powder*
- *1 cup coconut cream*
- *1 package cream cheese, room temperature*
- *1 tablespoon vanilla extract*
- *1 tablespoons butter*

Directions: Preheat the oven for 5 mins.

In a mixing bowl, combine all ingredients. Use a hand mixer to mix everything until fluffy. Pour into greased mugs. Bake for 15 mins at 350°F.

Place in the fridge to chill before serving.

Nutrition: Cal: 744; Fat: 69.7 g; Protein: 13.9 g

751. Strawberry Cake

Prep Time: 5 mins
Serving: 4

Cook Time: 30 mins

Ingredients:
- ¼ cup butter, melted
- 1 cup powdered erythritol
- 1 teaspoon strawberry extract
- 12 egg whites
- 2 teaspoons cream of tartar
- A pinch of salt

Directions: Preheat the air fryer for 5 mins.

Mix the egg whites and cream of tartar.

Use a hand mixer and whisk until white and fluffy.

Add the rest of the ingredients except for the butter and whisk for another minute.

Pour into a baking dish.

Place in the air fryer basket and cook for 30 mins at 400°F or if a toothpick inserted in the middle comes out clean.

Drizzle with melted butter once cooled.

Nutrition: Cal: 65; Fat: 5 g; Protein: 3.1 g

752. Fried Peaches

Prep Time: 130 mins
Serving: 4

Cook Time: 15 mins

Ingredients:
- 4 ripe peaches (1/2 a peach = 1 serving)
- 1 ½ cups flour
- Salt
- 2 egg yolks
- ¾ cups cold water
- 11/2 tablespoons olive oil
- 2 tablespoons brandy
- 4 egg whites
- Cinnamon

Directions: Combine the flour, egg yolks and salt in a mixing bowl. Stir in the water and then add the brandy. Set the mixture aside for 2 hours and make something for 1 hour and 45 mins.

Boil a large pot of water and cut and X in the bottom of each peach. While the water is boiling, fill another bowl with water and ice. Boil each peach for about a minute and then submerge it in the ice bath. Now the peels should fall off the peach. Beat the egg whites and mix them into the butter mixture. Dip each peach into the mixture to coat it.

Pour the coated peach into the oven basket. Place the basket on the center oven rack of the air fryer. Set the temperature to 360°F and set the time to 10 mins.

Prepare a plate with the cinnamon, roll the peaches in the mixture.

Nutrition: Cal: 306; Fat: 3 g; Protein: 10 g

753. Apple Dumplings

Prep Time: 10 mins
Serving: 4

Cook Time: 25 mins

Ingredients:
- 2 tbsp. melted coconut oil
- 2 puff pastry sheets
- 1 tbsp. brown sugar
- 2 tbsp. raisins
- 2 small apples of choice

Directions: Preheated your Air Fryer to 356 degrees F.

Core and peel apples and mix with raisins and sugar.

Place a bit of apple mixture into puff pastry sheets and brush sides with melted coconut oil.

Cook 25 mins, we were turning halfway through. It will be golden when done.

Nutrition: Cal: 367; Fat: 7 g; Protein: 2 g

754. Apple Pie

Prep Time: 5 mins
Serving: 4

Cook Time: 35 mins

Ingredients:
- ½ teaspoon vanilla extract
- 1 beaten egg
- 1 large apple, chopped
- 1 Pillsbury Refrigerator pie crust
- 1 tablespoon butter
- 1 tablespoon ground cinnamon
- 1 tablespoon raw sugar
- 2 tablespoon sugar
- 2 teaspoons lemon juice
- Baking spray

Directions: Lightly grease baking pan of air fryer oven with cook spray. Spread the pie crust on the bottom of the pan up to the sides.
In a bowl, mix cinnamon, lemon juice, vanilla, sugar, and apples. Pour on top of pie crust.
Top apples with butter slices.
Cover apples with the other pie crust. Pierce with the knife the tops of the pie.
Spread beaten egg on top of crust and sprinkle sugar.
Cover with foil.
For 25 mins, cook at 390°F.
Remove foil cook for 10 mins at 330°F until tops are browned.

Nutrition: Cal: 372; Fat: 19 g; Protein: 4.2 g

755. Air Fryer Chocolate Cake

Prep Time: 5 mins
Serving: 9

Cook Time: 35 mins

Ingredients:
- ½ C. hot water
- 1 tsp. vanilla
- ¼ C. olive oil
- ½ C. almond milk
- 1 egg
- ½ tsp. Salt
- ¾ tsp. Baking soda
- ¾ tsp. baking powder
- ½ C. unsweetened cocoa powder
- 2C. almond flour
- 1C. brown sugar

Directions: Preheat your air fryer oven to 356 degrees F.
Stir all dry ingredients together. Then stir in wet ingredients. Add hot water last.
Pour cake batter into a pan that fits into the fryer. Cover with foil and poke holes into the foil.
Bake 35 mins. Discard foil and then bake another 10 mins.

Nutrition: Cal: 378; Fat: 9 g; Protein: 4 g

756. Banana Chocolate Muffins (Vegan)

Prep time: 5 mins
Servings: 1-2

Cook time: 20 mins

Ingredients:
- 1/3 cup oil
- 1/3 lb. brown sugar
- Three ripe bananas
- ½ lb. flour
- 3 tsp. yeast
- ½ lb. chocolate and hazelnut cream

Directions: Peel the bananas and chop them. Put them in a bowl and cook them with the help of a fork. Add the oil, sugar and stir until everything is integrated.
Add the flour with the yeast sifted and continue stirring until you obtain a homogeneous dough.
Arrange muffin capsules on the plate and fill them with the batter to 2/3 full. Pour 1 tsp of cocoa cream on top and stir with a toothpick to blend well.
Bake and cook the muffins for 20 mins in the air fryer preheated to 360 degrees F until they are done. Remove and cool on a wire rack.

Nutrition: Cal: 133.1 Carbs: 26. 3g Fat: 2.9 g

757. Banana-Choco Brownies

Prep Time: 5 mins
Serving: 12

Cook Time: 30 mins

Ingredients:
- 2 cups almond flour
- 2 teaspoons baking powder
- ½ teaspoon baking powder
- ½ teaspoon baking soda
- ½ teaspoon salt
- 1 over-ripe banana
- 3 large eggs
- ½ teaspoon stevia powder
- ¼ cup of coconut oil
- 1 tablespoon vinegar
- 1/3 cup almond flour
- 1/3 cup cocoa powder

Directions: Preheat the air fryer oven for 5 mins.
Combine all ingredients in a food processor and pulse until well-combined.
Pour into a baking dish that will fit in the air fryer.
Place in the air fryer basket and cook for 30 mins at 350°F or if a toothpick inserted in the middle comes out clean.

Nutrition: Cal: 75; Fat: 6.5 g; Protein: 1.7 g

758. Chocolate Donuts

Prep Time: 5 mins
Serving: 8-10

Cook Time: 20 mins

Ingredients:
- (8-ounce) can jumbo biscuits
- Cook oil
- Chocolate sauce, such as Hershey's

Directions: Separate the biscuit dough into eight biscuits and place them on a flat work surface. Use a small circle cookie cutter to cut a hole in each biscuit center. You can also cut the holes using a knife.
Spray the air fryer basket with cook oil.
Place four donuts in the oven. Do not stack. Spray with cook oil. Set temperature to 350°F. Cook for 4 mins.
Open the air fryer and flip the donuts—Cook for an additional 4 mins.
Remove the cooked donuts from the oven, and then repeat for the remaining four donuts.
Drizzle chocolate sauce over the donuts and enjoy while warm.

Nutrition: Cal: 181; Fat: 98 g; Protein: 3 g

759. Air Fryer Donuts

Prep Time: 5 mins
Serving: 8

Cook Time: 5 mins

Ingredients:
- Pinch of allspice
- 4 tbsp. dark brown sugar
- ½ – 1 tsp. cinnamon
- 1/3 C. granulated sweetener
- 3 tbsp. melted coconut oil
- 1 can of biscuits

Directions: Mix all spice, sugar, sweetener, and cinnamon.
Take out biscuits from can and with a circle cookie cutter, cut holes from centers, and place into the air fryer.
Cook 5 mins at 350 degrees F. As batches are cooked, use a brush to coat with melted coconut oil and dip each into sugar mixture.

Nutrition: Cal: 209; Fat: 4 g; Protein: 0 g

760. Chocolate Soufflé

Prep Time: 5mins
Serving: 2

Cook Time: 14 mins

Ingredients:
- 2 tbsp. Almond flour
- ½ tsp. vanilla
- 3 tbsp. sweetener
- 2 separated eggs
- ¼ C. melted coconut oil
- 3 ounces of semi-sweet chocolate, chopped

Directions: Brush coconut oil and sweetener onto ramekins.
Melt coconut oil and chocolate together.
Beat egg yolks well, adding vanilla and sweetener. Stir in flour and ensure there are no lumps.
Preheat the air fryer oven to 330 degrees F.
Whisk egg whites till they reach peak state and fold them into chocolate mixture.
Pour batter into ramekins and place them into the air fryer oven. Cook 14 mins.
Serve with powdered sugar dusted on top.

Nutrition: Cal: 238; Fat: 6 g; Protein: 1 g; Sugar: 4 g

761. Fried Bananas with Chocolate Sauce

Prep Time: 10 mins
Serving: 2

Cook Time: 10 mins

Ingredients:
- *1 large egg*
- *¼ cup cornstarch*
- *¼ cup plain bread crumbs*
- *3 bananas halved crosswise*
- *Cook oil*
- *Chocolate sauce*

Directions: In a small bowl, beat the egg. In another bowl, place the cornstarch.
Place the breadcrumbs in a third bowl.
Dip the bananas in the cornstarch, then the egg, and then the breadcrumbs.
Spray the air fryer basket with cook oil. Place the bananas in the basket and spray them with cook oil.
Set temperature to 360°F and cook for 5 mins. Open the air fryer and flip the bananas—Cook for an additional 2 mins. Transfer the bananas to plates. Drizzle the chocolate sauce over the bananas and serve.

Nutrition: Cal: 203; Fat: 6 g; Protein: 3 g

762. Chocolate Banana Muffins

Prep Time: 5 mins
Serving: 12

Cook Time: 25 mins

Ingredients:
- *¾ cup whole wheat flour*
- *¾ cup plain flour*
- *¼ cup of cocoa powder*
- *¼ teaspoon baking powder*
- *1 teaspoon baking soda*
- *¼ teaspoon salt*
- *2 large bananas, peeled and mashed*
- *1 cup sugar*
- *1/3 cup canola oil*
- *1egg*
- *½ teaspoon vanilla essence*
- *1 cup mini chocolate chips*

Directions: In a bowl, mix flour, cocoa powder, baking powder, baking soda, and salt.
In another bowl, add bananas, sugar, oil, egg, and vanilla extract and beat till well combined.
Add flour mixture to egg mixture and mix till just combined. Fold in chocolate chips.
Preheat the air fryer oven to 345 degrees F. Grease 12 muffin molds.
Transfer the mixture into prepared muffin molds evenly and cooks for about 20-25 mins.
Remove the Air fryer's muffin molds and keep on a wire rack to cool for about 10 mins. Carefully turn on a wire rack to cool completely before serving.

763. Air Fryer Apple Pies

Prep Time: 10 mins
Serving: 4

Cook Time: 25 mins

Ingredients:
- *4 tbsp butter*
- *6 tbsp brown sugar*
- *1 tsp ground cinnamon*
- *2 medium Granny Smith apples, diced*
- *1 tsp cornstarch*
- *2 tsp cold water*
- *½ (14 oz.) package pastry to get a 9-inch double-crust pie*
- *cook spray*
- *½ tablespoon grapeseed oil*
- *¼ cup powdered sugar*
- *1 tsp milk, or more as required*

Directions: Combine the apples, butter, brown sugar and cinnamon in a skillet. Cook over medium heat for about 5 mins.

Dissolve cornstarch in cold water. Stir into apple mixture and cook until sauce thickens, for about 1 minute. Remove the apple pie filling from the heat and set aside to cool while you prepare the crust.

Unroll the crust on a lightly floured surface and roll out lightly to smooth the surface of the dough. Cut dough into small enough rectangles so that two can fit on the air fryer at the same time. Repeat with the remaining crust until you have eight equal rectangles, rolling back a few pieces of dough if necessary.

Wet with water the outside edges of 4 rectangles and then put some apple filling in the center about ½ inch into the edges. Roll out the rest of the rectangles so that they are slightly more significant than the ones being served. Place them on top of the filling; crimp the edges with a fork to seal. Cut 4 small slits in the top of the cupcakes.

Spray the basket of an air fryer with cook spray. Brush the tops of two tablespoons with grapeseed oil and then move the cupcakes to the basket of the air fryer using a spatula.

Insert the tin and then set the temperature to 385 degrees F. Bake until golden brown, about 8 mins. Remove the cakes to the basket and then repeat with the other two cakes.

Mix the milk powder and sugar in a small bowl. Brush frosting over hot cakes and allow to dry. Drink the pops warm or at room temperature.

764. Air Fryer Churros

Prep Time: 8 mins
Serving: 4

Cook Time: 15 mins

Ingredients:
- ¼ cup butter
- ½ cup milk
- 1 pinch salt
- ½ cup flour
- 2 eggs
- ¼ cup white sugar
- ½ teaspoon ground cinnamon

Directions: Melt the butter in a saucepan over medium-high water. Pour in the milk and then add the salt. Reduce heat to gentle and bring to a boil, always stirring with a wooden spoon. Immediately add the flour all at once. Continue stirring until the mixture comes together.

Remove from heat and let cool for 5-7 mins. Stir in eggs with wooden spoon until choux paste comes together. Spoon dough into a pastry bag fitted with a large star tip-pipe dough pieces directly into the air fryer bowl.

Fry churros in air at 340 degrees F for 5 mins.

Meanwhile, mix the sugar and cinnamon in a small bowl and then pour onto a dish.

Remove the fried churros from the air fryer and roll out of the cinnamon and sugar mixture.

765. Spicy Cardamom Crumb Cake

Prep Time: 10 Mins
Servings: 15

Cook Time: 1 hour 15 mins

Ingredients:

For the Topping:
- 2 cups pecans
- 2 sticks unsalted butter melted
- ¾ cup light brown sugar
- ½ cup granulated sugar
- 2 2/3 cups all-purpose flour
- ½ teaspoon ground cardamom
- ½ teaspoon salt

For the Cake:
- 3 cups all-purpose flour
- ¼ cups sugar
- large eggs
- cup whole milk
- ½ sticks unsalted butter, melted
- teaspoons pure vanilla extract
- ½ teaspoons baking powder
- teaspoon salt

For the Glaze:
- ½ cup confectioners' sugar
- 2 tablespoons unsalted butter, melted
- 2 teaspoons whole milk
- ½ teaspoon pure vanilla extract

Directions: Grease the baking dish with butter.

Add the pecans to the baking dish. Select Bake mode and set the temperature to 350 F and the time to 8 mins.

Remove from oven, chop pecans and set aside.

Combine the melted butter, light brown sugar, granulated sugar, cardamom, flour, chopped nuts and salt in a medium bowl. Mix well.

In another bowl, combine the flour, baking powder, sugar, and salt.

Beat the eggs, milk, melted butter and vanilla in a separate bowl, add this mixture to the dry ingredients and pour this batter into the greased baking dish. Add the layer of walnut crumbs on top.
Select Bake mode and the temperature to 350 F and the time to 55 mins.
Meanwhile, in a separate bowl, whisk together the frosting ingredients and pour over the cooled cake.

Nutrition: 216 cal; 16 g Fat; 17 g Carbs; 1 g Protein

766. Peach Cobbler

Prep Time: 10 Mins   **Cook Time: 50 mins**
Servings: 8

Ingredients:
- 8 fresh peaches, peeled and sliced
- ½ cup packed light brown sugar
- ¼ cup cornstarch
- ½ cup butter, melted
- 1 ¼ cups all-purpose flour
- ½ cup sugar
- 2 tablespoons lemon juice
- 1 teaspoon grated ginger
- 1 teaspoon baking powder
- 1 teaspoon lemon zest
- 2 tablespoons milk
- ½ teaspoon salt

Directions: Prepare a baking pan by greasing it with non-stick cook spray.
Combine the sliced peaches, brown sugar, cornstarch, lemon juice and ginger. Mix well until cornstarch is dissolved. Pour this mixture into the greased baking pan.
In a separate bowl, combine flour, sugar, baking powder, lemon zest and salt. Slowly add milk and butter to this mixture.
Pour this mixture over the peaches in the baking pan.
Select the Bake mode, set the temperature to 350 F and the time to 45 mins.

Nutrition: 54 Cal; 0 g Fat; 12 g Carbs; 1 g Protein

767. Apple Cider Donuts

Prep Time: 10 Mins   **Cook Time: 50 mins**
Servings: 18

Ingredients:
- Two cups apple cider
- Three cups all-purpose flour
- ½ cup packed light brown sugar
- ½ cup cold milk
- One stick unsalted butter, grated
- Two teaspoons baking powder
- One teaspoon ground cinnamon
- One teaspoon ground ginger
- ½ teaspoon baking soda
- ½ teaspoon kosher salt
- ¼ cup all-purpose flour
- 8 tablespoons unsalted butter, melted
- One cup granulated sugar
- One teaspoon ground cinnamon

Directions: Place a pan over medium heat. Add 2 cups apple cider and bring to a boil for about 12 mins. Set aside to cool.
Combine flour, light brown sugar, baking soda, cinnamon, baking powder, ginger and salt in a bowl. Mix well.
Add grated butter to the flour mixture. Mix, make a well in the center and add the apple cider and milk. Mix well to form dough.
Knead the dough for about 5 mins on a floured surface. Shape it into a 9x13-inch rectangle, about ½ an inch thick.
Use a doughnut cutter to cut donuts out of the dough, place them on a baking pan. Refrigerate for 30 mins.
In a bowl, mix cinnamon and granulated sugar. To another bowl, add the melted butter.
Add donuts to the air fry basket. Set the temperature to 375° F and the time to 12 mins. Flip once halfway.
Dip cooked donuts in the melted butter, then in the cinnamon mixture.

Nutrition: 318 Cal; 12.4 g Fat; 49.1 g Carbs; 3.5 g Protein

768. Apple Pudding

Prep Time: 10 Mins   **Cook Time: 40 mins**
Servings: 6

Ingredients:
- 1 cup brown sugar
- 1 cup all-purpose flour
- ½ cup 2% milk
- 2 cups boiling water
- 3 apples, peeled and chopped
- 2 teaspoons baking powder
- ½ teaspoon ground cinnamon
- 2 tablespoons butter, cubed
- ½ teaspoon salt

Directions: In a bowl, combine flour, sugar, baking powder, cinnamon and salt.

Add milk and the apples. Mix well and transfer the mixture to a greased baking pan.

Rub the dough with butter. Add boiling water.

Select the Bake mode, set the temperature to 400° F and the time to 45 mins.

Remove from the oven and set aside to cool for 15 mins. Serve with ice cream.

Nutrition: 291 Cal; 5 g Fat; 61 g Carbs; 3 g Protein

769. Cinnamon Rolls

Prep Time: 10 Mins   **Cook Time: 30 mins**
Servings: 6

Ingredients:
- 1/3 cup packed brown sugar
- 1/3 cup all-purpose flour, for surface
- 8-oz. tube refrigerated Crescent rolls
- 2 tablespoons melted butter, plus more for brushing
- ½ teaspoon ground cinnamon
- A pinch of salt
- 2 oz. cream cheese, softened
- ½ cup powdered sugar
- 1 tablespoon milk

Directions: Line the air fry basket with parchment paper and grease with butter.

Combine butter, brown sugar, cinnamon, salt and mix well in a bowl. Roll out the crescent rolls on a floured surface.

Top the rolls with butter mixture and roll them up, seam the edges. Place the pieces into the air fryer leaving some space between the rolls.

Set the temperature to 350 F and the time to 10 mins.

Meanwhile, combine cream cheese, powdered sugar and milk in a separate bowl. Spread glaze over the cinnamon rolls.

Nutrition: 74 Cal; 2 g Fat; 13 g Carbs; 1 g Protein

770. Lava Cake

Prep Time: 10 Mins   **Cook Time: 20 mins**
Servings: 4

Ingredients:
- 3 ½ oz. unsalted butter
- 3 ½ oz. dark chocolate, chopped
- 2 eggs
- 1 ½ tablespoon self-rising flour
- 3 ½ tablespoons sugar

Directions: Grease and flour 4 oven safe ramekins.

Add chocolate and butter to a microwave safe bowl and melt for 3 mins, stirring frequently to make sure it doesn't burn.

In a separate bowl, whisk the eggs and sugar until frothy. Add melted chocolate mixture.

Add flour and mix well. Pour this into the ramekins. Place them into the air fry basket.

Set the temperature to 375° F and the time to 10 mins.

Let ramekins cool for 3 mins, turn upside down onto.

Nutrition: 244 Cal; 12 g Fat; 13 g Carbs; 21 g Protein

771. Cheesecake Egg Rolls

Prep Time: 10 Mins   **Cook Time: 20 mins**
Servings: 4

Ingredients:
- 1 block (16 oz) cream cheese, at room temperature
- 8 ½ oz. fig jam
- 15 ready-made egg roll wrappers, refrigerated
- 2 tablespoons unsalted butter, melted
- 1 egg, beaten
- 1 tablespoon water
- ¾ cup sugar
- 1 teaspoon ground cinnamon
- 1 tablespoon lemon juice
- 1 teaspoon vanilla extract

Directions: Combine sugar, cream cheese, lemon juice and vanilla extract in an electric mixer. Whip well on medium speed until combined. Add to a pastry bag.

Place egg roll wrapper on the working surface, pipe 2 tablespoons cream cheese at the center, top with 1 tablespoon jam. Brush the edge of the roll with egg and water. Fold and roll the wrap, spray with a cook spray. Add them to the air fry basket. Set the temperature to 370° F and the time to 7 mins.

Meanwhile, combine sugar and cinnamon in a bowl. Brush the cooked egg rolls with butter and sprinkle with cinnamon mix.

Nutrition: 170 Cal; 13 g Fat; 6 g Carbs; 7 g Protein

772. Brazilian Pineapple

Prep Time: 10 Mins   Cook Time: 20 mins
Servings: 4

Ingredients:
- *1 pineapple, peeled, cored and sliced*
- *½ cup brown sugar*
- *2 teaspoons ground cinnamon*
- *3 tablespoons butter, melted*

Directions: Combine brown sugar and cinnamon in a bowl. Set aside.
Place the pineapple slices on a plate, brush with butter and sprinkle with cinnamon mix.
Place the pineapples in the air fryer basket. Set the temperature to 400° F and the time to 10 mins.
Brush with more butter halfway through.

Nutrition: 295 Cal; 8 g Fat; 57 g Carbs; 1 g Protein

773. Chocolate Chunk Walnut Blondies

Prep Time: 10 Mins   Cook Time: 30 mins
Servings: 12

Ingredients:
- *1 cup butter, melted*
- *2 cups packed brown sugar*
- *2 cups all-purpose flour*
- *½ cup ground walnuts*
- *1 cup walnuts, chopped, toasted*
- *1 cup semisweet chocolate chunks*
- *2 eggs*
- *2 teaspoons vanilla extract*
- *1 teaspoon baking powder*
- *1/8 teaspoon baking soda*
- *A pinch of salt*

Directions: Grease a baking dish. Combine butter, brown sugar and vanilla in a bowl.
Gradually add eggs, one at a time. In a separate bowl combine flour, ground walnuts, baking powder, baking soda and salt.
Fold in the chopped walnuts and chocolate chunks. Spread on the prepared dish.
Select the Bake mode, set the temperature to 350 F and the time to 35 mins.
Remove from the oven and place on the cooling rack. Slice into bars.

Nutrition: 260 Cal; 15 g Fat; 32 g Carbs; 3 g Protein

774. Mexican Brownies

Prep Time: 10 Mins   Cook Time: 30 mins
Servings: 24

Ingredients
- *1 package fudge brownie mix*
- *¾ cup dark chocolate chips*
- *2 teaspoons ground cinnamon*
- *1 teaspoon ground ancho chili pepper*
- *½ cup canola oil*
- *¼ cup water*
- *2 eggs*

Directions: Combine the brownie mix, cinnamon and chili pepper. Add the mix to a glass jar and top with chocolate chips.
Grease a baking dish. In a separate bowl whisk eggs, oil, and water. Add the chocolate mix and stir thoroughly.
Spread batter into the greased baking dish.
Select the Bake mode, set the temperature to 350° F and the time to 25 mins.

Nutrition: 173 Cal; 10 g Fat; 21 g Carbs; 2 g Protein

775. Chocolate Chip Cookie Blondies

Prep Time: 10 Mins
Servings: 4

Cook Time: 35 mins

Ingredients:
- 2 cups all-purpose flour
- ¾ cup packed brown sugar
- ¾ cup sugar
- 1 cup semisweet chocolate chips
- 1 teaspoon baking soda
- 1 teaspoon salt
- ¾ cup canola oil
- 2 eggs
- 1 teaspoon vanilla extract

Directions: Combine baking soda, flour, and salt in a bowl. Add sugars and chocolate chips. Grease a baking dish with non-stick cook spray.
In a separate bowl combine the oil, eggs, and vanilla. Add the flour mix on top, mix well. Spoon the mixture onto the baking dish in the shape of cookies.
Select the Bake mode, set the temperature to 350° F and the time to 20 mins.

Nutrition: 190 Cal; 10 g Fat; 26 g Carbs; 2 g Protein

776. Blueberry Bars

Prep Time: 10 Mins
Servings: 24

Cook Time: 40 mins

Ingredients:
- 1 1/3 cups butter, softened
- 2/3 cup sugar
- ½ teaspoon vanilla extract
- 3 ¾ cups all-purpose flour
- 1 egg
- ¼ teaspoon salt
- 3 cups blueberries
- 1 cup sugar
- 3 tablespoons cornstarch

Directions: In a bowl, mix cream butter, sugar and salt and beat until light and fluffy.
Add in the egg and vanilla and beat it well. Gradually add in the flour, mix well, shape into a ball, wrap the dough in a plastic wrap and refrigerate for 2-8 hours.
Grease a baking dish with non-stick cook spray.
Place a sauce dish over medium heat. Add blueberries, sugar and cornstarch. Bring to a boil, stir until the sauce thickens and set aside to cool.
Place dough on a working surface and roll out. Shape into a rectangle and freeze for 10 mins.
Place one rectangle onto the baking dish and add the filing on top. Cut the remaining rectangle into strips and place over filling.
Select the Bake mode, set the temperature to 375° F and the time to 35 mins.
Remove from the oven and set aside to cool.

Nutrition: 233 Cal; 11 g Fat; 32 g Carbs; 3 g Protein

777. Potato Cream Cheese Bars

Prep Time: 10 Mins
Servings: 24

Cook Time: 50 mins

Ingredients:
- 1 package white cake mix
- 1 cup chopped pecans, toasted
- ½ cup cold butter, cubed
- 8 oz. cream cheese, softened
- ½ cup sugar
- 3 eggs, divided
- 14 oz. sweetened condensed milk, divided
- 3 cups sweet potatoes, cooked and mashed
- 2 teaspoons pumpkin pie spice

Directions: Grease a baking pan with non-stick cook spray.
In a bowl combine cake mix, pecans and butter. Transfer the mix to the baking dish.
In a separate bowl mix well the cream cheese, sugar, 1 egg and 2 tablespoons milk.
Mix together potatoes, 2 eggs, remaining milk and pie spice. Pour this mixture on top of the pecan mix. Top with a dollop of cream cheese.
Select the Bake mode, set the temperature to 350° F and the time to 45 mins.
Remove from the oven and let it cool. Cut into bars.

Nutrition: 304 Cal; 15 g Fat; 40 g Carbs; 5 g Protein

778. Raspberry Crumble Cake

Prep Time: 10 Mins
Servings: 12

Cook Time: 40 mins

Ingredients:
- 2 cups raspberries, frozen
- ¼ cup butter, softened
- ¾ cup sugar
- ¾ cup 2% milk
- 2 ¼ cups all-purpose flour
- 2 eggs, room temperature
- 2 teaspoons baking powder
- 1 teaspoon salt
- 3 egg whites
- 1 cup sugar
- ½ cup boiling water
- 1/3 cup almonds, sliced
- 1/8 teaspoon cream of tartar
- ¼ teaspoon almond extract

Directions: Grease a baking dish with non-stick cook spray. Whisk the cream butter and sugar in a bowl until fluffy. Add eggs and continue to whisk.
In a separate bowl, mix flour, baking powder and salt. Add the cream mixture and milk, mix well.
Fold in frozen berries and spread in the baking dish.
Select the Bake mode, set the temperature to 350 F and the time to 30 mins.
Combine egg whites, sugar, cream of tartar and place in a heatproof bowl. Place bowl over boiling water. Remove from heat and beat it on high speed until stiff peaks form.
Fold in almond extract, spread frosting over the cake. Sprinkle with almonds.

Nutrition: 266 Cal; 5 g Fat; 51 g Carbs; 5 g Protein

779. Carrot Cake

Prep Time: 10 Mins
Servings: 12

Cook Time: 50 mins

Ingredients:
- 2 cups all-purpose flour
- 2 cups sugar
- 1 ½ cups canola oil
- 2 cups carrots, grated
- 1 cup pineapple, crushed
- 1 cup sweetened coconut, shredded
- 1 cup nuts, chopped
- 3 eggs
- 2 teaspoons ground cinnamon
- 1 teaspoon baking soda
- 1 teaspoon vanilla extract
- A pinch of salt
- 6 oz. cream cheese, softened
- 3 cups confectioners' sugar
- 6 tablespoons butter, softened
- 1 teaspoon vanilla extract

Directions: Combine flour, sugar, cinnamon, baking soda, salt, eggs, carrots and vanilla in a bowl. Stir well.
Fold in the pineapple, coconut and chopped nuts. Pour the mix into a baking pan greased with non-stick cook spray.
Select the Bake mode, set the temperature to 350 F and the time to 60 mins.
Meanwhile, beat the cream cheese and butter. Add confectioner's sugar and vanilla and mix until smooth. Spread this frost on top of the cooled cake.

Nutrition: 819 Cal; 49 g Fat; 91 g Carbs; 8 g Protein

780. Pineapple Orange Cake

Prep Time: 10 Mins
Servings: 15

Cook Time: 25 mins

Ingredients:
- 1 package yellow cake mix
- 11 oz. mandarin oranges, undrained
- 4 egg whites
- ½ cup unsweetened applesauce
- 20 oz. crushed pineapple, undrained
- 1 oz. sugar-free instant vanilla pudding mix
- 8 oz. reduced-fat whipped topping

Directions: Mix oranges, egg whites and applesauce on low speed using the hand mixer in a bowl. Pour dough in a baking dish greased with non-stick cook spray.
Place in the oven and bake for ½ an hour at 350 degrees F.
In a separate bowl mix the toppings ingredients and spread over the cooled cake.
Place cake in refrigerator for 60 mins.

Nutrition: 231 Cal; 5 g Fat; 43 g Carbs; 3 g Protein

781. Chocolate Strawberry Cobbler

Prep Time: 10 Mins
Servings: 12

Cook Time: 35 mins

Ingredients:
- 1 cup butter, cubed, melted
- 1 ½ cups self-rising flour
- 2 ¼ cups sugar, divided
- ¾ cup 2% milk
- 1/3 cup baking cocoa
- 4 cups fresh strawberries, quartered
- 2 cups boiling water
- Whipped cream
- 1 teaspoon vanilla extract

Directions: Add butter to a baking dish to grease it.
In a separate bowl, combine flour, 1 cup sugar, milk and vanilla. Mix well.
Combine cocoa and remaining sugar in a separate bowl.
Sprinkle the baking dish with cocoa mixture. Pour boiling water on top.
Select the Bake mode, set the temperature to 350° F and the time to 40 mins.
Set aside to cool for 10 mins. Serve the cake with whipped cream.

Nutrition: 368 Cal; 16 g Fat; 55 g Carbs; 3 g Protein

782. Leches Cake

Prep Time: 10 Mins
Servings: 20

Cook Time: 30 mins

Ingredients:
- 1 package yellow cake mix
- 3 eggs
- 2/3 cup 2% milk
- ½ cup butter, softened
- 1 teaspoon vanilla extract
- 14 oz. sweetened condensed milk
- 12 oz. evaporated milk
- 1 cup heavy whipping cream
- 1 cup heavy whipping cream
- 3 tablespoons confectioners' sugar
- 1 teaspoon vanilla extract

Directions: Grease a baking dish with cook spray.
Mix cake mix, eggs, milk, butter and vanilla in a large bowl, beat with a hand mixer on low speed for ½ a minute. Beat on medium for 2 more mins.
Select the Bake mode, set the temperature to 350 F and the time to 35 mins.
Remove from the oven and let it cool for 20 mins.
Poke holes in the cake, mix the topping ingredients and slowly pour it over the cake, filling the holes. Refrigerate the cake for 4-8 hours.
Beat cream in a bowl until thick. Add confectioners' sugar and vanilla. Beat until soft peaks form. Spread the frostin over the cake.

Nutrition: 343 Cal; 20 g Fat; 36 g Carbs; 6 g Protein

783. Caramel Apple Crisp

Prep Time: 10 Mins
Servings: 12

Cook Time: 45 mins

Ingredients:
- 3 cups old-fashioned oats
- 2 cups all-purpose flour
- 1 ½ cups packed brown sugar
- 1 cup butter, cold, cubed
- 8 cups apples, peeled and sliced
- 14 oz. caramels, halved
- 1 cup apple cider
- 1 teaspoon ground cinnamon

Directions: Grease the baking pan with non-stick cook spray.
Combine oats, flour, brown sugar, cinnamon, butter in a bowl and mix well. Press the dough into the baking pan.
Layer half of each of the following ingredients on top: apples, caramel, remaining oats.
Repeat layers and drizzle with ½ cup cider.
Select the Bake mode, set the temperature to 350° F and the time to 30 mins.
Drizzle with the remaining cider and continue to bake for 20 mins. Remove from the oven.

Nutrition: 564 Cal; 20 g Fat; 94 g Carbs; 7 g Protein

784. Gingerbread with Lemon Cream

Prep Time: 10 Mins
Servings: 20

Cook Time: 35 mins

Ingredients:
- 1 cup shortening
- 1 cup sugar
- 1 cup molasses
- 2 eggs
- 3 cups all-purpose flour
- ½ teaspoons baking soda
- 1 teaspoon ground ginger

- 1 teaspoon ground cinnamon
- 1 cup hot water
- A pinch of salt
- ½ cup sugar
- 1 cup half-and-half cream
- 2 large egg yolks, beaten
- 2 teaspoons cornstarch

- 2 tablespoons butter
- 4 tablespoons lemon juice
- 1 teaspoon grated lemon zest
- 1 dash nutmeg
- 1 dash salt

Directions: Grease a baking dish. Combine shortening, sugar, molasses and eggs in a bowl and set aside.
Combine flour, baking powder, ginger, baking soda, cinnamon and salt. Stir well in a separate bowl.
Add the flour mixture to the molasses mix alternating with hot water, stir until dough is formed. Place the dough on the baking pan.
Select the Bake mode, set the temperature to 350° F and the time to 40 mins.
Meanwhile place a small sauce pan over medium high heat, add the lemon sauce ingredients except for egg yolks, butter, lemon juice and zest to the sauce pan. Cook until thickened, remove from heat.
Add a bit of the hot filling to the egg yolks, return the mix to the pan and stir well.
Bring to a boil and cook for 2 mins. Remove from heat. Add in butter, lemon juice and zest.
Serve cake with lemon cream.

Nutrition: 283 Cal; 12 g Fat; 41 g Carbs; 3 g Protein

785. Tiramisu Cheesecake

Prep Time: 10 Mins
Servings: 12

Cook Time: 40 mins

Ingredients:
- 32 oz. cream cheese, softened
- 12 oz. vanilla wafers
- 1 cup sugar

- 1 cup sour cream
- 5 teaspoons instant coffee
- 3 tablespoons hot water

- 4 eggs, beaten
- 1 cup whipped cream topping
- 1 tablespoon cocoa powder

Directions: Grease a baking dish with non-stick cook spray. Dissolve 2 teaspoons coffee granules in 2 tablespoons hot water in a bowl.
Layer half wafers at the bottom of the baking pan, brush with 1 tablespoon of coffee mix.
Beat sour cream cheese and sugar until smooth. Add eggs and continue to beat on low speed. Set aside half of the filling.
Dissolve remaining coffee granules in the remaining water, add it to half of the filling. Spread the filling over wafers.
Layer the remaining wafers on top, brush with coffee mix and spread the other half of the filling on top.
Select the Bake mode, set the temperature to 325° F and the time to 45 mins.
Set aside to cool. Spread whipped topping on top and slice.

Nutrition: 536 Cal; 37 g Fat; 43 g Carbs; 10 g Protein

786. Pumpkin Cheesecake

Prep Time: 10 Mins
Servings: 24

Cook Time: 45 mins

Ingredients:
- 1 ½ cups gingersnaps, crushed
- ¼ cup butter, melted
- 40 oz. cream cheese, softened
- 1 cup sugar

- 15 oz. solid-pack pumpkin
- 1 teaspoon ground cinnamon
- 1 teaspoon vanilla extract
- 5 eggs, beaten

- 1 pinch ground nutmeg
- Maple syrup

Directions: Grease a baking pan with non-stick cook spray.
Combine gingersnaps crumbs and butter in a bowl, press this mix into the bottom of the baking pan.
Beat cream cheese and sugar in another separate bowl until smooth with a hand mixer.
Add pumpkin, cinnamon, vanilla and eggs. Beat on low speed. Pour this mix over the crust and sprinkle with nutmeg.

Select the Bake mode, set the temperature to 350 F and the time to 45 mins. Slice the cake.

Nutrition: 276 Cal; 20 g Fat; 20 g Carbs; 5 g Protein

787. Cinnamon Bread Pudding

Prep Time: 10 Mins
Servings: 2

Cook Time: 35 mins

Ingredients:
- *1 cup cinnamon-raisin bread, cubed*
- *1 egg*
- *2/3 cup 2% milk*
- *1/3 cup raisins*
- *3 tablespoons brown sugar*
- *1 tablespoon butter, melted*
- *½ teaspoon ground cinnamon*
- *¼ teaspoon ground nutmeg*
- *A pinch of salt*

Directions: Grease a baking pan with non-stick cook spray.
Place bread cubes into the baking pan. Combine egg, milk, brown sugar, butter, cinnamon, nutmeg and salt in a bowl. Mix well. Add in the raisins, pour the mixture over the cubed bread, set aside for 15 mins.
Select the Bake mode, set the temperature to 350° F and the time to 40 mins.

Nutrition: 337 Cal; 11 g Fat; 54 g Carbs; 9 g Protein

788. Chocolate Croissant Pudding

Prep Time: 10 Mins
Servings: 15

Cook Time: 1 hour

Ingredients:
- *6 croissants, at least 1 day old*
- *1 cup semisweet chocolate chips*
- *5 eggs*
- *12 egg yolks*
- *5 cups half-and-half cream*
- *1 ½ cups sugar*
- *1 ½ teaspoons vanilla extract*
- *1 tablespoon coffee liqueur*

Directions: Grease a baking dish. Arrange croissant bottoms in the baking pan, sprinkle with chocolate chips and place croissant tops on top.
Whisk together the eggs, egg yolks, cream, sugar, coffee liqueur and vanilla. Pour the mix over croissants, set aside for 15 mins.
Select the Bake mode, set the temperature to 350 F and the time to 60 mins.
Set aside to cool.

Nutrition: 400 Cal; 21 g Fat; 41 g Carbs; 9 g Protein

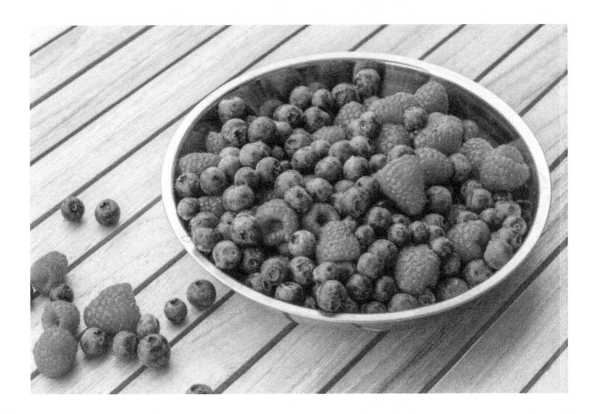

789. Cocoa and Coconut Bars (Vegan)

Prep time: 10 mins   **Cook time: 14 mins**
Servings: 12

Ingredients:

- 6 ounces coconut oil, melted
- Three tbsp. Flax meal combined with three tbsp. water
- 3 ounces of cocoa powder
- Two tsp. vanilla
- ½ tsp. baking powder
- 4 ounces coconut cream
- Five tbsp. coconut sugar

Directions: In a blender, mix the flax meal with oil, vanilla, cream, cocoa powder, baking powder, and sugar and pulse. Pour this into a lined baking dish that fits your air fryer, introduce in the fryer at 320 degrees F, bake for 14 mins, slice into rectangles and serve.

Nutrition: Cal 178 Fat 14 g Carbs 12 g Protein 5 g

790. Vanilla Cake

Prep time: 10 mins   **Cook time: 25 mins**
Servings: 12

Ingredients:

- Six tbsp. black tea powder
- 2 cups almond milk, heated
- 2 cups of coconut sugar
- Three tbsp. Flax meal combined with three tbsp. water
- Two tsp. vanilla extract
- ½ cup of vegetable oil
- Three and ½ cups whole wheat flour
- One tsp. baking soda
- Three tsp. baking powder

Directions: In a bowl, mix heated milk with tea powder, stir and leave aside for now.

In another bowl, mix the oil with sugar, baking powder, flax meal, vanilla extract, baking soda and flour.

Add tea and milk mix, stir well and pour into a greased cake pan.

Introduce in the fryer, cook at 330 degrees F for 25 mins, leave aside to cool down, slice and serve it.

Nutrition: Cal 180 Fat 4 g Carbs 6 g Protein 2 g

791. Vegan Apple Cupcakes

Prep time: 10 mins
Servings: 4

Cook time: 20 mins

Ingredients:
- Four tbsp. vegetable oil
- Three tbsp. Flax meal combined with three tbsp. water
- ½ cup pure applesauce
- Two tsp. cinnamon powder
- One tsp. vanilla extract
- One apple, cored and chopped
- Four tsp. maple syrup
- ¾ cup whole wheat flour
- ½ tsp. baking powder

Directions: Heat a pan put the vegetable oil over medium heat, add flax meal, applesauce, vanilla, maple syrup, stir, take off the heat and cool down.

Add flour, cinnamon, baking powder and apples, whisk, pour into a cupcake pan, introduce in your air fryer at 350 degrees F and bake for 20 mins.

Nutrition: Cal 200 Fat 3 g Carbs 5 g Protein 4 g

792. Vegan Orange Bread and Almonds

Prep time: 20 mins
Servings: 8

Cook time: 40 mins

Ingredients:
- One orange, peeled and sliced
- Juice of 2 oranges
- Three tbsp. vegetable oil
- Two tbsp. flax meal combined with two tbsp. water
- ¾ cup coconut sugar+ 2 tbsp.
- ¾ cup whole wheat flour
- ¾ cup almonds, ground

Directions: Grease a loaf pan with some oil, sprinkle two tbsp. of sugar and arrange orange slices on the bottom.

In a bowl, mix the oil with ¾ cup sugar, almonds, flour and orange juice, stir, spoon this over orange slices, place the pan in your air fryer and cook at 360 degrees F for 40 mins.

Nutrition: Cal 202 Fat 3 g Carbs 6 g Protein 6 g

793. Vegan Tangerine Cake

Prep time: 10 mins
Servings: 8

Cook time: 20 mins

Ingredients:
- ¾ cup of coconut sugar
- 2 cups whole wheat flour
- ¼ cup olive oil
- ½ cup almond milk
- One tsp. cider vinegar
- ½ tsp. vanilla extract
- Juice and zest of 2 lemons
- Juice and zest of 1 tangerine

Directions: In a prepared bowl, mix flour with sugar and stir.

In another bowl, mix oil with milk, lemon juice and zest, tangerine zest, flour, vinegar, vanilla extract, and whisk very well, pour this into a cake pan, introduce in the fryer and cook at 360 degrees F for 20 mins.

Nutrition: Cal 210 Fat 1 g Carbs 6 g Protein 4 g

794. Maple Tomato Bread (Vegan)

Prep time: 10 mins
Servings: 4

Cook time: 30 mins

Ingredients:

- One and ½ cups whole wheat flour
- One tsp. cinnamon powder
- One tsp. baking powder
- One tsp. baking soda
- ¾ cup maple syrup
- One cup tomatoes, chopped
- ½ cup olive oil
- Two tbsp. apple cider vinegar

Directions: In a bowl, mix flour with baking powder, cinnamon, maple syrup, and baking soda, and stir well.
In another bowl, mix tomatoes with olive oil and vinegar and mix well.
Combine the two mixtures, stir well, pour into a greased loaf pan, introduce in the fryer and cook at 360 degrees F for 30 mins.
Leave the cake to cool down, slice and serve.

Nutrition: Cal 203 Fat 2 g Carbs 12 g Protein 4 g

795. Vegan Lemon Squares

Prep time: 10 mins
Servings: 6

Cook time: 30 mins

Ingredients:

- One cup whole wheat flour
- ½ cup of vegetable oil
- One and ¼ cups of coconut sugar
- One medium banana
- Two tsp. lemon peel, grated
- Two tbsp. lemon juice
- Two tbsp. Flax meal combined with two tbsp. water
- ½ tsp. baking powder

Directions: In a bowl, mix flour with ¼ cup sugar and oil, stir well, press on the bottom of a pan, introduce in the fryer and bake at 350 degrees F for 14 mins.
In another prepared bowl, mix the rest of the sugar with lemon juice, lemon peel, banana, baking powder, stir using your mixer and spread over baked crust.
Bake for 15 mins more, leave aside to cool down, cut into medium squares and serve cold.

Nutrition: Cal 140 Fat 4 g Carbs 12 g Protein 1 g

796. Dates and Cashew Sticks (Vegan)

Prep time: 10 mins
Servings: 6

Cook time: 15 mins

Ingredients:

- 1/3 cup stevia
- ¼ cup almond meal
- One tbsp. almond butter
- One and ½ cups cashews, chopped
- Four dates, chopped
- ¾ cup coconut, shredded
- One tbsp. chia seeds

Directions: In a bowl, mix stevia with almond meal, coconut, almond butter, cashews, dates and chia seeds and stir well again.
Spread this on a lined baking pan, press well, introduce in the fryer and cook at 300 degrees F for 15 mins.
Leave the mix to cool down, cut into medium sticks and serve.

Nutrition: Cal 162 Fat 4 g Carbs 5 g Protein 6 g

797. Vegan Grape Pudding

Prep time: 10 mins
Servings: 6

Cook time: 40 mins

Ingredients:

1 cup grapes curd
3 cups grapes
Three and ½ ounces maple syrup

Three tbsp. Flax meal combined with three tbsp. water
2 ounces coconut butter, melted

Three and ½ ounces of almond milk
½ cup almond flour
½ tsp. baking powder

Directions: In a bowl, mix half of the fruit curd with the grapes, stir and divide into six heatproof ramekins.
In a prepared bowl, mix the flax meal with maple syrup, melted coconut butter, the rest of the curd, baking powder, milk and flour and stir well.
Divide this into the ramekins and introduce in the fryer and cook at 200 degrees F for 40 mins.

Nutrition: Cal 230 Fat 22 g Carbs 17 g Protein 8 g

798. Pumpkin and Coconut Seeds Bars (Vegan)

Prep time: 10 mins
Servings: 4

Cook time: 35 mins

Ingredients:

- 1 cup coconut, shredded
- ½ cup almonds
- ½ cup pecans, chopped

- Two tbsp. coconut sugar
- ½ cup pumpkin seeds
- ½ cup sunflower seeds

- Two tbsp. sunflower oil
- One tsp. nutmeg, ground
- One tsp. pumpkin pie spice

Directions:
In a bowl, mix almonds and pecans with pumpkin seeds, coconut, sunflower seeds, nutmeg and pie spice and mix well.
Heat a pan put the sunflower oil over medium heat, add sugar, stir well, pour this over nuts and coconut mix and stir well.
Spread this on a lined baking pan, introduce in your air fryer and cook at 300 degrees F and bake for 25 mins.

Nutrition: Cal 252 Fat 7g Carbs 12 g Protein 7 g

799. Vegan Cinnamon Bananas

Prep time: 10 mins
Servings: 4

Cook time: 15 mins

Ingredients:

- Three tbsp. coconut butter
- Two tbsp. flax meal combined with two tbsp. water

- Eight bananas, peeled and halved
- ½ cup of cornflour
- Three tbsp. cinnamon powder

- 1 cup vegan breadcrumbs

Directions: Heat a pan with the butter over medium-high heat, add breadcrumbs, stir and cook for 4 mins and then transfer to a bowl.
Roll each banana in flour, flax meal and breadcrumbs mix.
Arrange bananas in your air fryer's basket, dust with cinnamon sugar and cook at 280 degrees F for 10 mins.

Nutrition: Cal 214 Fat 1 g Carbs 12 g Protein 4 g

800. Coffee Pudding

Prep time: 10 mins
Servings: 4

Cook time: 10 mins

Ingredients:

- 4 ounces coconut butter
- 4 ounces dark vegan chocolate, chopped
- Juice of ½ orange
- One tsp. baking powder
- 2 ounces whole wheat flour
- ½ tsp. instant coffee
- Two tbsp. Flax meal combined with two tbsp. water
- 2 ounces of coconut sugar

Directions: Heat a pan with the coconut butter over medium heat, add chocolate and orange juice, stir well and take off the heat. In a bowl, mix sugar with instant coffee and flax meal, beat using your mixer, add chocolate mix, salt, baking powder, and flour. Pour this into a greased pan, introduce in your air fryer, cook at 360 degrees F for about 10 mins, divide between plates and serve.

Nutrition: Cal 189 Fat 6 g Carbs 14 g Protein 3 g

801. Vegan Blueberry Cake

Prep time: 10 mins
Servings: 6

Cook time: 30 mins

Ingredients:

- ½ cup whole wheat flour
- ¼ tsp. baking powder
- ¼ tsp. stevia
- ¼ cup blueberries
- 1/3 cup almond milk
- One tsp. olive oil
- One tsp. flaxseed, ground
- ½ tsp. lemon zest, grated
- ¼ tsp. vanilla extract
- ¼ tsp. lemon extract
- Cook spray

Directions: In a bowl, mix flour with baking powder, milk, oil, flaxseeds, lemon zest, stevia, blueberries, vanilla extract and lemon extract and whisk well.
Spray a cake pan with cook spray, line it with parchment paper, pour cake batter, introduce in the fryer and cook at 350 degrees F for 30 mins.

Nutrition: Cal 210 Fat 4 g Carbs 10 g Protein 4 g

802. Peach Cinnamon Cobbler

Prep time: 10 mins
Servings: 4

Cook time: 30 mins

Ingredients:

- 4 cups peaches, peeled and sliced
- ¼ cup of coconut sugar
- ½ tsp. cinnamon powder
- One and ½ cups vegan crackers, crushed
- ¼ cup stevia
- ¼ tsp. nutmeg, ground
- ½ cup almond milk
- One tsp. vanilla extract
- Cook spray

Directions: In a bowl, mix peaches with coconut sugar and cinnamon and stir.
In a separate bowl, mix crackers with stevia, nutmeg, almond milk and vanilla extract and stir.
Spray a pie pan with cook spray and spread peaches on the bottom.
Add crackers mix, spread, introduce into the fryer and cook at 350 degrees F for 30 mins

Nutrition: Cal 201 Fat 4 g Carbs 7 g Protein 3 g

Conversion Tables

Volume

Imperial	Metric	Imperial	Metric
1 tbsp	15ml	1 pint	570 ml
2 fl oz	55 ml	1 ¼ pints	725 ml
3 fl oz	75 ml	1 ¾ pints	1 liter
5 fl oz (¼ pint)	150 ml	2 pints	1.2 liters
10 fl oz (½ pint)	275 ml	2½ pints	1.5 liters
		4 pints	2.25 liters

Weight

Imperial	Metric	Imperial	Metric	Imperial	Metric
½ oz	10 g	4 oz	110 g	10 oz	275 g
¾ oz	20 g	4½ oz	125 g	12 oz	350 g
1 oz	25 g	5 oz	150 g	1 lb.	450 g
1½ oz	40 g	6 oz	175 g	1 lb. 8 oz	700 g
2 oz	50 g	7 oz	200 g	2 lb.	900 g
2½ oz	60 g	8 oz	225 g	3 lb.	1.35 kg
3 oz	75 g	9 oz	250 g		

Oven temperatures

Gas Mark	Fahrenheit	Celsius	Gas Mark	Fahrenheit	Celsius
1/4	225	110	4	350	180
1/2	250	130	5	375	190
1	275	140	6	400	200
2	300	150	7	425	220
3	325	170	8	450	230
			9	475	240

Metric cups conversion

Cups	Imperial	Metric
1 cup flour	5oz	150g
1 cup caster or granulated sugar	8oz	225g
1 cup soft brown sugar	6oz	175g
1 cup soft butter/margarine	8oz	225g
1 cup sultanas/raisins	7oz	200g
1 cup currants	5oz	150g
1 cup ground almonds	4oz	110g
1 cup oats	4oz	110g
1 cup golden syrup/honey	12oz	350g
1 cup uncooked rice	7oz	200g
1 cup grated cheese	4oz	110g
1 stick butter	4oz	110g
¼ cup liquid (water, milk, oil etc.)	4 tablespoons	60ml
½ cup liquid (water, milk, oil etc.)	¼ pint	125ml
1 cup liquid (water, milk, oil etc.)	½ pint	250ml

INDEX:

3-Ingredients: Banana Bread	32
Air Fried Asparagus	194
Air Fried Beef Schnitzel	150
Air Fried Blackened Chicken Breast	112
Air Fried Brussels Sprouts	194
Air Fried Cajun Salmon	164
Air Fried Carrots, Squash & Zucchini	195
Air Fried Cheesy Chicken Omelet	64
Air Fried Chicken Fajitas	111
Air Fried Empanadas	152
Air Fried Fish Fillet	158
Air Fried Kale Chips	195
Air Fried Maple Chicken Thighs	109
Air Fried Shrimp with Chili-Greek Yogurt Sauce	167
Air Fried Steak with Asparagus	151
Air Fry Catfish	158
Air Fry Rib-Eye Steak	153
Air Fry Salmon	182
Air Fryer Apple Fritter	266
Air Fryer Apple Pies	275
Air Fryer Avocado Fries	60
Air Fryer Bacon-Wrapped Jalapeno Poppers	59
Air Fryer Blueberry Muffins Recipe	264
Air Fryer Breaded Pork Chops	86
Air Fryer Breakfast Toad-in-the-Hole Tarts	64
Air Fryer Brown Rice Chicken Fried	114
Air Fryer Buffalo Cauliflower	53
Air Fryer Buffalo Cauliflower	57
Air Fryer Chicken & Broccoli	108
Air Fryer Chicken Nuggets	54
Air Fryer Chocolate Cake	273
Air Fryer Churros	276
Air Fryer Cookies	266
Air Fryer Crab Cakes	167
Air Fryer Crisp Egg Cups	61
Air Fryer Delicata Squash	56
Air Fryer Donuts	274
Air Fryer Egg Rolls	53
Air Fryer Fish & Chips	162
Air Fryer Hamburgers	152
Air Fryer Kale Chips	57
Air Fryer Lemon Cod	161

Air Fryer Lemon Slice & Bake Cookies	265
Air Fryer Lemon-Garlic Tofu	61
Air Fryer Meatloaf	151
Air Fryer Mini Pizza	53
Air Fryer Nuts	52
Air Fryer Olives	52
Air Fryer Onion Rings	55
Air Fryer Pork Chop & Broccoli	87
Air Fryer Roasted Corn	56
Air Fryer Salmon	171
Air Fryer Salmon (2nd Version)	188
Air Fryer Salmon Fillets	161
Air Fryer Salmon Patties	188
Air Fryer Salmon with Maple Soy Glaze	164
Air Fryer Shrimp Scampi	164
Air Fryer Spanakopita Bites	55
Air Fryer Spicy Chickpeas	65
Air Fryer Steak Kabobs with Vegetables	152
Air Fryer Sushi Roll	168
Air Fryer Sweet Potato Fries	57
Air Fryer Tasty Egg Rolls	86
Air Fryer Tuna Patties	167
Air Fryer Walnuts	65
Air-Fried British Breakfast	18
Air-Fried Crumbed Fish	163
Air-Fried Fish Nuggets	162
Air-Fried Lemon and Olive Chicken	107
Air-Fried Spinach Frittata	56
Allspice Chicken Wings	66
Almond Asparagus	197
Almond Flour Coco-Milk Battered Chicken	117
Almond-Crusted Chicken	118
Apple Bread	32
Apple Chips	65
Apple Cider Donuts	277
Apple Cider Vinegar Donuts	268
Apple Dumplings	272
Apple Pastries	271
Apple Pie	273
Apple Pudding	277
Artichokes Dish	232
Artichokes with Oregano	247

Asparagus and Prosciutto	201		Basil Chicken Bites	90
Asparagus Frittata	18		Basil Crackers	67
Asparagus Frittata	59		Basil Pesto Chicken	119
Avocado Chips	65		Basil Tomatoes	202
Avocado Egg Rolls	60		Basil-Garlic Breaded Chicken Bake	119
Avocado Rolls	66		Basil-Parmesan Crusted Salmon	160
Baby Potatoes	198		BBQ Chicken Wings	119
Bacon and Garlic Pizzas	32		BBQ Spicy Chicken Wings	120
Bacon Chicken Lasagna	118		Bean Burger	68
Bacon Shrimps	186		Bean Dish	102
Bacon Wrapped Shrimp	85		Bean Soup	261
Bacon-Wrapped Shrimp	171		Beef and Pasta Casserole	157
Bagels	22		Beef Casserole	157
Baguette Bread	66		Beef in Almond and Eggs Crust	157
Baked Almonds	67		Beef Roast in Worcestershire-Rosemary	155
Baked Bread	33		Beef Soup	261
Baked Chicken	120		Beef with Honey and Mustard	156
Baked Chicken & Potatoes	118		Beefsteak with Olives And Capers	153
Baked Chicken Breasts	146		Beet Salad	202
Baked Egg Tomato	199		Beet Salad and Parsley	202
Baked Eggplant with Marinara and Cheese	198		Beets and Arugula Salad	203
Baked Macaroni with Cheese	200		Beets Chips	68
Baked Potato with Cream Cheese (Vegan)	199		Bell Peppers and Kale Leaves	203
Baked Potatoes	251		Bell Peppers Frittata	110
Baked Salad (Vegan)	200		Berry Cheesecake	266
Baked Salmon Rolls	171		Blueberry Bars	280
Baked Sweet Potatoes	200		Blueberry Cobbler	19
Baked Tilapia	175		Blueberry Tacos	270
Baked Vegan Eggplant	199		Brazilian Pineapple	279
Baked Zucchini Egg	225		Bread with Lentils and Millet (Vegan)	45
Baked Zucchini with Cheese	200		Breaded Chicken Tenderloins	107
Balsamic Cabbage	201		Breaded Mushrooms	89
Balsamic Mushrooms	201		Breakfast Berry Pizza	49
Balsamic Vinaigrette on Roasted Chicken	89		Breakfast Bombs	64
Banana & Raisin Bread	67		Breakfast Potatoes	19
Banana & Walnut Bread	68		Broccoli Salad	205
Banana Bread (Vegan)	44		Broccoli Stew	90
Banana Chips	67		Broccoli Stuffed Peppers	20
Banana Muffins in Air Fryer	268		Broccoli with Cream Cheese	213
Banana Slices	269		Brown Rice, Spinach and Frittata	204
Banana Split	262		Brown Sugar Banana Bread	69
Banana with Tofu 'n Spices	218		Brownies	265
Banana-Choco Brownies	274		Brussels Sprouts And Tomatoes	205
Bang Panko Breaded Fried Shrimp	89		Brussels Sprouts with Pine Nuts	205
Bang Panko Breaded Fried Shrimp	189		Buffalo Chicken Tenders	120

Buffalo Chicken Wings	120	Cheesecake Egg Rolls	278
Buffalo Sauce Cauliflower	220	Cheesy Asparagus and Potatoes	210
Burritos	206	Cheesy Bacon Bread	35
Buttermilk Chicken in Air-Fryer	113	Cheesy Bell Pepper Eggs	60
Butternut Squash with Thyme	69	Cheesy Broccoli Casserole	209
Buttery Potatoes	206	Cheesy Chicken Rice	123
Cabbage Rolls	69	Cheesy Dip	74
Cajun Asparagus	206	Cheesy Garlic Bread	35
Cajun Catfish Fillets	172	Cheesy Garlic Dip	70
Cajun Mushrooms and Beans	207	Cheesy Macaroni Balls	210
Cajun Salmon	172	Cheesy Meatloaf	122
Cajun Shrimp in Air Fryer	161	Cheesy Pork Chops in Air Fryer	87
Cajuned Salmon	186	Cheesy Spinach	211
Caprese Sandwiches (Vegan)	51	Cheesy Tuna Patties	173
Caramel Apple Crisp	282	Cherry Tarts	24
Caribbean Chicken	121	Cherry Tomato Salad	210
Carne Asada Tacos	121	Cherry Tomatoes Skewers	209
Carrot & Potato Mix	85	Chicken & Pepperoni Pizza	48
Carrot Bread	34	Chicken and Asparagus	106
Carrot Cake	281	Chicken and Beans	90
Carrot Fries	76	Chicken and Broccoli Soup	260
Carrot Mix	207	Chicken Bites in Air Fryer	115
Carrot, Raisin & Walnut Bread	34	Chicken Breasts & Spiced Tomatoes	122
Carrots and Zucchinis with Mayo Butter	219	Chicken Casserole	123
Catfish with Green Beans	169	Chicken Cheesey Quesadilla in Air Fryer	114
Cauliflower Chickpea Tacos	208	Chicken Coconut Meatballs	123
Cauliflower Crackers	70	Chicken Drumsticks	101
Cauliflower Hummus	73	Chicken Drumsticks with Garlic & Thyme	132
Cauliflower in an Almond Crust with Avocado Ranch Dip	195	Chicken Fajita Casserole	148
Cauliflower Pizza Crusts	35	Chicken Fajitas	124
Cauliflower Rice	196	Chicken Fillets, Brie & Ham	124
Cauliflower, Chickpea, and Avocado Mash	208	Chicken Kabab	124
Cauliflower, Olives, and Chickpeas	255	Chicken Lasagna	122
Chard Salad	248	Chicken Meatballs	125
Cheddar Muffins	207	Chicken Meatballs	146
Cheddar Turkey Bites	121	Chicken Mushrooms Bake	125
Cheese and Bacon Muffins	27	Chicken Paillard	125
Cheese and Bean Enchiladas	208	Chicken Parmesan	126
Cheese and Veggie Air Fryer Egg Cups	63	Chicken Parmesan	134
Cheese Brussels Sprouts	70	Chicken Pasta Parmesan	91
Cheese Onion Dip	71	Chicken Pizza Crust	126
Cheese Soufflés	20	Chicken Pizza Crusts	126
Cheese Spinach Dip	71	Chicken Pizza Rolls	36
Cheesecake Bites	270	Chicken Pram	127
		Chicken Soup	259

Chicken Stir-Fry	127	Cod and Endives	174
Chicken Tenders	54	Cod and Tomatoes	174
Chicken Thighs	132	Coffee Pudding	289
Chicken Thighs Smothered Style	113	Collard Green Mix	212
Chicken with Oregano Chimichurri	127	Collard Wraps with Satay Dipping Sauce	128
Chicken with Potatoes	98	Corn and Cabbage Salad	212
Chicken with Vegetables	139	Corn Bread	46
Chicken Zucchini Casserole	139	Corn Fritters	72
Chicken with Mixed Vegetables	112	Cornish Game Hens	92
Chickpea, Fig, and Arugula Salad	223	Courgettes Casserole	92
Chickpeas Snack	71	Crab Cakes	174
Chili Potatoes	211	Crab Dip	75
Chili Tuna Casserole	173	Crab Dip	175
Chimichanga	95	Cranberry Bread	36
Chimichurri Turkey	128	Creamed Cod	187
Chinese Beans	211	Creamy Cauliflower and Broccoli	93
Chinese Cauliflower Rice	232	Creamy Chicken Wings	129
Chinese Chicken Drumsticks	91	Creamy Spinach Quiche	213
Chinese Chicken Wings	140	Crisp Chicken with Mustard Vinaigrette	129
Chocolate Banana Bread	71	Crispy & Spicy Chicken Thighs	137
Chocolate Banana Muffins	275	Crispy Air Fryer Brussels Sprouts	58
Chocolate Bites	270	Crispy Air Fryer Fish	161
Chocolate Bread	38	Crispy Chicken Thighs	129
Chocolate Chip Cookie Blondies	280	Crispy Fat-Free Spanish Potatoes	62
Chocolate Chunk Walnut Blondies	279	Crispy Fish Sandwiches	166
Chocolate Croissant Pudding	284	Crispy Honey Garlic Chicken Wings	130
Chocolate Donuts	274	Crispy Paprika Fillets	175
Chocolate Mug Cake	271	Crispy Potatoes	78
Chocolate Soufflé	274	Crunchy Almond and Salad with Roasted Chicken	130
Chocolate Strawberry Cobbler	282	Crust-less Meaty Pizza	37
Chocolate-Filled Doughnuts	21	Curried Chicken, Chickpeas and Raita Salad	93
Cilantro-Lime Fried Shrimp	92	Curried Coconut Chicken	93
Cinnamon Banana Bread	72	Curried Coconut Chicken	130
Cinnamon Bread Pudding	284	Date & Walnut Bread	72
Cinnamon Chickpeas	82	Date Bread	73
Cinnamon Rolls	278	Dates and Cashew Sticks (Vegan)	287
Cinnamon Sugar Toast	36	Delicious Chicken Pie	115
Cinnamon Toast	271	Delicious Curried Chicken	140
Cocoa and Coconut Bars (Vegan)	285	Delicious Potato Fries	226
Coconut & Spinach Chickpeas	255	Dijon Salmon	175
Coconut Artichokes	197	Easy Air Fryer Omelet	63
Coconut Chili Shrimp	186	Easy Air Fryer Zucchini Chips	59
Coconut Mix	211	Easy Brussels Sprouts	219
Coconut Shrimp	159	Egg and Bell Pepper with Beef	155
Coconut Shrimp	173		

Egg Roll Wrapped with Cabbage and Prawns	75	Greek Chicken Meatballs	131
Eggless & Vegan Cake	268	Greek Pesto Salmon	177
Eggplant and Garlic Sauce	249	Greek Potato	228
Eggplant Bake	94	Green Beans	224
Eggplant Fries	94	Green Beans and Tomatoes	249
Fajita Chicken	141	Green Beans Casserole	232
Fennel and Tomato Stew	94	Green Beans with Shallot	238
Fennel Chicken	131	Green Cayenne Cabbage	246
Fennel Cod	188	Green Paneer Ginger Cheese Balls	255
Fish And Chips	178	Green Salad	229
Fish Finger Sandwich	168	Green Veggies	247
Fish Sticks in Air Fryer	160	Grilled Ham and Cheese	19
Fishless Tacos With Chipotle Cream	239	Grilled Pork in Cajun Sauce	153
Fitness Bread	37	Grilled Salmon	177
Flat Bread with Olive and Rosemary	50	Grilled Salmon	189
Flavored Green Beans	248	Grilled Salmon with Lemon-Honey Marinade	162
Flying Fish	189	Hash Browns	21
French Mushroom	230	Hasselback Potatoes	250
French Toast Sticks	23	Healthy Veggies	252
Fried Bananas with Chocolate Sauce	275	Herb Garlic Meatballs	142
Fried Chicken Roast Served with Fruit Compote	134	Herbed Chips	239
Fried Peaches	272	Herbed Eggplant and Zucchini	248
Fried Potatoes	23	Herbed Roasted Chicken	95
Fried Ravioli	76	Herb-Marinated Chicken Thighs	111
Fruit and Vegetable Skewers	256	Honey & Sriracha Tossed Calamari	170
Garlic Beans	245	Honey Chicken Breasts	131
Garlic Cauliflower Florets	76	Honey Glazed Chicken Drumsticks	96
Garlic Lemon Shrimp	187	Honey Mustard Sauce Chicken	140
Garlic Lime Shrimp	176	Honey Seasoned Vegetables	218
Garlic Parmesan Chicken Tenders	112	Honey-Glazed Salmon	160
Garlic Parsnips	245	Hot Chicken Wings	142
Garlic Rosemary Prawns	163	Indian Cilantro Potatoes with Pepper	212
Garlic Tilapia	176	Indian Fish Fingers	178
Garlic Tomatoes	249	Italian Chicken Soup	260
Garlicky Cauliflower	224	Italian Eggplant Parmesan	244
Garlicky Chicken Wings	141	Italian Frittata	29
Garlicky Pork Stew	95	Italian Turkey	142
Ginger Tofu Sushi Bowl	243	Jackfruit Taquitos	243
Gingerbread with Lemon Cream	283	Jalapeno Muffins	25
Gingered Chicken Drumsticks	95	Jalapeno Poppers	74
Glazed Tuna and Fruits	176	Jalapeño Poppers	204
Gold Ravioli	221	Jalapeno Spinach Dip	76
Golden Beer-Battered Cod	177	Jamaican Jerk Pork in Air Fryer	88
Grain-Free Cakes	267	Juicy Air Fryer Salmon	166
Granola	23	Juicy Baked Chicken Wings	142

Juicy Garlic Chicken	143	Mushroom and Pepper Pizza Squares	238
Kale & Celery Crackers	54	Mushroom Cakes	229
Kale Salad Sushi Rolls	242	Mushroom Oatmeal	109
Korean Chicken Wings	132	Mushroom Pizza	78
Lamb Kebabs	150	Mushroom-Onion Eggplant Pizzas	39
Lava Cake	278	Mushrooms Frittata	25
Leches Cake	282	Mushrooms with Mascarpone	222
Leek, Rice, and Potato Soup	259	Mustard Turkey Bites	133
Lemon Bread	38	Mustard-Crusted Sole Fillets	178
Lemon Garlic Shrimp in Air Fryer	165	New York Pizza	40
Lemon Lentils and Fried Onion	96	No-breaded Turkey Breast	117
Lemon Pepper Chicken Breast	111	No-Breading Chicken Breast in Air Fryer	110
Lemon Pepper Chicken Legs	133	Nuggets with Parmesan Cheese	79
Lemon Pepper Drumsticks	133	Nutmeg Chicken Thighs	134
Lemon Pepper Shrimp in Air Fryer	165	Nutty Bread Pudding	40
Lemon Rosemary Chicken	108	Okra and Corn Salad	248
Lemon Rosemary Chicken	144	Okra Casserole	97
Lemon-Butter Shortbread	39	Old Bay Chicken	144
Lemon-Garlic Chicken	113	Old Bay Crab Cakes	191
Lemongrass Chicken	138	Olive Bread and Rosemary	34
Lemony Pear Chips	239	Olive Tomato Chicken	145
Lemony Tuna	96	Omelet	26
Lemony Tuna	190	Onion Pie	233
Lime Broccoli	246	Onion Rings with Almond Four Battered	197
Lime Endives	247	Orange Chicken Wings	114
Lime-Garlic Shrimp Kebabs	168	Oregano Eggplants	245
Low Carb Air Fryer Baked Eggs	63	Paella	180
Low Carb Peanut Butter Cookies	264	Paneer Pizza	103
Lunch Pizzas	42	Panettone Bread Pudding	38
Mac and Cheese	37	Paprika Cod	97
Macaroni Samosa	228	Paprika Onion	254
Mahi Fillets	172	Parmesan Asparagus	258
Maple Tomato Bread (Vegan)	287	Parmesan Breaded with Zucchini Chips	252
Maple-Glazed Doughnuts	22	Parmesan Broccoli Florets	251
Marinated Beef BBQ	154	Parmesan Chicken & Vegetables	145
Masala Gallettes	226	Parmesan Chicken Meatballs	108
Meat Lovers' Pizza	48	Parmesan Cod	179
Mediterranean Vegetables	221	Parmesan Garlic Crusted Salmon	163
Mexican Brownies	279	Parmesan Green Beans	252
Mexican Chicken Lasagna	141	Parmesan Pesto Chicken	145
Mexican Stuffed Potatoes	97	Parmesan Potatoes	226
Mixed Berry Muffins	25	Parmesan Shrimp	166
Mozzarella Flatbread	40	Parmesan Walnut Salmon	179
Mozzarella, Bacon & Turkey Calzone	48	Parmesan-Crusted Halibut Fillets	179
Mushroom and Kale Soup	260	Parmesan-Crusted Salmon Patties	180

Parsnip & Potato Bake with Parmesan	254	Pumpkin and Coconut Seeds Bars (Vegan)	288
Pasta with Artichoke Pesto and Chickpeas (Vegan)	196	Pumpkin Bread	41
Peach Cinnamon Cobbler	289	Pumpkin Cheesecake	283
Peach Cobbler	277	Pumpkin Chicken Lasagna	146
Peanut Butter Banana Bread	77	Pumpkin Oatmeal	250
Pepper Lemon Baked Chicken Legs	143	Radish Hash Browns	26
Pepper Lemon Chicken	144	Ranch Potatoes	78
Pepper Lemon Chicken Breasts	143	Raspberry Crumble Cake	281
Pesto Tomatoes	257	Ratatouille	236
Philo Pasta Rolls	41	Ribs with Cajun and Coriander	153
Pineapple Bites	269	Rice and Eggplant	222
Pineapple Orange Cake	281	Rice and Eggplant	238
Pineapple Sticky Ribs	75	Rice Balls	79
Pistachio-Crusted Lemon-Garlic Salmon	191	Ricotta Dip	83
Pita Bread	49	Roasted Apple Potatoes	223
Pizza	33	Roasted Asparagus	252
Pizza Bombs	41	Roasted Balsamic Vegetables	257
Pizza Crust	39	Roasted Broccoli	225
Polenta Biscuits	77	Roasted Carrots	251
Polenta Roll with Cheese	217	Roasted Carrots with Garlic	257
Polenta Roll with Cheese Sauce	198	Roasted Chicken	135
Pomegranate and Florets	246	Roasted Chickpeas	98
Popcorn (Vegan)	241	Roasted Potatoes with Rosemary	256
Popcorn Chicken in Air Fryer	115	Roasted Salmon with Fennel Salad	169
Pork Dumplings in Air Fryer	87	Roasted Veggie Pasta Salad	42
Pork Rind Nachos	88	Rosemary Grilled Chicken	98
Pork Taquitos in Air Fryer	86	Rosemary Russet Potato Chips	99
Pork Tenderloin with Mustard Glazed	88	Sago Galette	227
Potato Air Fried Hash Browns	242	Salmon and Cauliflower Rice	180
Potato and Beans Dip	77	Salmon and Dill Sauce	181
Potato and Broccoli with Tofu Scramble	236	Salmon Cakes in Air Fryer	159
Potato Casserole	224	Salmon Dill Patties	181
Potato Cauliflower Patties	100	Salmon Noodles	191
Potato Chips	78	Salmon Patties	181
Potato Cream Cheese Bars	280	Salmon Quiche	99
Potato Croquettes	82	Salmon Quiche	192
Potato Samosa	227	Salmon with Coconut Sauce	180
Potato Tots	82	Salmon with Shrimp & Pasta	42
Potato Wedges	83	Salsa Cheesy Dip	79
Potato with Cheese	217	Salsa Chicken	138
Potatoes with Tofu	220	Salted Caramel Banana Muffins (Vegan)	43
Potatoes with Tofu	237	Sausage and Cream Cheese Biscuits	27
Potatoes with Zucchini	235	Sausage and Egg Burrito	27
Puffed Egg Tarts	26	Scallops and Vegetables	192
		Scallops with Creamy Tomato Sauce	170

Scramble Casserole	20	Stew of Okra and Eggplant	231
Sesame Garlic Chicken Wings	80	Sticky Hoisin Tuna	183
Sesame Seeds Fish Fillet	165	Stir-Fried Chicken with Water Chestnuts	136
Sesame Shrimp	182	Strawberry Bread	44
Shortbread Sticks	271	Strawberry Cake	272
Shrimp Fajitas	184	Strawberry Tarts	24
Shrimp Pasta	43	Strawberry Turkey	136
Shrimp Po Boy	190	Stuffed Eggplant	241
Shrimp Spring Rolls in Air Fryer	170	Stuffed Peppers	249
Simple Chicken Thighs	147	Stuffed Peppers Baskets	228
Simply Baked Chicken	147	Stuffed Potatoes	244
Soda Bread	80	Stuffed Tomatoes	257
Sole and Cauliflower Fritters	182	Sugar-Free Air Fried Carrot Cake	263
Soufflé	21	Sugar-Free Chocolate Donut Holes	264
Sour Cream Banana Bread	80	Sugar-Free Chocolate Soufflé	263
Southwest Chicken in Air Fryer	110	Sugar-Free Low Carb Cheesecake Muffins	263
Soy Salmon Fillets	190	Sugar-Free Pumpkin Bread	45
Spanish Rice Casserole with Beef and Cheese	155	Summer Rolls	236
Spiced Chicken	99	Sunflower Seed Bread	81
Spiced Chicken Breasts	135	Sweet & Spicy Parsnips	258
Spiced Duck Legs	135	Sweet and Savory Breaded Shrimp	184
Spicy Broccoli with Garlic	256	Sweet and Sour Chicken	136
Spicy Brussels Sprouts	81	Sweet Chicken	139
Spicy Butternut Squash	258	Sweet Potato Fries	74
Spicy Cardamom Crumb Cake	276	Taco Stuffed Bread	45
Spicy Cauliflower	243	Tahini Oatmeal Chocolate Chunk Cookies	267
Spicy Cauliflower Florets	81	Tamarind Glazed Potatoes	100
Spicy Cheese Lings	254	Tandoori Chicken Legs	102
Spicy Chicken Legs	100	Teriyaki BBQ Recipe	156
Spicy Chicken Meatballs	147	Teriyaki Chicken Wings	136
Spicy Chicken Wings	147	Teriyaki Duck Legs	137
Spicy Potato Fries	253	Texas Beef Brisket	156
Spicy Shrimp	183	Thai-Style Crab Cakes	240
Spicy Tilapia	183	The Cheesy Sandwich (Vegan)	101
Spinach and Lentils	231	Thyme Eggplant and Beans	102
Spinach and Olives	101	Tilapia and Salsa	184
Spinach and Shrimp	101	Tilapia with Vegetables	185
Spinach Dish	235	Tiramisu Cheesecake	283
Spinach Frittata	28	Tomato and Avocado	103
Squash Stew	230	Tomato and Balsamic Greens	246
Sriracha Cauliflower	223	Tomato and Beef Sauce	103
Sriracha Honey Brussels Sprouts	250	Tomato Chili and Black Beans	204
Steak and Eggs	22	Tomatoes and Cabbage Stew	104
Steak with Chimichurri Sauce	154	Tomatoes Salad	229
Steamed Broccoli	196	Tortilla Chips	81

Tortilla with Bell Pepper-Corn Wrapped	203	Vegetable Egg Cups	28
Trout with Mint	185	Vegetable Egg Soufflé	28
Tuna Stuffed Potatoes	192	Vegetable Spring Rolls	58
Tuna Veggie	185	Vegetable Stew	234
Turkey and Bok Choy	104	Vegetable Tots	225
Turkey and Broccoli Stew	105	Vegetables Lasagna	233
Turkey and Mushroom Stew	105	Vegetables Pizza	234
Turkey and Quinoa Stuffed Peppers	105	Vegetables with Tandoori Spice	218
Turkey Breast with Mustard Maple Glaze	116	Vegetarian Frittata	253
Turkey Fajitas Platter in Air Fryer	116	Veggie Burger with Spices	220
Turkey Juicy Breast Tenderloin	116	Veggie Kebab	227
Turkey Turnovers	137	Veggie Sticks	83
Turmeric Cauliflower Steaks	245	Waffles and Chicken	28
Vanilla Cake	285	Walnut Bread with Cranberries	46
Veg Rolls	221	Walnut Zucchini Bread	46
Veg Rolls	237	White Beans Stew	231
Vegan Apple Cupcakes	286	Whole Wheat Toast	47
Vegan Beer Bread	33	Winter Green Beans	231
Vegan Blueberry Cake	289	Wontons	83
Vegan Breakfast Sandwich	62	Yellow Lentil	233
Vegan Cauliflower Rice	90	Yellow Squash 'n Zucchini	219
Vegan Cinnamon Bananas	288	Yellow Squash, Zucchini and Carrots	250
Vegan Grape Pudding	288	Yogurt Banana Bread	50
Vegan Lemon Squares	287	Yogurt Bread	50
Vegan Mashed Potato Bowl	61	Yogurt Pumpkin Bread	47
Vegan Orange Bread and Almonds	286	Zingy & Nutty Chicken Wings	138
Vegan Spelled Bread	43	Zucchini and Pumpkin Salad	230
Vegan Spicy Sourdough Bread	44	Zucchini Chips	74
Vegan Spring Rolls	240	Zucchini Gratin	58
Vegan Tangerine Cake	286	Zucchini Muffins	29
Vegan Taquito	104	Zucchini Noodles	30
Vegan Wholegrain Bread	47	Zucchini Parmesan Chips	56
Vegetable and Beef Soup	260	Zucchini Turkey Burgers	117
Vegetable Burger	235		

Made in United States
North Haven, CT
13 December 2021

12670542R00167